International Geophysics Series

EDITORS

J. VAN MIEGHEM

Royal Belgian Meteorological Institute
Uccle, Belgium

ANTON L. HALES

Australian National University
Canberra, A.C.T., Australia

CLIMATE AND LIFE

CLIMATE
AND LIFE

M. I. BUDYKO

Corresponding Member of the
U.S.S.R. Academy of Sciences
Main Geophysical Observatory
Leningrad

English Edition Edited by

DAVID H. MILLER

University of Wisconsin
Milwaukee, Wisconsin

1974

ACADEMIC PRESS   New York   San Francisco   London

A Subsidiary of Harcourt Brace Jovanovich, Publishers

ACADEMIC PRESS, INC.
111 Fifth Avenue, New York, New York 10003

United Kingdom Edition published by
ACADEMIC PRESS, INC. (LONDON) LTD.
24/28 Oval Road, London NW1

Library of Congress Cataloging in Publication Data

Budyko, Mikhail Ivanovich.
   Climate and life.

   (International geophysics series, 18)
   Translation of Klimat i zhizň.
   Includes bibliographical references.
   1.   Heat budget (Geophysics)   2.   Climatology.
3.   Bioclimatology.   I.   Title.   II.   Series.
QC809.E6B813   551.6   73-801
ISBN 0-12-139450-6

CLIMATE AND LIFE. Translated from the original Russian
edition entitled КЛИМАТ и ЖИЗНЬ, published by
ГИДРОМЕТЕОРОЛОГИЧЕСКОЕ ИЗДАТЕЛЬСТВО,
ЛЕНИНГРАД, 1971.

Contents

I. Solar Radiation and Its Transformations

II. Methods for Determining the Components of the Heat Balance

III. Heat Balance of the Globe

Editor's Foreword

This work warranted translation because (i) it is an authoritative statement of the new concepts of climatic analysis that are based on the laws of conservation of mass and of energy that have developed in many parts of the world in the past 25 years, but nowhere as comprehensively as in the great Voeikov Geophysical Observatory in Leningrad [GGO], and (ii) it applies these energy-budget concepts to important questions in the biology of the planet. The book can be termed authoritative because its author, Mikhail Ivanovich Budyko, the director of the Observatory, has led its energy-mass budget investigations, and has himself explored many of the implications of the seemingly simple concept of the budget.

The first English-language summary of the research at the Voeikov Observatory was based on the Russian work of 1956 that Budyko brought to a conference in Washington of the Committee on Climatology of the World Meteorological Organization. The importance of the book was immediately recognized and it was translated into English by the Office of Climatology of the U.S. Weather Bureau with support from the U.S. Army Natick Laboratories and the Cold Regions Research and Engineering Laboratory, three groups that were then getting involved in energy research and applications. (A translation into Japanese was published the next year.)

In many areas of geophysics in North America (including climatology, hydrology, and meteorology) energy-mass budget work then under way was powerfully strengthened by the methods and the global-scale data published in this translation ("The Heat Balance of the Earth's Surface," Washington, 1958). It has since repeatedly served as the base level on which further investigations have built—some at the micro- and mesoscales, others at the world scale.

"Climate and Life" surpasses the contributions of the 1956 book and its two associated atlases. Larger than the book of 1956, it goes from a recapitulation of methodology and the time and space distributions of the energy fluxes to an examination of contemporary questions, biological as well as geophysical, in the light of the relevant energetics.

As a long-time believer in the efficacy of energy analysis to get at the roots of refractory problems in geophysics, geography, and biology, I find Budyko's analyses logical and compelling. These analyses offer new insights, whether applied to photosynthetic productivity of the earth's vegetation, the heat balance of man and other organisms, or to such emerging global questions as climatic change. The culminating chapter unites small-scale biological and large-scale geophysical phenomena as could be done only by an individual with a firm grasp of processes operating at both scales could do.

Professor Budyko wrote many years ago that application of the energy–water balance can bring about a rapprochement of the rapidly diverging sciences of the earth by providing a conceptual base for sound interdisciplinary investigations. In this book he demonstrates the even more fundamental rapprochement between the physics and the biology of this man-occupied planet.

I hope that other readers will find this synthesis and the separate analyses as challenging as I have. The unusually complete citations at the end of each chapter should be helpful to the interested reader, and where possible I have added information about translations of general availability. I also have given (by MGA) the call numbers of abstracts published in Meteorological and Geoastrophysical Abstracts (Boston, 1950).

I take this opportunity to thank my wife for help over rough spots. I want to dedicate my own small contribution here to the shining memory of a gentleman and a scholar: Светлой памяти Бориса Львовича Дзердзеевского, 1898–1971.

DAVID H. MILLER

Preface to the Russian Edition

Since the 1940's, investigations of the transformations of solar energy at the earth's surface have been carried out in the Voeikov Main Geophysical Observatory in Leningrad. The results of these investigations have been used to solve various problems in climatology, hydrology, oceanography, physical geography, and other disciplines. The first summary of these investigations was published in 1956 in the author's book, "Тепловои Баланс Земной Поверхности" ("The Heat Balance of the Earth's Surface"). In the years since this book was published, many newer works on energy balance embracing a wider range of problems have been written.

The principles that govern the heat balance of both the earth's surface and the atmosphere have been studied in these works. In recent years much attention has been paid to the problem of the effect of climatic energetic factors on biological processes. In the course of these studies a number of basic concepts have been found that connect the activity of living organisms with climatic conditions.

The present book is a new summary of investigations in the field of solar energy transformations at the earth's surface and in the atmosphere. Its title indicates that special attention is paid to the problems of bioclimatology. As the book covers a wide array of problems relating to several fields of natural sciences, the statements are necessarily brief and limited to the data of investigations conducted in the Main Geophysical Observatory.

It should be noted that the variety of problems discussed are united by a common approach, which is the study of energetic processes forming the geographical conditions on our planet.

The author would like to thank his collaborators, with whom he has for many years analyzed the problems set forth in this book. The author also thanks all those who have read this material and made comments on it.

ix

Introduction

The available data concerning contemporary climatic conditions on our planet have been obtained as a result of the work of meteorological observational systems, which embrace all the regions of the globe. This system includes the world network of constantly operating surface meteorological stations, which are situated on all the continents (Antarctica included) and on many islands. The network includes more than ten thousand climatological stations and several tens of thousands of meteorological posts. These stations carry out daily observations on temperature and humidity of the air, atmospheric precipitation, cloudiness, wind, pressure, and other meteorological elements. The observational program at meteorological posts is more limited than this, and is often reduced to observations of atmospheric precipitation.

In recent decades, the world network of actinometric and aerological stations has been brought into the general system of surface meteorological observations. The actinometric network includes about a thousand stations at which observations of solar radiation and its transformation are conducted. The aerological network also comprises about a thousand stations, where, with the aid of radiosondes and other instruments, observations of the meteorological regime in the free atmosphere up to altitudes of 30 to 40 km are carried out.

Observations obtained at surface meteorological stations are supplemented by observations on the oceans, where a number of weather ships are always at work in given regions. As weather ships are comparatively few in number, meteorological observations conducted on board merchant ships during their trips to different destinations are also of great importance for studying the climates of the oceans.

During recent years, observational data from the earth's satellites have begun to be used in climatological work. These observations permit us to learn more about the environment of clouds, the radiational fluxes at the altitudes of the satellites' movement, and some parameters of the physical condition of the lower layers of the atmosphere.

The data from meteorological observations give us information about the meteorological elements for the period of existence of the observational system. As the world network of the principal meteorological stations was formed in the middle of the last century, this period is now approximately equal to one century.

On the basis of analyzing the results of meteorological observations and studying the climates of the past, it has been established that although the climatic conditions on our planet are changing these changes are comparatively slow and, as a rule, hardly noticeable during intervals comparable in length with the duration of a man's life.

This permits us to consider the contemporary climate as being more or less stable and to characterize it by means of norms of the meteorological elements (i.e., by mean values) for different seasons and geographical regions. The values of such norms and the variability characteristics of meteorological elements from year to year are given in reference books on climatology and are shown on climatic maps.

The meteorological regime observed in the contemporary epoch is characterized by a strongly pronounced latitudinal thermal zonality. If in the tropics the air temperature near the earth's surface remains high during the whole year, then in moderate latitudes it decreases noticeably in winter time, the difference between summer and winter temperatures being especially great in continental regions remote from the oceans. The mean annual temperature in the middle latitudes is thus noticeably lower than the mean annual temperature in the low latitudes.

In polar latitudes with noticeable seasonal changes of temperature, the temperature of the air remains low during the whole year, promoting a wide spreading of ice cover on land and ocean.

The cause of differences between the earth's climates attracted the attention of the thinkers of antiquity. As long ago as that time it was established that there is a close relationship between climatic conditions and the mean altitude of the sun, i.e., the latitude of the terrain. This relationship explains the origin of the term climate (from the Greek verb κλινειν (to tilt), characterizing the angle of the solar rays).

Although in the 18th century M. V. Lomonosov, Benjamin Franklin, and other scientists expressed some ideas concerning the regularities of formation of climate, the ways of studying the genesis of climate were indicated only at the end of the 19th century in the works of a distinguished climatologist and geographer, A. I. Voeikov (1842–1916). He pointed out in his works that for explaining the mechanism of climate formation it is necessary to investigate the transformation of solar energy incident upon our planet.

In the monograph, "Климаты Земного Шара, в Особенности России" ("Climates of the World, Especially Russia") (1884), Voeikov wrote:

> *I believe that one of the most important tasks of physical sciences at present is keeping an account book of solar heat received by the globe with its air and water envelope.*
>
> *We want to know how much solar heat is received near the upper boundaries of the atmosphere, how much it takes for heating the atmosphere, for changing the state of water vapor added to it, then what amount of heat reaches the land and water surface, what amount it takes for heating various bodies, what for changing their state (from solid to liquid and from liquid to gaseous), in chemical reactions especially connected with organic life; then we must know how much heat the earth loses owing to radiation into space and how this loss occurs, i.e., to what extent by lowering the temperature and to what extent by changing the state of bodies, especially water.*
>
> *Difficulties connected with reaching the goal cannot discourage scientists who are able to understand the great aims of science. It cannot be reached in one century. Therefore I thought it useful to set forth the task in all its breadth without obscuring the great difficulties connected with its solution.*

For a better appreciation of these thoughts it will be recalled that in the time when "Climates of the World" was written, the problem of solar energy transformation was but little developed. However, Voeikov not only formulated correctly the main tasks of studying the earth's heat balance but also expressed the conviction that the great difficulties connected with the solution of these tasks will be successfully overcome.

Further development of meteorology has confirmed the fact that an explanation of regularities in climate formation is possible only on the basis of studying the transformation of solar energy, which is practically the only source of energy for all atmospheric processes. It has therefore proved necessary to have data on solar energy absorption and its further transformations at the earth's surface, in the atmosphere, and in the hydrosphere for investigating the genesis of climate. Such data have been obtained during the process of studying the heat balance of the earth.

Next to the problem of explaining the genesis of climate, the second important task of climatology is the study of the relations between climate and other natural processes.

It is known that climatic conditions produce a deep and often determining influence upon the whole complex of natural processes developing in the geographical envelope of the earth (the term "geographical envelope" [or mantle] unites the atmosphere, the hydrosphere, and the upper layers of the lithosphere). In the 19th century it was found that the hydrological regime of the land depends largely on climatic factors; for this reason Voeikov called rivers "a product of climate." A similar conclusion relating to soils, the distribution of which proved to be closely connected with climatic conditions, was drawn by Dokuchaev. The dependence of geographical distributions of plants and animals on climate has been established in works on geobotany and zoogeography. A little later such dependency was found for indices of exogenous geomorphological processes, changing the surface of the continents.

It was pointed out in the works of the outstanding geographer, A. A. Grigor'ev (1883–1968), that all the natural processes developing in the geographical envelope are closely interconnected and represent a single complex, including climatic, hydrologic, soil, biological, and exogenous geomorphological processes. Grigor'ev considered this complex to be a single physico-geographical process, forming the geographical envelope of the earth.

Grigor'ev noted that climatic factors play a leading part in the physico-geographical process as they determine the conditions for transforming solar energy, the main source of energy for all the processes in the geographical envelope. He pointed out that interrelations between processes developing within the geographical envelope are, to a considerable extent, based on the exchange of energy and a number of substances (water, carbon dioxide, nitrogen, and others) between the atmosphere, the hydrosphere, the lithosphere, and living organisms. For the purpose of studying these interrelations Grigor'ev suggested that data on energy balances and the mass balances of various categories of mineral and organic substances should be used.

During the process of investigations aimed at studying geographical processes in various regions, Grigor'ev applied the method of balances for characteristic features of geographical zones. Notwithstanding the great difficulty associated with the lack of factual material, Grigor'ev managed to present in these works not only a general picture of income and expenditure of energy and some categories of matter in various geographical regions, but also established, on the basis of this picture, the general regularities of geographical zonality.

Grigor'ev's works suggested the great possibilities of quantitative study of the whole complex of geographical processes on the basis of investigations of the balances of energy and different kinds of mineral and organic substances. Investigations of this kind are of great importance for the development of physical geography as a single science.

During recent decades the descriptive sections of the geographical disciplines reached a certain degree of completeness, and therefore a problem of further development of the physico-geographical sciences arose. This problem has been more successfully solved by particular geographical disciplines, which have gradually turned from describing the external features of natural processes and phenomena to explaining their internal regularities, using for this purpose the materials of adjacent sciences (namely, geophysics, geochemistry, biology, and others). Such a reorientation of the geographical sciences has been accompanied by their increasing differentiation and separation, which together with some positive results have led to difficulty in studying complex problems and to a certain disparity between the rapid progress in the field of the separate geographical disciplines and the lag in studying the problem of physical geography as a whole. It is probable that this lag has appeared not only as a result of the objective difficulty of studying complicated interdisciplinary regularities of geographical processes, but also to some extent is an inevitable consequence of a progressive fundamental specialization of particular geographical disciplines. This specialization has led to an enormous accumulation of factual material within the limits of each geographical discipline and to a considerable complication of investigative methods. Therefore it has become difficult for individual scientists to use actively the materials of adjacent geographical sciences. This situation has made it difficult to study the general problems of physical geography.

The ways of overcoming the difficulty indicated in the works of Grigor'ev have pointed out the perspectives of reorientation of physical geography, which are being realized in contemporary investigations.

Proceeding from the concept of a single complex of geographical processes connected with different forms of energy and materials exchange, it is possible to pose the question of quantitative explanation of the fundamental features of these processes on the basis of general laws of the exact sciences.

The first step in solving this question is the working out of a theory of climate that permits us to investigate the transformation of solar energy in the geographical mantle and to connect the geographical distribution of meteorological elements with the climate-forming factors. Modern investigations have given a series of results on this problem, relating both to climatic conditions of our time and to the climates of the geological past.

Another direction in working out a physical theory of geographical processes aims at creating a theory of the hydrologic regime, which for land conditions must explain the regularities of the spatial-temporal distributions of such water-balance components as run-off and evaporation. The basis of this theory is the relationship of water-balance components with climatic factors, which have long been studied in hydrology. In works that have been done recently, the relations of components of the water balance to components of the heat balance have been established, both for mean annual values and for changes during the annual cycle. The use of these relations permits us to determine from climatic data the annual values of evaporation and run-off in areas that differ in their climatic conditions.

The task of explaining physically the geographical distribution of the vegetation cover is very difficult because for its solution it is necessary to take into account complex biological laws. In earlier investigations, the analysis of this problem was reduced to establishing relations between the boundaries of geobotanical zones and climatological factors, including the components of the heat and water balances. More recently, the possibility of studying the dependence of the productivity of vegetation cover on climatological factors has been elucidated on the basis of the physical laws of photosynthesis. Analysis of this problem may be important not only for illuminating the physical mechanism of zonal changes in vegetation cover but also for explaining the quantitative regularities of soil formation, because productivity of vegetation is one of the important factors in the soil-forming process. This manner of investigation would be a supplement to numerous works that aim at establishing quantitative relations between zonal characteristics of soil properties and climatic factors.

We should also indicate that special attention paid recently to quantitative regularities that connect geographical features of a process with external factors, particularly climatological ones, has become characteristic of investigations of other geographical processes (e.g., in studying the problems of zoogeography).

All this permits us to hope that relatively soon we may obtain a complete system of quantitative interrelations determining the main features of the whole complex of natural processes, on the basis of an accounting of incoming solar energy and the properties of mineral and organic substances in the geographical envelope. This system will include the equations of the theory of climate and the theory of hydrologic processes. The solutions of these equations, by determining conditions of the heat and water regime, would become a base for quantitative study of soil, biogeographical, and other geographical processes.

In this system of quantitative relationships, semiempirical and empirical relations will take an important place along with the established methods of physical deduction, especially when studying processes that are substantially influenced by biological factors. It should be borne in mind that physical methods of investigation can also be widely used when studying the bio-geographical processes, since these processes depend to a great extent upon external physical conditions, especially climatic factors. When studying such cross-discipline generalities, geophysical methods of investigation must be well coordinated with an accounting of the influence of biological factors.

Working out a complete system of quantitative relations interconnecting the characteristics of geographical processes will be of great importance for the further progress of physical geography. Such a system of relations can be used for many a practical purpose, particularly for calculating the changes in the whole complex of natural conditions resulting from action affecting individual geographical processes.

The system can also be applied in working out problems of paleogeography, by introducing into the system of relations the additions necessary for calculating the nonstationary character of the processes under investigation.

We think that the development of such investigations will further the conversion of physical geography from a descriptive science into an exact science.

Although a general solution of the problem of constructing a system of quantitative relations determining the dynamics of the whole complex of natural processes in the geographical envelope is a thing of the future, we have at present a number of investigations in which individual parts of this problem are considered.

In this monograph are set forth the results of such investigations, based mainly on the results of research accomplished in the Voeikov Main Geophysical Observatory.

In the opening chapters, the regularities of solar radiation transformation in the geographical envelope are considered, and some data concerning the heat balance of the earth are presented. In the following chapters are given the results of investigations into the genesis of climate, based upon studies of the heat balance. The concluding part of the book is dedicated to investigations of the influence of climatic factors on natural processes, in which data on the balances of water, energy, carbon dioxide, and organic matter are used.

I

Solar Radiation and Its Transformations

1. Solar Radiation

The sun is the star closest to the earth and belongs to a class of yellow stars—dwarfs. The diameter of the sun equals 1.4 million kilometers, and the mean distance between the sun and the earth is 149.5 million kilometers. As a result of nuclear reactions that occur in the sun, the temperature of its surface is approximately 6000°, which causes the radiation of a considerable amount of energy by the sun.

The radiation coming from the sun to the earth is the only form of incoming radiant energy that determines the heat balance and the thermal regime of the earth. Radiational energy incident upon the earth from all other celestial bodies is so small that it does not noticeably influence the processes of heat exchange occurring upon the earth.

The spectrum of solar radiation corresponds to that of a black body, which is described by Planck's formula. In accordance with the temperature of the sun's radiating surface, the maximum radiation flux is observed at the wavelength of approximately 0.45 μm, and most of the energy radiated by the sun falls in the wavelength interval from 0.3 to 2.0 μm.

Moving away from the sun, the intensity of radiation decreases in inverse proportion to the square of the distance. As the earth moves around the sun in its elliptical orbit, the intensity of solar radiation falling on the external boundary of the atmosphere changes during the year according to the change of distance between the earth and the sun.

The smallest distance between the earth and the sun is observed at the beginning of January, when it equals 147 million kilometers. The greatest distance, reached at the beginning of July, equals 152 million kilometers.

The flux of solar energy in one minute across an area of 1 cm² placed perpendicular to the sun's rays, beyond the atmosphere, and located at the mean distance between the earth and the sun, is called the solar constant. With the changes in the distance between the earth and the sun, the actual values of the solar energy flux at the outer boundary of the atmosphere vary from the value of the solar constant. This variation amounts to 3.5%.

For a long time, the value of the solar constant was considered approximately equal to 1.9 cal cm^{-2} min^{-1}. Then it was established that a noticeable amount of solar energy is absorbed in the upper layers of the atmosphere, and as a result the value of the solar constant was considered to be near 2.0 cal cm^{-2} min^{-1}. In organizing the International Geophysical Year, it was decided to consider the value of the solar constant to be equal to 1.98 cal cm^{-2} min^{-1} (Radiation Instruments and Measurement, 1958). Observations made recently (Kondrat'ev and Nikolskii, 1968; Drummond and Hickey, 1968) give a slightly smaller value of the solar constant, namely, 1.94–1.95 cal cm^{-2} min^{-1}.

We should indicate that for many investigations it is more important to know, not the true value of the solar constant, but its conditional value, corresponding to the amount of radiation that reaches the upper layers of the troposphere. In contemporary studies, this value of the conditional solar constant is usually considered equal to 1.90–1.92 cal cm^{-2} min^{-1}.

The question of the stability of the solar constant with time is of great interest. This question has been discussed in a number of studies—many authors considering that if changes in the solar constant do occur, they do not exceed the accuracy of the available measurements [refer to Allen (1958), and others]. In addition, it should be borne in mind that small variations of the solar constant of the order of 1% or even 0.1% from its value may produce a certain influence on weather and climate. For this reason, the question of the stability of the solar constant deserves greater attention.

Knowing the value of the solar constant, one can calculate how much energy penetrates to the earth's surface in different latitudes in the absence of atmospheric influences upon radiation. We shall consider here the main points of such a calculation [refer to Milankovich (1930)].

The flux of solar energy reaching the earth's orbit equals S_0/l^2, where S_0 is the solar constant, and l is the ratio of the distance between the earth and the sun at a given moment of time to the mean value of this distance.

Upon an element of the horizontal surface of the earth there falls an amount of radiation equal to

$$Q_s = \frac{S_0}{l^2} \cos z_\odot,$$ (1.1)

where $z_\odot$ is the angle between the direction of the sun and the zenith (the zenith angle).

The value of the zenith angle depends on latitude, time of day, and season. In order to establish these dependence relations, we shall use a scheme presented in Fig. 1.

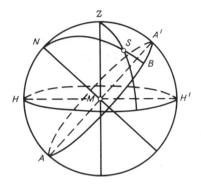

Fig. 1   The celestial sphere.

The position of the point for which the calculation of radiation is being performed corresponds in this picture to the center of the sphere M. The point S represents the position of the sun, Z is the zenith, and the line MN shows the direction of the earth's axis. The plane of the circle HH' represents the horizon apparent to the observer at point M. The circle AA', perpendicular to the line MN, lies in the plane of the celestial equator. The arc passing through points N and S cuts the celestial equator at point B, with its section BS corresponding to the angle of the sun's declination $\delta_\odot$.

As is seen from this figure, the arc NS in the spherical triangle NSZ corresponds to angle $\frac{1}{2}\pi - \delta_\odot$, the arc ZS to the angle $z_\odot$, and the arc ZN to the angle $\frac{1}{2}\pi - \phi$, where ϕ is the latitude of the point in question. Designating the spherical angle ZNS by the letter ω (the hour angle of the sun), we derive the relation

$$\cos z_\odot = \sin \phi \sin \delta_\odot + \cos \phi \cos \delta_\odot \cos \omega. \tag{1.2}$$

Thus

$$Q_s = \frac{S_0}{l^2} (\sin \phi \sin \delta_\odot + \cos \phi \cos \delta_\odot \cos \omega). \tag{1.3}$$

It follows from this relation that $Q_s = 0$ with

$$\cos \omega_0 = -\tan \phi \tan \delta_\odot. \tag{1.4}$$

This formula can be used for calculating the time of sunrise and sunset and the duration of daylight. Equation (1.4) also permits us to determine a position of the great circle separating the illuminated part of the earth from the dark part.

The amount of energy received by the earth as a whole is equal to the product of the area of this circle multiplied by the value of the radiational flux at a given distance, i.e., $(S_0/l^2)\pi r_e{}^2$, where r_e is the earth's radius. To determine the mean quantity of energy incident upon a unit area of the earth's surface, one must divide the last value by the surface area, which is equal to $4\pi r_e{}^2$. Thus, the mean value of the incoming solar energy upon the unit area of surface is equal to $\frac{1}{4}(S_0/l^2)$.

In order to determine the solar energy income in different latitudinal zones, one must calculate the sums of the right side of Eq. (1.3) for different intervals of time.

From Eq. (1.3) we define

$$dQ_s = (M + N \cos \omega) \, dt, \qquad (1.5)$$

where

$$M = \frac{S_0}{l^2} \sin \phi \sin \delta_\odot, \qquad N = \frac{S_0}{l^2} \cos \phi \cos \delta_\odot, \qquad t = \text{time}.$$

Taking into account the fact that $\omega = (2\pi/\tau)t$ (τ is the duration of daylight), we get the equation

$$dQ_s = (M + N \cos \omega) \frac{\tau}{2\pi} \, d\omega. \qquad (1.6)$$

Integrating the left and right sides of this equation from $-\omega_0$ to $+\omega_0$, we define the diurnal sums of radiation incident upon the earth's surface under a transparent atmosphere,

$$Q_{s\tau} = \frac{\tau}{2\pi} \int_{-\omega_0}^{\omega_0} (M + N \cos \omega) \, d\omega, \qquad (1.7)$$

from which it follows that

$$Q_{s\tau} = \frac{\tau}{\pi} \frac{S_0}{l^2} (\omega_0 \sin \phi \sin \delta_\odot + \sin \omega_0 \cos \phi \cos \delta_\odot) . \qquad (1.8)$$

In calculations of $Q_{s\tau}$ by this formula, the value of ω_0 is determined from Eq. (1.4).

For high latitudes, during the twenty-four hours when the sun does not set, one should consider $\omega_0 = \pi$. Then

$$Q_{s\tau} = \tau \frac{S_0}{l^2} \sin \phi \sin \delta_\odot. \qquad (1.9)$$

One can calculate the diurnal amounts of incoming solar radiation at various latitudes in different seasons by Eqs. (1.8) and (1.9). Some results of such calculations made for $S_0 = 2$ cal cm^{-2} min^{-1} are given in Table 1.

As seen from Table 1, the largest diurnal quantities of radiation occur over the poles at the summer solstice. It should be noted that at these periods with a shift toward lower latitude, there is some reduction of quantity of radiation,

TABLE 1

DIURNAL TOTALS OF SOLAR RADIATION INCIDENT UPON THE SURFACE
OF THE EARTH UNDER A COMPLETELY TRANSPARENT ATMOSPHERE (kcal cm^{-2})

Latitude (degrees)	Mar. 21	May 6	June 22	Aug. 8	Sept. 23	Nov. 8	Dec. 22	Feb. 4
90 N	—	0.80	1.11	0.79	—	—	—	—
80	0.16	0.78	1.09	0.78	0.16	—	—	—
70	0.32	0.77	1.04	0.76	0.31	0.02	—	0.02
60	0.46	0.83	1.01	0.83	0.46	0.15	0.05	0.15
50	0.59	0.89	1.02	0.89	0.59	0.30	0.18	0.30
40	0.71	0.94	1.02	0.93	0.70	0.44	0.33	0.45
30	0.80	0.96	1.00	0.95	0.79	0.58	0.48	0.59
20	0.87	0.95	0.96	0.94	0.86	0.71	0.62	0.71
10	0.91	0.92	0.90	0.91	0.90	0.81	0.76	0.82
0	0.92	0.86	0.81	0.86	0.91	0.90	0.87	0.90
10	0.91	0.78	0.71	0.78	0.90	0.96	0.96	0.96
20	0.87	0.68	0.58	0.67	0.86	0.99	1.03	1.00
30	0.80	0.56	0.45	0.56	0.79	0.99	1.07	1.00
40	0.71	0.43	0.31	0.42	0.70	0.97	1.09	0.98
50	0.59	0.28	0.17	0.28	0.59	0.93	1.09	0.94
60	0.46	0.14	0.05	0.14	0.46	0.87	1.08	0.87
70	0.32	0.02	—	0.02	0.31	0.80	1.11	0.81
80	0.16	—	—	—	0.16	0.81	1.17	0.82
90 S	—	—	—	—	—	0.83	1.18	0.83

then a small secondary maximum. This gives way to the zones in which the quantity of radiation steadily declines to zero. At the equinoxes, the maximum quantity of radiation falls on the equator; with increasing latitude, the quantities of radiation decrease at first slowly and then more and more rapidly.

For calculating the monthly, seasonal, and annual quantities of radiation, one can use the formulas above, taking into account that $\delta_\odot$ and l must be considered variable in this case. An appropriate calculation requires rather bulky computations; therefore, we shall here give an account only of the results of determining the quantities of radiation in the summer and winter half-years at various latitudes (Table 2). It should be borne in mind that the quantity of radiation in each half-year at a given latitude of the Northern Hemisphere equals the quantity of radiation at the same latitude in the Southern Hemisphere.

In reality, the atmosphere is not a completely transparent medium for solar radiation. A noticeable part of the radiation coming from the sun is absorbed and scattered in the atmosphere, and also is reflected into space. Solar radiation is especially influenced by clouds; but even when cloudiness is absent, solar radiation is changed greatly in the atmosphere.

TABLE 2

SUMS OF SOLAR RADIATION INCIDENT UPON THE SURFACE OF THE EARTH
UNDER A COMPLETELY TRANSPARENT ATMOSPHERE (kcal cm^{-2})

	Latitude									
	0°	10°	20°	30°	40°	50°	60°	70°	80°	90°
Summer half-year	160.5	170	175	174	170	161	149	139	135	133
Winter half-year	160.5	147	129	108	84	59	34	13	3	0
Year	321	317	304	282	254	220	183	152	138	133

Solar radiation is absorbed in the atmosphere by water vapor, water droplets, carbon dioxide, ozone, and dust. Diffusion of solar radiation is affected both by the molecules of air and by various admixtures—dust, water drops, and so forth.

The flux of direct solar radiation that passes through the atmosphere depends on the transparency of the atmosphere and the sun's altitude, which defines the length of the path of the solar rays in the atmosphere.

For a quantitative accounting of this effect, the following considerations are usual.

Let us consider that the reduction of the flux of direct solar radiation S_λ of wavelength λ, over the path segment dx is proportional to its initial value, i.e.,

$$dS_\lambda = -k_\lambda S_\lambda \, dx, \tag{1.10}$$

where k_λ is the coefficient of reduction, taking into account the effect of absorption and scattering processes.

Hence, after integrating for values of x from 0 to ∞, one can derive a formula

$$S_\lambda = Q_{s\lambda} \exp\left(-\int_0^\infty k_\lambda \, dx\right), \tag{1.11}$$

where $Q_{s\lambda}$ is the corresponding flux of radiation at the external boundary of the atmosphere.

This formula defines the conditions of reduction of the solar radiation flux of a given wavelength when it passes through the atmosphere. Equation (1.11) can be written in the form

$$S_\lambda = Q_{s\lambda}P_\lambda, \tag{1.12}$$

the value of P_λ (equal to $\exp[-\int_0^\infty k_\lambda \, dx]$) being called the coefficient of atmospheric transparency.

If a flux of radiation is directed at a slant with an angle of $z_\odot$ to the vertical, then the element of the ray's path dx equals $\sec z_\odot \, dh$, where h is the vertical coordinate. From this we derive the formula

$$S_\lambda = Q_{s\lambda} \exp\left(-\sec z_\odot \int_0^\infty k_\lambda \, dh\right), \tag{1.13}$$

or

$$S_\lambda = Q_{s\lambda}P_\lambda^{\sec z_\odot}. \tag{1.14}$$

In real conditions, as a consequence of the earth's sphericity, the angle between the solar ray and the vertical turns out to be different in different latitudes. Besides, the ray usually becomes distorted in the atmosphere because of refraction. Therefore, the two last formulas are approximate and in more accurate calculations must be replaced by the expression

$$S_\lambda = Q_{s\lambda}P_\lambda^{m(z_\odot)}, \tag{1.15}$$

where $m(z_\odot)$ is the optical mass of the atmosphere.

At zenith angles from 0 to 60°, the optical mass is close to the value of $\sec z_\odot$, but at large angles, its values are noticeably smaller than the secant.

As observational results show, values of transparency coefficients are different for different wavelengths.

In actinometric investigations, the mean value of the transparency coefficient for the total flux of solar energy is often used. In this case, the following formula is applied:

$$S = Q_s P^{m(z_\odot)}. \tag{1.16}$$

In contrast to the value of P_λ, the value of P turns out to depend noticeably on optical mass (Forbes effect). This dependence is explained by the fact that when solar rays pass through the atmosphere, their spectral composition changes in accordance with the differential reduction of rays of different wavelengths. Therefore, the value of P increases with the increase of path length in the atmosphere.

More satisfactory results are obtained in calculating the reduction of solar radiation in the atmosphere from a simple formula of Kastrov (1928),

$$S = \frac{Q_s}{1 + cm(z_\odot)},$$ (1.17)

where c is a dimensionless coefficient defining atmospheric transparency.

The mean values of the coefficient P in middle latitudes at small values of m are usually equal to 0.7 to 0.8. The coefficient c in Kastrov's formula is a more sensitive index of transparency and changes over much wider limits.

For evaluating atmospheric transparency, the index of turbidity, proposed by Makhotkin (1957), which corresponds to the number of normal atmospheres and which provides an observed value of radiation flux at a given altitude of the sun, deserves attention.

As has been pointed out above, in addition to conditions of atmospheric transparency, cloudiness also greatly influences the value of direct radiation reaching the earth's surface. With more or less dense clouds covering the sun, direct radiation is zero.

The greatest value of the direct radiation flux is observed with a cloudless sky and a highly transparent atmosphere. In such conditions, the flux of direct radiation incident on a perpendicular surface (the intensity of solar radiation) at sea level can amount to 1.5–1.7 cal cm^{-2} min^{-1}. Average afternoon values of this flux in middle latitudes usually equal 1.0–1.4 cal cm^{-2} min^{-1}.

As the altitude of the sun decreases during the diurnal cycle, the direct solar radiation is noticeably reduced in accordance with the increase in optical mass.

The amount of scattered radiation reaching the earth's surface changes within wide limits, mainly in accordance with conditions of cloudiness and the sun's altitude. The theoretical calculation of this radiation flux is rather complicated and does not give precise results. The available observational data permit us to think that in many cases the flux of scattered radiation is comparable in value with the flux of direct radiation incident on a horizontal surface. The greatest values of scattered radiation are observed when cloudiness is present. Scattered radiation is greatly influenced by the reflectivity of the earth's surface. In particular, scattered radiation increases appreciably in the presence of snow cover, which reflects a considerable amount of solar energy.

The spectral composition of solar radiation reaching the earth's surface differs greatly from that of radiation outside the atmosphere.

The energy distribution in the solar spectrum obtained from the ground observational data is represented by the curve B in Fig. 2. For comparison, the energy distribution in the spectrum outside the atmosphere is given (curve *A*). Comparison of these two curves shows that ultraviolet radiation (wavelengths less than 0.4 μm) is to a considerable extent absorbed in the atmosphere and does not reach the earth's surface. It is known that the absorption of the ultraviolet radiation is mainly caused by atmospheric ozone. As seen in Fig. 2, the absorption of solar radiation in the domain of large wavelengths is very uneven, which indicates the heterogeneity of the spectral transparency of the atmosphere.

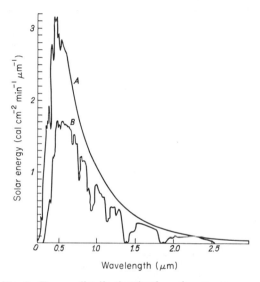

Fig. 2 Energy distribution in the solar spectrum.

The greatest amount of energy in the solar spectrum falls in the domain of the visible part of the spectrum (the wavelengths from 0.40 to 0.74 μm). Along with this, a considerable amount of energy is transmitted in the form of infrared radiation (wavelengths exceeding 0.74 μm). Ultraviolet radiation is relatively small; however, it has a large influence on various biological processes.

The general picture of the basic solar energy transformations in the geographical envelope of the earth is as follows.

The flux of solar radiation at a mean distance of the earth from the sun is approximately equal to 1000 kcal cm^{-2} yr^{-1}. Because of the spherical shape of the earth, there comes to the unit area of the external atmospheric boundary, on the average, one fourth of the total flux—about 250 kcal cm^{-2} yr^{-1}, of which approximately 170 kcal cm^{-2} yr^{-1} are absorbed by the earth as a planet. It is significant that the greater part of the total amount of absorption represents absorption by the earth's surface, while the atmosphere absorbs a considerably smaller fraction.

The earth's surface, heated by absorbing solar radiation, is a source of emitted long-wave radiation, which heats the atmosphere. Water vapor in the atmosphere, dust, and various gases absorbing long-wave radiation hamper the long-wave radiation going out from the earth's surface. Thus, a great part of the emission from the earth's surface is compensated by the counter-radiation of the atmosphere.

The difference between the earth's surface emission itself and the counter-radiation of the atmosphere is called the net long-wave radiation. The value of net long-wave radiation is usually several times smaller than the flux of long-wave emission from the earth's surface that would be observed if the atmosphere were completely transparent to long-wave radiation.

The algebraic sum of the radiative energy fluxes coming to the earth's surface and going out from it is called the radiation budget or balance at the earth's surface. It is evident that the value of the radiation budget is equal to the difference between the amount of direct and scattered short-wave radiation absorbed by the surface and the value of the net long-wave radiation.

On the average for the whole surface of the earth, the net long-wave radiation is much less than the absorbed short-wave radiation. This is a consequence of the so-called greenhouse effect, that is, the result of a relatively great transparency of the atmosphere for short-wave radiation in comparison to a smaller transparency for long-wave emission. Therefore, the mean radiation balance at the earth's surface is a positive value.

The energy in the radiation budget or balance at the earth's surface is expended on heating the atmosphere by means of turbulent heat conductivity, on evaporation, on heat exchange with the deeper layers of the hydrosphere or lithosphere, and so on. The quantitative characteristics of all the forms of solar energy transformation at the earth's surface are comprised in the equation of the heat balance at the earth's surface, which includes the algebraic sum of energy fluxes incident upon and outgoing from the earth's surface. According to the law of conservation of energy, this sum is equal to zero.

The radiation and heat balances at the earth's surface are definitely connected with the radiation and heat balances of the atmosphere. The earth as a planet receives heat from space and gives it back only in the form of radiation. As the mean temperature of the earth changes little in time, it is evident that the radiation balance of the earth (the difference between absorbed radiation and radiation emitted into space) is equal to zero.

Therefore, the radiation budget of the atmosphere, which equals the difference between the planet Earth's radiation balance and the radiation budget at the earth's surface, turns out, on the average, to be negative, and is equal in absolute value to the radiation budget at the earth's surface.

In the heat balance of the atmosphere, the negative radiation budget is compensated by a supply of energy resulting from condensation of water vapor in the formation of clouds and precipitation, and by a supply of [sensible] heat from the earth's surface resulting from the turbulent heat conductivity of the lower layers of the atmosphere.

Along with the processes of redistributing solar energy in the vertical direction, strong processes of horizontal redistribution of heat are developed in the geographical envelope. Especially important among these processes is the transfer of thermal energy in the atmosphere and the hydrosphere between high and low latitudes, determined by the heterogeneity of radiative heating of the spherical surface of the earth. This transfer is carried out in the form of macroturbulent heat exchange and heat transfer by mean motion, and also (in the atmosphere) in the form of phase transformations of water.

The enumerated processes of solar energy transformation, dependent on radiative factors, in their turn significantly change the radiation regime, which depends substantially on circulations in the atmosphere and hydrosphere, phase transformations of water, and so forth. Cloudiness and snow (or ice) cover on the earth's surface produce an especially great effect on the radiation regime.

Beside the "first order" processes of transformations of solar energy, which substantially change the radiation and heat regimes, a number of solar-energy transformations, involving comparatively small amounts of heat, and not influencing the radiation and heat regimes directly, are developed in the geographical envelope. These processes are usually of less importance for meteorological investigations; however, some of them are very interesting for other natural sciences, such as, for example, the process of photosynthesis connected with transformation of radiant energy into a comparatively stable form of chemical energy and formation of organic matter.

The basic source of data for studying all the forms of solar-energy transformation in the geographical envelope is the material from the radiation and heat balances. Especially important for investigation of transformations of solar energy are data on the radiation and heat balances at the earth's surface, which are the main source of energy for the geographical envelope.

2. The Radiation Balance

The radiation balance (or budget) of the earth's surface R is equal to the difference between the absorbed solar radiation and the net long-wave radiation,

$$R = Q(1 - \alpha) - I, \tag{1.18}$$

where Q is the total short-wave radiation (the sum of direct and scattered radiation), α is the albedo (the reflectivity of the earth's surface for total short-wave radiation, expressed in fractions of unity), and I is the net long-wave radiation, i.e., the difference between the radiation emitted by the earth's surface itself and the absorbed counterradiation of the atmosphere.

One can similarly determine the radiation balance of the earth–atmosphere system R_s, i.e., the radiation balance of the vertical column through the whole thickness of the atmosphere to the earth's surface.

We obtain in this case

$$R_s = Q_s(1 - \alpha_s) - I_s, \tag{1.19}$$

where Q_s is the solar radiation incident on the outer boundary of the atmosphere, α_s is the albedo of the earth–atmosphere system, and I_s is the long-wave emission from the outer boundary of the atmosphere into space (outgoing emission).

The radiation balance or budget of the atmosphere R_a equals the difference between the values of R_s and R. Using Eqs. (1.18) and (1.19), we get

$$R_a = Q_s(1 - \alpha_s) - Q(1 - \alpha) - (I_s - I). \tag{1.20}$$

It has often been indicated [Budyko (1956), and elsewhere] that the term "radiation balance" [for "radiation surplus" or "radiation deficit"] is not quite satisfactory because the expression "balance" is not used here in a conventional sense, and means calculation of income and expenditure of only one category of energy—that of radiation. Application of this expression is especially awkward when studying the heat balance, as these similar terms have an entirely different physical content. However, it is difficult now to give up this expression, because it is generally used in all the hydrometeorological disciplines.

The conditions of reflection of solar radiation from the earth's surface are defined by the value of albedo, which is equal to the ratio of the value of reflected radiation to incoming. Theoretically, the values of albedo might vary from one for a completely white and reflective surface to zero for an absolutely black surface, which completely absorbs the sun's rays.

Available observational materials show that the albedo of natural underlying surfaces does vary within wide limits, their variations embracing almost the full possible range of values of reflective ability of various surfaces.

In experimental investigations of reflection of solar radiation, values of albedo for all more or less widespread natural underlying surfaces have been found. First of all, it follows from these investigations that the conditions of solar radiation absorption on land and water differ notably.

The greatest values of albedo are observed for clean and dry snow, where they may reach 0.90–0.95. As snow cover is rarely absolutely clean, the mean values of snow albedo are in most cases less than the noted value, and equal to 0.70–0.80. The albedo of wet or dirty snow may be still less, often reduced to 0.40–0.50.

In the absence of snow, the largest albedo on the land surface is observed in desert regions where the surface of the soil is covered by a layer of crystal salts (the bottoms of dry salt lakes). In these conditions, the value of albedo may reach 0.50. Slightly lesser values of albedo have been observed in the areas of deserts barren of any vegetation, with light-colored sandy soils. It must be indicated, however, that the albedo of deserts may vary within wide limits according to the color of soil.

The albedo of a damp soil is usually less than that of a similar dry soil. For damp chernozem soils, the albedo is reduced to very small values, in some cases as low as 0.05.

The albedo of natural surfaces with a dense vegetation cover varies within comparatively small limits, basically from 0.10 to 0.20–0.25. Some observational data show that the albedo of forest (especially needleleaf forest) is in most cases slightly less than the albedo of low vegetation of the meadow type. Such a phenomenon is probably explicable by better conditions of absorption within the limits of deep vegetation cover, where there is an increased probability that solar radiation fluxes having penetrated the vegetation will be absorbed after their first reflection from elements of the vegetation.

It follows from these data of albedo for various natural surfaces that albedo in many climatic regions must vary noticeably during the annual cycle. Such variations are important for the annual cycle of the radiation balance.

The conditions of solar radiation absorption by water bodies differ from those of absorption at the land surface. More or less clean water is comparatively transparent for short-wave radiation, and so the sun's rays penetrating the upper layers of a water body are widely scattered and then to a considerable extent absorbed.

It is easily understood that the process of solar radiation absorption in such conditions should depend on the solar altitude. If the sun stands high, a great part of the incoming radiation penetrates the upper layers of water and is in general absorbed there. At low altitudes of the sun, the rays incident on the water surface at small angles are specularly reflected and do not penetrate into the depths of the water body. This leads to an abrupt increase of the albedo.

As theoretical calculations and experimental investigations show [refer to Kondrat'ev (1965)], the albedo of water surfaces for direct radiation varies within a wide limit, in dependence on the sun's altitude.

The character of this dependence is seen from the graph in Fig. 3. At large altitudes of the sun, the albedo for direct radiation does not exceed several hundredths, while with the sun approaching the horizon the albedo reaches values of the order of several tenths. The albedo of a water surface for scattered radiation apparently varies much less. Its value is about 0.10.

The albedo of the earth–atmosphere system is of a more complicated nature than that of the earth's surface.

Solar radiation received by the atmosphere is partially reflected as a result of back-scattering. With clouds present, a considerable fraction of radiation can be reflected from their upper surfaces. With complete or partial absence of clouds, the albedo of the earth–atmosphere system depends essentially on the albedo of the earth's surface.

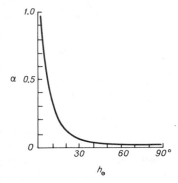

Fig. 3   Dependence of water-surface albedo for direct-beam radiation on the altitude of the sun.

The albedo of clouds depends on the thickness of their layers, its mean value being equal to 0.40–0.50. The albedo of the earth–atmosphere system without clouds is usually greater than that of the earth's surface. With clouds present, it is also usually greater than the albedo of the earth's surface, except in those cases when the surface is covered by more or less clean snow.

Together with the reflection of short-wave radiation, long-wave radiation is a no less important form of radiative energy outgo. The basic features of the process of heat transfer by long-wave radiation can be presented in the following form.

Radiation from an absolutely black body according to the Stefan–Boltzmann law equals σT^4, where T is the temperature in the Kelvin scale, and σ is the Stefan–Boltzmann constant (equal to 8.14×10^{-11} cal cm^{-2} min^{-1} deg^{-4}).

Available experimental data show that radiation from the earth's natural surfaces is, in general, rather close to radiation from a black body at the corresponding temperature, the ratio of the observed values of radiation to black-body radiation in most cases amounting to 0.90–1.00.

The greatest intensity of long-wave radiation from the earth's surface occurs in different wavelengths, depending on the temperature of the radiating surface. The principal part of the radiated energy occurs in wavelengths from five to several tens of micrometers.

A considerable part of the long-wave radiation flux emitted by the earth's surface is compensated by the counterradiation of the atmosphere.

The long-wave emission of the atmosphere without clouds present is, in general, determined by the presence of water vapor and carbon dioxide. The effect of the atmospheric ozone is usually less important.

Water vapor, as well as carbon dioxide, absorbs long-wave radiation mainly in certain spectral areas. In accordance with this pattern, the long-wave emission from the atmosphere is also rather heterogeneous in spectral distribution.

The most intensive absorption of radiation by water vapor takes place in the range of wavelengths from 5 to 7.5 μm, while in the spectral range from 9 to 12 μm, absorption of radiation is relatively small. Carbon dioxide has several bands of absorption, of which the band with wavelengths from 13 to 17 μm is of greatest importance.

It must be indicated that the carbon dioxide content in the atmosphere varies comparatively little, while the amount of water vapor may vary by a large amount in dependence on meteorological conditions. Therefore, variation of atmospheric humidity turns out to be a substantial factor influencing radiation from the atmosphere.

Usually the counterradiation of the atmosphere increases greatly with the presence of clouds. The clouds of lower and middle layers are, as a rule, sufficiently dense and radiate like an absolutely black body at the same temperature. Under such conditions, the net long-wave radiation is mainly defined by the difference between the temperature of the earth's surface and that of the lower surface of the clouds. If this difference is small, the net radiation also approaches zero.

High clouds, because of their small density, usually radiate less than a black body. Taking into account the fact that the temperature of such clouds is comparatively low, one can conclude that their effect on net long-wave radiation is negligible in comparison with the clouds of lower and middle layers.

Thus, the net long-wave radiation at the earth's surface depends primarily on the temperature of the earth's surface, the water content of the air, and cloudiness. In response to these factors, its value may vary from close to zero up to several tenths of a calorie per square centimeter per minute.

Radiation from the earth–atmosphere system is formed by that part of the radiation emitted by the earth's surface that passes through the atmosphere, and by radiation from the atmosphere. Without clouds, emission from the earth's surface at wavelengths from 9 to 12 μm plays a significant role in the radiation from the system. Under conditions of complete cloudiness, radiation from the upper surface of the clouds, which depends on their surface temperature, comes to be of principal importance. As this temperature is usually much lower than the temperature of the earth's surface, it is evident that cloudiness considerably reduces the loss of heat to space by long-wave radiation.

3. The Heat Balance

Equations of the heat balance represent a particular formulation of one of the principal laws of physics—the law of the conservation of energy. These equations can be derived for various volumes and surfaces in the atmosphere, the hydrosphere, and the lithosphere. The heat-balance equations for the earth's surface and for the earth–atmosphere system, i.e., for the vertical column passing through the whole geographical envelope, are most frequently used in modern investigations.

The heat-balance equation of the earth's surface includes the fluxes of energy between the surface element and surrounding space. These fluxes include the radiative fluxes of heat, whose sum is equal to the radiation balance.

Positive or negative values of the radiation balance are compensated by several fluxes of heat. As the temperature of the earth's surface is usually not equal to the air temperature, a flux of heat takes place between the underlying surface and the atmosphere, and is dependent on the turbulent heat conductivity.

A similar flux of heat is observed between the earth's surface and deeper layers of the lithosphere or hydrosphere, if the temperature of the surface differs from that of the deeper layers. In this case, a flux of heat in soil is determined by molecular heat conductivity, while the heat conductivity in water bodies is as a rule of a more or less turbulent character.

The conversion of heat for evaporation is very important for the heat balance at the earth's surface. The amount of evaporation depends on the moistness of the earth's surface, its temperature, atmospheric humidity, and the intensity of turbulent exchange in the lowest layer of air, which determines the rate of water-vapor transfer from the earth's surface to the atmosphere. With regard to this factor, the regularities of heat conversion in evaporation turn out to be similar in many respects to those of the turbulent exchange of sensible heat between the earth's surface and the atmosphere.

The conversion of heat in evaporation changes sign with the change in the direction of the water-vapor flux. If the flux of water vapor is directed from the atmosphere to the earth's surface, then the outgo of heat for evaporation is changed into an input of the heat of condensation of water vapor.

To derive the heat-balance equation, we shall designate the radiative flux of heat by R, the turbulent flux of heat between the underlying surface and the atmosphere by P, the heat flux between the underlying surface and the lower layers by A, and the conversion of heat in evaporation (or the release of heat in condensation) by LE (L is the latent heat of vaporization; E is the rate of evaporation). Since all other components of heat balance are usually much smaller than the fluxes of heat listed here, we may write, in the first approximation, the heat-balance equation in the form

$$R = LE + P + A. \tag{1.21}$$

The value of the radiative flux (the radiation balance) R is considered to be positive if it designates an income of heat to the underlying surface, and all other values are considered positive if they designate the disbursal of heat from the surface. It must be noted that, in a number of papers, another system of signs for the components of heat balance is used, according to which all the balance components have the same sign in accordance with the disbursal or income of heat. Such a system of designations is more logical, but it leads to difficulties connected with the fact that the expenditure of heat for evaporation and the turbulent loss of [sensible] heat from the earth's surface to the atmosphere must be considered as negative values, which is at variance with established practice.

The scheme of heat fluxes included in the equation of the heat balance is shown in Fig. 4.

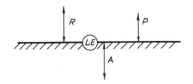

Fig. 4 Model of the heat balance at the earth's surface.

Regarding those components of heat balance that have not been included in Eq. (1.21), a considerable size can be attributed to the expenditure of heat for melting snow or ice on the earth's surface (or to the gain of heat from the freezing of water). Although for longer averaging periods (a year or so), the latter value, as a rule, is considerably smaller than the main components of the balance, however, in some cases (for instance, periods of snow melting in the middle and high latitudes) this value should be included in Eq. (1.21) as an additional term.

Other components of the heat balance—heat fluxes due to the dissipation of the mechanical energy of wind, wind waves, tides, and currents, the heat flux (positive or negative) transferred by the fall of precipitation that has a different temperature from that of the underlying surface, as well as the conversion of energy in photosynthesis and the gain from oxidation of biological substances—are usually considerably smaller than the chief components of the balance, for averages obtained for periods of any length.

Exceptions to this rule are possible (as for instance in case of a forest fire, when great quantities of energy previously accumulated by the process of photosynthesis are rapidly released), but are relatively rare.

Because of the linearity of Eq. (1.21), the balance components designating the heat fluxes may be substituted for their sums for any given period of time. In this case, the form of the equation remains unchanged.

The value of heat flux A going from the earth's surface to lower layers can be determined by the other heat-balance components of the upper layers of the lithosphere or hydrosphere. If we derive a heat-balance equation for the vertical column with the upper boundary at the earth's surface and the base at a depth where the flux of heat is negligible, we get an equation

$$A = B + F_0, \qquad (1.22)$$

where F_0 is the income of heat resulting from heat exchange between the column and the ambient space of the lithosphere or hydrosphere in a horizontal direction, and B is the change in amount of heat within the column during the given period of time (refer to Fig. 5).

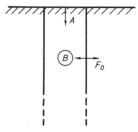

Fig. 5   Model of the heat balance of the upper layer of the lithosphere or hydrosphere.

The vertical flux of heat passing through the base of the column can be assumed to be equal to zero, since the heat flow from the depths of the earth is usually negligible in comparison with the' principal components of the heat balance.

The value of F_0 is equal to the difference between the heat fluxes entering and leaving through the sides of the column in question. The F_0 component becomes very important in large water bodies where currents exist and great horizontal heat conductivity takes place, conditioned by the effects of macro-turbulence.

In the lithosphere, the F_0 value is, as a rule, insignificant because of the small heat conductivity of soil. Therefore, for the land, we have $A = B$. Because, on the average over the year, the upper layers of soil are neither warmed nor cooled, we must assume that long-term annual mean values for the land are $A = B = 0$.

In the heat balance of water bodies that are more or less insignificant as to area and analyzed as whole bodies, the values of A are also very close to B, because the heat exchange between the water and ground is usually small in comparison with the principal components of the heat balance.

However, for some portions of the oceans and other water bodies (lakes and seas), the values of A and B might be very different. Therefore, in such conditions, the mean annual value of heat exchange between the active surface and the underlying layers is equal, not to zero, but to the amount of heat received or lost by the vertical column through the hydrosphere because of the activity of currents and macroturbulence (that is, $A = F_0$).

Thus, the equation of heat balance for the land over the mean annual period will be

$$R = LE + P, \qquad (1.23)$$

and, for the ocean,

$$R = LE + P + F_0. \qquad (1.24)$$

In some cases, both these equations can be simplified. Thus, in deserts, where the amount of evaporation is close to zero, Eq. (1.23) will simply be $R = P$. For the world ocean as a whole, where the general redistribution of heat by sea currents is self-compensatory and sums up to zero, Eq. (1.24) is transformed into $R = LE + P$.

Concluding our analysis of the heat-balance equations for the earth's surface, we must note that when these equations are applied one must bear in mind that the concept of the "earth's surface" (sometimes called the "active surface" or the "underlying surface") is somewhat conventionalized.

Actually, the "surface" processes of solar-energy transformation are developed, not on a two-dimensional surface, but in a layer of some thickness, as for example when the processes of heat conversion for evaporation on land takes place, or when water bodies absorb solar energy, and so on. The "active layer" reaches a considerable thickness in places having tall vegetation (especially so in forests).

However, even when dealing with an active layer of considerable thickness, we can use the concept of the active surface, which will not lead us into any noticeable inaccuracies, especially in studies of the balance components where long periods of time are averaged. But in individual cases (studying rapid changes in the components, etc.), it is more suitable to use the concept of an active layer instead of the active surface.

To derive a heat-balance equation for the earth–atmosphere system, we must analyze the gains and losses of heat energy in the vertical column that extends through the whole atmosphere and the upper layers of the hydro- and lithosphere down to the levels where seasonal (or diurnal) variations in temperature cease.

The exchange of heat between the column and outer space will be characterized by its radiation balance R_s, which equals the difference between solar radiation absorbed by the whole column and the total long-wave outgoing radiation from the column (refer to Fig. 6). We will consider the value of R_s as being positive when it shows that heat is gained by this system.

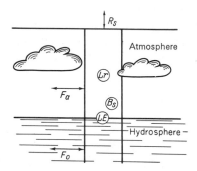

Fig. 6   Model of the heat balance of the earth–atmosphere system.

Extending the column deep into the lithosphere or hydrosphere, down to those layers where the thermal regime is no longer affected by variations of meteorological factors, we may assume that the flux of heat through the base of the column is practically equal to zero.

The fluxes of heat passing through the lateral surfaces of the column are determined by the horizontal transfer of heat in the atmosphere and hydrosphere. The difference between the income and outgo of heat due to heat transfer in the atmosphere is presented in Fig. 6 by the arrow F_a, and the similar characteristic for the hydrosphere by arrow F_0.

It must be indicated that F_a is similar in its physical meaning to F_0. This value defines the input or outgo of heat in the air column owing to the activity of atmospheric advection and macroturbulence.

Besides the heat exchange that occurs through the surfaces of the column, there are other factors that also affect its heat balance, namely, sources of heat (positive or negative) located inside the column. Among these, basic significance is attributed to the sources or sinks of heat associated with phase changes of water and especially the process of evaporation and condensation.

The gain of heat from condensation in the atmosphere is equal to the difference between the income and outgo of heat connected with condensation and evaporation of water droplets in clouds and fog. Over a sufficiently homogeneous surface for long periods of time, the averaged difference between the values of condensation and evaporation in the atmosphere is equal to total precipitation r. The income of heat in this case is equal to Lr. The corresponding component of the heat balance represents the difference between the income of heat from condensation and the expenditure of heat in evaporating droplets. It might, however, differ from the value Lr in conditions of broken country and also in individual short intervals of time.

The expenditure of heat for evaporation (the difference between the loss of heat for evaporation from the surface of water bodies, from vegetation and soil, and the gain of heat from condensation on these objects) is equal to LE. The general influence of condensation and evaporation on the heat balance of the column can be approximately expressed by the value $L(r - E)$.

Among the other heat-balance components of the column, the change in heat content inside the column B_s that occurs during the period for which the values have been summarized should be taken into account. The other components of the balance (the gain of heat from dissipation of mechanical energy, the difference between the amount converted in melting ice and the gain from ice formation, the difference between the loss of heat in photosynthesis processes and the gain in oxidation of organic matter, and so on) are usually insignificant in the heat balance of the earth–atmosphere system and need not be calculated.

Writing down the equation of the heat balance of the earth–atmosphere system in the form

$$R_s = F_s + L(E - r) + B_s \qquad (1.25)$$

where $F_s = F_a + F_0$, we will assume that all the terms on the right side are positive if they show an outgo of heat. For the average annual period, the B_s value will be close to zero and Eq. (1.25) will be transformed into

$$R_s = F_s + L(E - r). \qquad (1.26)$$

For land, this equation has the form

$$R_s = F_a + L(E - r). \qquad (1.27)$$

Since, for the earth as a whole, $E = r$ and the horizontal heat transfer in the atmosphere and hydrosphere in total is approximately equal to zero, the heat-balance equation for the whole geographical envelope assumes the simple form

$$R_s = 0. \tag{1.28}$$

The heat-balance equation of the atmosphere can be obtained by summing up the relevant heat fluxes, or simply by taking the difference between the heat balance of the earth–atmosphere system and the earth's surface.

Assuming that the radiation balance of the atmosphere R_a is equal to $R_s - R$, and that the change in heat content in the atmosphere B_a is equal to $B_s - B$, we find that

$$R_a = F_a - Lr - P + B_a \tag{1.29}$$

and, for the average annual period,

$$R_a = F_a - Lr - P. \tag{1.30}$$

Investigating the heat balance, it is necessary in many cases to take into account data on water balance.

The equation of water balance for the land is the expression of the condition when the algebraic sum of all forms of gain and loss of solid, fluid, and gaseous water received by a horizontal surface from ambient space during a certain interval of time is equal to zero.

This equation will be

$$r = E + f_w + G, \tag{1.31}$$

where r is the precipitation, E is the difference between evaporation and condensation on the earth's surface (usually just called evaporation), f_w is the surface run-off, and G is the flow of moisture from the earth's surface to the underlying layers.

The last value (G) is the algebraic sum of the gravitational flux of liquid water from the soil surface into deeper layers, the vertical flux of film moisture, the vertical flux of water vapor, the flux of water raised by the roots of plants, and so on, obtained in summing up these fluxes for the analyzed period of time.

Equation (1.31) is more often used in a modified form, which can be derived by considering the fact that the vertical flux of moisture G is equal to the sum of ground-water flow f_p and the change of water content in the upper layers of the lithosphere b. (This equality corresponds to the equation of water balance of the vertical column that extends through the upper layers of the lithosphere down to the depths where moisture exchange practically does not take place.)

Bearing in mind the fact that the sum of the surface run-off f_w and underground run-off f_p is equal to the total run-off f, we find that

$$r = E + f + b. \tag{1.32}$$

Equation (1.32) can also be used for calculating the water balance in water bodies or in separate parts of them. In this case, the value of f will characterize the redistribution of water in a horizontal direction for the analyzed period in the water body itself and underlying layers of the ground (if there is any noticeable redistribution of moisture). Similarly, the value of b, if taken for the water body, is equal to the total change in water quantity in the reservoir itself, and underlying layers as well, if there is a noticeable change in moisture content. Practically, in many cases the value of b is determined for water bodies by the change in water level. For the average annual period, the value of b is often very small, and the equation of the water balance changes into the form

$$r = E + f. \tag{1.33}$$

Over the whole globe, the horizontal redistribution of moisture does not matter, and therefore the equation of water balance has the simple form

$$r = E. \tag{1.34}$$

The equation of water balance has the same form for the mean annual period for conditions of land areas without run-off, including deserts.

In closing, we will give the equation of water balance in the atmosphere. By adding up all the categories of the gain and loss of moisture in the vertical column that extends through the atmosphere, we easily obtain the equation

$$E = r + c_\mathrm{a} + b_\mathrm{a}, \tag{1.35}$$

where c_a is the quantity of moisture that is gained or lost by the vertical column by the action of air currents and horizontal turbulent exchange, and b_a is the change in the quantity of water in the column.

Since the atmosphere can contain only relatively small quantities of water in any of its phases, the value of b_a is usually much smaller than the other components of the balance. Its average annual value is close to zero.

4. General Review of Investigations on the Transformation of Solar Energy

The formulation of the problem of heat-balance investigations was made by the outstanding climatologist Voeikov, who analyzed in his many works various concrete questions associated with the study of the heat balance. For instance, in "Климаты земного шара, в особенности России (The Climate of the Earth, Especially Russia")" (1884), Voeikov paid much attention to the calculation of the annual regime in the heat content of lakes. These calculations permitted him to draw conclusions about the influence of water bodies on climatic conditions in various regions.

In his work "Кругооборот тепла в оболочке земного шара (The Circulation of Heat in the Mantle of the Globe") (1904), the question about the climate-forming effect of the heat exchange in soil and water bodies is analyzed in detail. Many ideas of Voeikov outlined in this work had great influence on investigations of the genesis of climate. It is enough to remember, for one thing, Voeikov's statement about the exceptionally important concept of the active surface, and his analysis of the relation between heat exchange and the annual and diurnal marches of temperature.

However, it is obvious that any more or less comprehensive investigations of the heat balance at the earth's surface could be started only after establishment of an effective methodology for determining its principal components.

Let us consider first some investigations on heat balance at the earth's surface.

The development of methods for determining the components of the heat balance started in two principal directions: (1) designing special instruments for measuring the separate components of the balance; and (2) developing methods for calculating the balance components, based on the general regularities of the physics of the atmosphere and employing the data of mass hydrometeorological observations.

The first stage in the development of methods for determining the balance components, based on application of special instruments, was closely connected with the development of actinometric investigations. These investigations began in the first half of the 19th century, when instruments for measuring direct solar radiation were designed. One of the first instruments of the kind was based on the thermostat principle, heating by solar rays permitting the determination of the incoming radiative energy (Pouillet, 1838).

Systematic observations of direct solar radiation were started in the second half of the 19th century. The actinometer of Khvol'son, with which the observations of direct solar radiation were started in Pavlovsk in 1890, played a great role in the development of actinometry in Russia. The possibilities for measuring solar shortwave radiation were greatly expanded when Mikhel'son, Ångström, and Abbot invented more perfect actinometers. Later on, instruments that permitted more accurate measurements of scattered radiation were invented. The progress achieved in improvements of actinometric instruments contributed to a rather rapid expansion of the actinometric observational network.

The data on expansion of the network of actinometric stations are presented in Fig. 7. It is seen from this figure that the development of the world actinometric network was especially accelerated during the 1950s—the period of preparation for and conducting the International Geophysical Year.

Although the number of actinometric stations now available is noticeably less than that of the meteorological stations that carry out observations of the principal meteorological elements, it is possible even now to generalize the available data of actinometric observations to obtain a number of conclusions of a climatological character.

However, it must be noted that up to the present time, actinometric observations at most stations have been limited to measurements of the flux of short-wave radiation. Measurements of long-wave radiation, and especially net long-wave radiation, involved considerable methodological difficulties and therefore were started much later than the measurements of short-wave radiation.

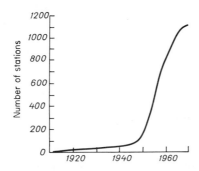

Fig. 7 Development of the world actinometric network.

The first instrument used for more or less systematic measurements of the net long-wave radiation was the pyrgeometer of K. Ångström, designed in 1916. Subsequently, it was established that observations made with this instrument contained significant errors.

Later, instruments were constructed that permitted measurements of net long-wave radiation without major errors, not only at night but also during daylight hours. Among these instruments are the effective pyranometer of Ianishevskii, the vibrational balance-meter of Falkenberg, and others.

More or less reliable instruments for direct measurement of the radiation balance have been designed comparatively recently. Among them there are the balance-meters of Ianishevskii, Aizenshtat, Courvoisier, Schulze, Gier and Dunkle, and other workers.

In the USSR, the improvement of balance-meters has been accomplished by Ianishevskii. As a result of long years of investigation, he has designed a rather simple construction of a thermoelectric balance-meter that permits the measurement of radiation-balance values without large errors.

At present, balance-meters are largely used in stationary observations at the meteorological stations of the USSR. Since the end of the 1950s, observations of radiation balance have been carried out at more than 100 stations of this country. In other countries, however, such observations are organized at a much smaller number of points, which restricts the possibilities of using the data from observations of radiation balance in climatological investigations.

Methods for direct measurements of other components of the heat balance of the earth's surface, especially the exchanges of latent and sensible heat, are much less developed than those for measurements of the components of the radiation balance.

Since the latent heat of evaporation represents a well-known physical value, there is the possibility of finding the amount of heat lost in evaporation by measuring evaporation from the earth's surface.

Although the instruments for determining evaporation from the land surface (evaporimeters of several makes) have been developed over a long period of time, the available observational data from evaporimeters are relatively scarce and probably not free of appreciable systematic errors. Therefore, soil evaporimeters cannot be accepted as a universal method for determining evaporation from the land surface.

Various kinds of evaporimeters have been used to determine evaporation from water surfaces. However, these observations also contain some errors, and are insufficient to warrant larger climatological generalizations.

Because of the difficulty of applying evaporimeters, gradient methods for calculating evaporation from the vertical gradient of moisture, simultaneously taking into account the value of the turbulent exchange coefficient, have been used during recent decades to determine evaporation and the associated outgo of heat. Another variation of the gradient method for determining evaporation is the so-called balance method, which determines evaporation or the outgo of heat in it by measurements of vertical gradients of temperature and humidity in the air layer near the ground and by measurements of the radiation surplus and the heat flux in the soil.

The gradient method also permits us to determine the magnitude of the turbulent sensible-heat flux—one of the most difficult components of the heat balance for direct measurement. During the 1950s, systematic gradient observations were organized at several dozen stations in the USSR.

Omitting the mention of other instrumental methods for determining heat-balance components that, for various reasons, are not applied in the network of meteorological stations, we will point out that, as a result of progress achieved in experimental meteorology, there appears the possibility of measuring all the principal components of the heat balance under various natural conditions. Since specific balance observations (except measurements of radiation fluxes) are not yet in use on a mass basis, conclusions drawn from these observations are usually insufficient for more or less broad climatological generalization.

For this reason, calculation methods for determining the components of heat balance remain important at present. These permit us to compute the values of the terms of the heat balance, using data of mass meteorological observations.

First calculations of heat-balance components were aimed at determining the changes of heat content in closed water bodies and in the upper layers of the soil. Such calculations, which are comparatively simple from the point of view of procedure, were accomplished in the last century by Voeikov, Ferrel, and others.

The first fundamental investigations aimed at calculating solar energy transformation in the atmosphere were completed at the end of the 19th century. Among such works is the study of Angot (1883), in which the amount of short-wave radiation reaching the earth's surface in various latitudinal zones of the globe was determined.

However, the first calculations of all the components of the heat balance were accomplished only at the beginning of our century. The work of Schmidt, published in 1915, proved very important for investigation of the heat balance. Using calculation methods, Schmidt found annual mean values of the heat-balance components in latitudinal zones of the world ocean in the Northern and Southern Hemispheres, including the calculation of the mean quantities of heat in each latitude that are transferred in a horizontal direction in the ocean by the activity of ocean currents and macroturbulence.

Although the calculation methods used by Schmidt were rather approximate (especially in respect to determining the conversion of heat in evaporation and the sensible-heat exchange), he nevertheless obtained the right order of values of the principal components of the heat balance. It should be noted that Schmidt was the first to tie the calculated heat-balance components with a determination of the water balance of the world ocean.

Among the subsequent investigations of heat balance, the works of A. Ångström are worth mentioning. In a paper published in 1920, Ångström established all the components of heat balance in a closed water body— Vassijaure Lake in Sweden. For this purpose, he was able to improve considerably the calculation methods for determining the components of radiation and heat balances, although the problem of calculating the heat conversion in evaporation and the sensible-heat exchange could not be solved without using a rather provisional hypothesis.

In one of his next studies, Ångström (1925) calculated the principal heat-balance components in the region of Stockholm in all months and for the year. The shortcoming of this work was his neglect of reflected radiation when determining the radiation balance for the warm season.

In the calculations of Savinov, published in "Курс геофизики (Geophysics)" by Tverskoi (1934), the annual and monthly values of the radiation balance were found for a land region (Pavlovsk), taking into account the value of reflected radiation.

For development of the heat balance of individual seas, the work of Shuleikin (1935) turned out to be very important. It was in this work, on the basis of special observations and a series of computations, that the components of the radiation and heat balances for one of the seas (the Kara Sea) were first determined.

It should be mentioned that as a result of determining the heat-balance components, Shuleikin could show the importance of the role of currents in forming the thermal regime of the Kara Sea. This conclusion was later corroborated by the data of direct observations (Shuleikin, 1941).

Beginning in the 1940s, the number of investigations of the heat balance at the earth's surface started expanding rapidly. It was during these years that the investigations of the teams of scientists of the Main Geophysical Observatory were started, which aimed at a detailed study of the climatic regularities of the radiation and heat balances. In this program, much attention was paid to working out methods for independent determination of all the heat-balance components, which made it possible to check objectively the accuracy of the derived calculations in closing the balance equation. The last task was first solved for conditions at a single point (Budyko, 1946), and then for an extensive area of land, the southern areas of the European part of the USSR (Budyko, 1947). Having thus corroborated the reliability of the procedures developed to determine the balance components, we were first able in this work to construct maps of the heat-balance components at the land surface.

In subsequent works of members of the Main Geophysical Observatory, seasonal and annual maps of heat-balance components for the European part of the USSR (T. G. Berliand, 1948), annual maps of the balance components for the extratropical part of the Northern Hemisphere (T. G. Berliand, 1949), and annual maps of radiation balance for Western Europe and the eastern part of North America (Zubenok, 1949) were drawn, and calculations of latitudinal values of the heat-balance components in the Northern Hemisphere were completed (Budyko, 1949).

After these investigations, which were, in a sense, a preparation, the author, Berliand, and Zubenok accomplished the task of constructing world maps of the balance components for the annual period as well as for separate months. This series included maps of total short-wave radiation, radiation balance at the earth's surface, evaporation and flux of latent heat, sensible-heat flux from the underlying surface to the atmosphere, and also a map (for the year) of the amount of heat gained or lost by the ocean surface due to the action of sea currents. In all, this series included 66 maps, which gave a general representation of the geographical regularities of the transformations of solar energy at the earth's surface.

The annual maps from this series were published in 1953 in the second volume of the "Морской Атлас (Marine Atlas)" (Budyko et al., (1953). The whole series of maps was published in the first edition of the "Атлас теплового баланса (Atlas of Heat Balance)" (1955).

A summary of the material on the heat balance at the earth's surface that was available by the middle of the 1950s was presented in the book "Тепловой баланс земной поверхности (Heat Balance of the Earth's Surface)" (Budyko, 1956).

Later on, using observational data on the heat-balance components and applying an improved procedure of climatological calculations, the scientists in the Main Geophysical Observatory designed a new series of more detailed and accurate maps of the components of the heat balance.

This work resulted in preparation of the maps of total short-wave radiation, radiation balance, evaporation, potential evapotranspiration, latent-heat flux, sensible-heat flux, and also some components of the heat balance of the earth–atmosphere system. Some data of these investigations were published in the works of T. G. Berliand on the solar radiation regime on the continents (1961), Efimova on the radiation balance of land surfaces (1962), Zubenok on the heat balance of the continents (1962), Strokina on the heat balance of the oceans (1959, 1962), Efimova and Strokina on net long-wave radiation (1963), Zubenok and Strokina on evaporation from the surface of the globe (1963), and other authors. The new series of maps of heat balance was published in the "Атлас теплового баланса земного шара (Atlas of the Heat Balance of the Earth)" (1963).

In further works, members of the Main Geophysical Observatory constructed maps of Arctic and Antarctic radiation regimes [respectively, Gavrilova (1963), and Rusin et al. (1966)]; of the distribution of absorbed energy at the earth's surface (Berliand and Mukhenberg, 1963; Mukhenberg and Strokina, 1967); of albedo of the land surface of the globe (Mukhenberg, 1967).

In the works done in the Main Geophysical Observatory, much attention was paid to studying the radiation and heat balances of the territory of the Soviet Union and its various regions (Sapozhnikova, 1948; Ogneva, 1955, 1968; Berliand and Efimova, 1955; Barashkova et al., 1961; Pivovarova, 1960, 1963, 1966; Pivovarova and Pleshkova, 1962; Borzenkova, 1965; and others).

Together with the papers listed, a number of investigations of this kind were dedicated to problems of the climatology of the heat balance at the earth's surface. One of the first investigations in this direction was the work of Albrecht (1940), in which the means of components of the radiation and heat balances were found for several places—some of them various regions of land, others individual regions of the oceans.

Among the investigations aimed at studying the heat balance of different geographical regions, the following should be mentioned: the works on the heat balance of the Arctic (Marshunova and Chernigovskii, 1965, and other works; Doronin, 1963; Vowinkel and Orvig, 1964, and others; Fletcher, 1965, and others), on the Antarctic heat balance (Rusin, 1961, and others), on the radiation regime and heat balance of the Ukraine (Konstantinov et al. 1966), of Central Asia (Aizenshtat, 1966, and other papers), of the Caucasus (Shikhlinskii, 1963, and others; Tsutskiridze, 1964, and others; Borzenkova, 1965, and others), and so on.

In the above-mentioned works of Konstantinov and Aizenshtat, and also in the investigations of Rauner (1961 and elsewhere), experimental data were obtained on the heat balance of various natural landscapes and agricultural fields.

Not mentioning many other works studying the heat balance in various geographical regions, we will point to some investigations in which maps of heat-balance components were first drawn.

The first maps of the heat balance of water bodies were constructed in the works of Jacobs (1943) and Sverdrup (1945) for northern portions of the Atlantic and Pacific Oceans. Subsequently, in the investigations of Albrecht (1949, 1951, 1952, 1960), calculations of heat-balance components for oceans were carried out. On the basis of these calculations, he made up a series of maps of the balance components for single months and the year.

Maps of the heat-balance components for various oceanic regions were constructed in the works of Sauberer and Dirmhirn (1954), Privett (1960), Wyrtki (1965), Samoilenko (1966), Mani et al. (1967) and other authors.

In a number of investigations, maps of the components of the heat balance of individual seas were drawn up (Arkhipova, 1957; Aldoshina, 1957; Seriakov, 1959; Batalin, 1959; Zaitsev, 1960; Makerov, 1961; Soliankin, 1963; Smetannikova, 1963; Arsen'eva, 1964; Pomeranets, 1964; and others).

Along with maps of the heat balance of water bodies, maps of heat-balance components in different regions of the USSR have been prepared (Styro and Gritsiute, 1955; Verle and Svinukhov, 1958; Mezentsev, 1959; Shikhlinskii, 1963; "Атлас составляющих теплового и водного балансов Украины (Atlas of the Components of the Heat and Water Balances of the Ukraine", 1966; and others), and for other countries (Tomlain, 1964; Albrecht, 1965; "Atlas balanzu promienowania w Polsce (Atlas of the Radiation Balance in Poland)", 1966; and others).

In conclusion, we will point out that, besides the above-mentioned papers of scientists in the Main Geophysical Observatory, some papers also include world maps of elements of the radiation regime at the earth's surface (Bernhardt and Philipps, 1958, 1966; Landsberg, 1965; Löf *et al.*, 1966; and others).

Let us now turn to the problem of investigating the heat balance of the atmosphere. The available data on the geographical distribution of the heat-balance components of the atmosphere are much inferior, in respect to accuracy and detail, to available data on the heat balance at the earth's surface.

Direct measurement of terms of the atmospheric heat balance is associated with great difficulty compared to the measurement of the heat-balance components at the earth's surface. Because of this, information about regularities of the spatial distribution of the components of the heat balance of the atmosphere and the earth–atmosphere system have been obtained until recently only as a result of application of various calculation methods.

Of great significance for the study of the heat balance of the atmosphere was the paper by Simpson (1929), who carried out approximate calculations and constructed schematic world maps of the earth's radiation into space and of the radiation balance of the earth–atmosphere system. These maps, designed for two months—January and July—permitted us for the first time to get an idea of the spatial distribution of the radiation balance of the planet Earth.

Of later papers in this direction, it is worth mentioning the investigation of Baur and Philipps (1934, 1935), in which calculation of the mean latitudinal indices of the atmospheric heat balance was accomplished. It might be noted that a similar calculation was carried out by Trolle (1938) for the region of Pavlovsk at about the same time.

The calculations of Baur and Philipps as well as other contemporary works included considerable error, owing to the use of inaccurate data on the heat balance at the earth's surface. The absence of necessary data led Baur and Philipps, for example, not only to quantitative errors but also to the wrong qualitative conclusions about regularities of the heat balance. These authors concluded that for the whole earth the mean turbulent flux of sensible heat is directed from the atmosphere to the earth's surface. Accumulation of reliable data on the heat-balance components of the earth's surface has permitted the determination, in later investigations, of mean latitudinal values of the components of the atmospheric heat balance without the above-mentioned error (Budyko, 1949).

Further more detailed calculations of the heat balance of the atmosphere and the earth-atmosphere system were made. Among these investigations, the paper of T. G. Berliand (1956) is important. In it, maps of the components of the atmospheric heat balance for the Northern Hemisphere were constructed.

Houghton (1954), London (1957), and Möller (1960) gave the results of calculations of the mean values of radiation balance and heat balance of the atmosphere for latitudinal zones and for the earth as a whole.

World maps of the radiation balance of the earth–atmosphere system, of the heat gain from condensation in the atmosphere, and of heat transfer by air currents were designed by Vinnikov and published in "Атлас теплового баланса земного шара [Atlas of the Heat Balance of the Earth]" 1963).

D'iachenko and Kondrat'ev (1965), using calculation methods, determined the mean values of the long-wave balance of the atmosphere and designed world maps of its monthly and annual values.

In the 1960s, in connection with the development of observations from meteorological satellites, there appeared the possibility of constructing maps of components of the radiational regime of the earth–atmosphere system directly from observational data. The first map of the kind contained data for single periods of time (for example, Raschke et al., 1968). Later, on the basis of these data, maps of mean long-term values of elements of the radiation regime were constructed (Vonder Haar and Suomi, 1969, and others).

Correspondence of these maps of atmospheric heat fluxes to those that were constructed earlier by calculation methods is poorer than the correspondence of maps of components of the radiation balance at the earth's surface based on observational data to maps based on calculated values.

It is quite clear that the accuracy of calculations of radiation fluxes in the atmosphere and observations of these fluxes from satellites is inferior to the corresponding accuracies for fluxes at the earth's surface. Nevertheless, many substantial features of the radiation regime of the earth–atmosphere system found by calculation are in good conformity with observations from satellites.

In conclusion, we would like to note that, as is seen from recently published reviews (Miller, 1965; Sellers, 1965; and others), the number of investigations of the heat balance of the earth's surface and the atmosphere has been rapidly increasing. In the course of these investigations, the general picture of the transformation of solar energy in the geographical envelope of the earth has become clear.

REFERENCES

Айзенштат Б. А. (1966). Исследования теплового баланса Средней Азии Сб. «Современные проблемы климатологии». Гидрометеоиздат, Л.

Aizenshtat, B. A. (1966). Investigations of the heat balance of Central Asia. In "Sovremennye Problemy Klimatologii (Contemporary Problems of Climatology)" (M. I. Budyko, ed.), pp. 94–129. Gidrometeoizdat, Leningrad.

Алдошина Е. И. (1957). Тепловой баланс поверхности Японского моря. Труды ГОИН, вып. 35.

Aldoshina, E. I. (1957). The heat balance of the surface of the Sea of Japan. Tr. Gos. Okeanogr. Inst. 35, 119–159. MGA 13E-174.

Арсеньева Н. Я. (1964). Тепловой баланс Белого моря и его изменения во времени и пространстве. Труды ГОИН, вып. 81.

Arsen'eva, N. Ia. (1964). The heat balance of the White Sea and its distribution in time and space. *Tr. Gos. Okeanogr. Inst.* **81.**

Архипова Е. Г. (1957). Тепловой баланс Каспийского моря. Труды ГОИН, вып. 35.

Arkhipova, E. G. (1957). The heat balance of the Caspian Sea. *Tr. Gos. Okeanogr. Inst.* **35,** 3–101. MGA 13E-175.

Атлас составляющих тепловго и водного балансов Украины (1966). Под ред. А. Р. Константинова. Гидрометеоиздат, Л.

"Atlas Sostavliaiushchikh Teplovogo i Vodnogo Balansov Ukrainy (Atlas of the Components of the Heat and Water Balances of the Ukraine)" (A. R. Konstantinov and N. I. Goisa, eds.). Gidrometeoizdat, Leningrad, 1966.

Атлас теплового баланса. (1955). Под ред. М. И. Будыко. Изд. ГГО, Л.

"Atlas Teplovogo Balansa (Atlas of the Heat Balance)." (M. I. Budyko, ed.). Izdat. Gl. Geofiz. Observ., Leningrad, 1955. MGA 11A-25.

Атлас теплового баланса земного шара. (1963). Под ред. М. И. Будыко. Междуведомственный геофизический комитет, М.

"Atlas Teplovogo Balansa Zemnogo Shara (Atlas of the Heat Balance of the Earth." (M. I. Budyko, ed.). Akad. Nauk SSSR, Prezidium. Mezhvedomstvennyi Geofiz. Komitet, Moscow, 1963; Guide to the "Atlas of the Heat Balance of the Earth." U.S. Weather Bur., WB/T No. 106. U.S. Weather Bur., Washington, D.C., 1964.

Барашкова Е. П. [и др.]. (1961). Радиационный режим территории СССР. Гидрометеоиздат, Л.

Barashkova, E. P., Gaevskii, V. L., D'iachenko, L. N., Lugina, K. M., and Pivovarova, Z. I. (1961). Radiatsionnyi Rezhim Territorii SSSR (Radiation Regime of the USSR)." Gidrometeoizdat, Leningrad.

Баталин А. М. (1959). Тепловой баланс дальневосточных морей. Изв. АН СССР, сер. геофиз., №. 7.

Batalin, A. M. (1959). Heat balance of the seas of the Far East. *Izv. Akad. Nauk SSSR Ser. Geofiz.* **No. 7,** 1003–1010. MGA 13E-201; Transl. *Bull. Acad. Sci. USSR Geophys. Ser.* **No. 7** (1959).

Берлянд Т. Г. (1948). Радиационный и тепловой баланс Европейской территории СССР. Труды ГГО, вып. 10.

Berliand, T. G. (1948). Radiation and heat balance of the European area of the USSR. *Tr. Gl. Geofiz. Observ.* **10.**

Берлянд Т. Г. (1949). Радиационный и тепловой баланс поверхности суши внетропических широт северного полушария. Труды ГГО, вып. 18.

Berliand, T. G. (1949). Radiation and heat budgets of land surfaces of the extratropical latitudes of the Northern Hemisphere. *Tr. Gl. Geofiz. Observ.* **18.**

Берлянд Т. Г. (1956). Тепловой баланс атмосферы северного полушария. Сб «А. И. Воейков и современные проблемы климатологии». Гидрометеоиздат, Л.

Berliand, T. G. (1956). The heat balance of the atmosphere of the Northern Hemisphere. *In* "A. I. Voeikov i Sovremennye Problemy Klimatologii" (M. I. Budyko, ed.), pp. 226–252. Gidrometeoizdat, Leningrad; Translated in "A. I. Voeikov and Problems in Climatology: Selected Articles," pp. 57–83. Isr. Program Sci. Transl., Jerusalem, 1963.

Берлянд Т. Г. (1961). Распределение солнечной радиации на континентах. Гидрометеоиздат, Л.

Berliand, T. G. (1961). "Raspredelenie Solnechnoi Radiatsii na Kontinentakh (Distribution of Solar Radiation on the Continents)." Gidrometeoizdat, Leningrad. MGA 17.4-1.

Берлянд Т. Г., Ефимова Н. А. (1955). Месячные карты суммарной солнечнои радиации и радиационного баланса территории СССР. Труды ГГО, вып. 112.

Berliand, T. G., and Efimova, N. A. (1955). Monthly maps of insolation and radiation balance of the USSR. *Tr. Gl. Geofiz. Observ.* **112**.

Берлянд Т. Г., Мухенберг В. В. (1963). Роль поглощенной радиации в формировании радиационного баланса. Труды ГГО, вып. 139.

Berliand, T. G., and Mukhenberg, V. V. (1963). The role of absorbed radiation in formation of the radiation balance. *Tr. Gl. Geofiz. Observ.* **139**.

Борзенкова И. И. (1965). О некоторых закономерностях изменения составляющих радиационного и теплового балансов в горных районах. Труды ГГО, вып. 179.

Borzenkova, I. I. (1965). Some regular variations of the radiation- and heat-balance components in mountainous regions. *Tr. Gl. Geofiz. Observ.* **179**, 186–198. MGA 17.6-276.

Будыко М. И. (1946). Методы определения естественного испарения. Метеорология и гидрология, № 3.

Budyko, M. I. (1946). Methods of determining natural evaporation. *Meteorol. Gidrol.* No. 3.

Будыко М. И. (1947). О водном и тепловом балансах поверхности суши. Метеорология и гидрология, № 5.

Budyko, M. I. (1947). On the water and heat balances of the land surface. *Meteorol. Gidrol.* No. 5.

Будыко М. И. (1949). Тепловой баланс северного полушария. Труды ГГО, вып. 18.

Budyko, M. I. (1949). The heat balance of the Northern Hemisphere. *Tr. Gl. Geofiz. Observ.* **18**.

Будыко М. И. (1956). Тепловой баланс земной поверхности. Гидрометеоиздат, Л.

Budyko, M. I. (1956). "Teplovoi Balans Zemnoi Poverkhnosti." Gidrometeoizdat, Leningrad; "Heat Balance of the Earth's Surface," translated by N. A. Stepanova. U.S. Weather Bur., Washington, D.C., 1958. MGA 13E-286, 11B-25.

Будыко М. И., Берлянд Т. Г., Зубенок Л. И. (1953). Тепловой баланс земной поверхности. Морской Атлас, т. II, лист 41.

Budyko, M. I., Berliand, T. G., and Zubenok, L. I. (1953). Heat balance of the earth's surface. "Morskoi Atlas (Marine Atlas)," Vol. 2, sheet 41.

Верле Е. К., Свинухов Г. В. (1958). Радиационный баланс территории Приморского края. Труды ДВНИГМИ, вып. 6.

Verle, E. K., and Svinukhov, G. V. (1958). Radiation budget of the Primorskii Krai. *Tr. Dal'ne-Vostoch. Nauch.-Issled. Gidrometeorol. Inst.* **6**, 30–43; Translated by I. A. Donehoo. U.S. Weather Bur., Washington, D.C., 1960.

Воейков А. И. (1884). Климаты земного шара, в особенности России. СПб

Voeikov, A. I. (1884). "Klimaty Zemnogo Shara, v Osobennosti Rossii (The Climate of the Earth, especially Russia)." St. Petersburg. MGA 3.4-4, 11A-97.

Воейков А. И. (1904). Кругооборот тепла в оболочке земного шара. Сб. статей по физике, посвященный проф. Р. Ф. Петрушевскому.

Voeikov, A. I. (1904). The circulation of heat in the mantle of the globe. *Sb. Stat. Fiz. Posviashchennyi Prof. R. F. Petrushevskomu*, 111–147.

Гаврилова М. К. (1963). Радиационный климат Арктики. Гидрометеоиздат, Л.

Gavrilova, M. K. (1963). "Radiatsionnyi Klimat Arktiki." Gidrometeoizdat, Leningrad; "Radiation Climate of the Arctic." Isr. Program Sci. Trans., Jerusalem, 1966. MGA 18.11-4.

Доронин Ю. П. (1963). О тепловом балансе центральной Арктики. Труды ААНИИ, т. 253.

Doronin, Iu. P. (1963). On the heat balance of the central Arctic. *Tr. Arkt. Antarkt. Nauch. Issled. Inst.* **253**, 178–184; Res. Mem. RM-5003-PR, pp. 193–205. Rand Corp., Santa Monica, California, 1966. MGA 18.2-283.

Дьяченко Л. Н., Кондратьев К. Я. (1965). Распределение длинноволнового баланса атмосферы по земному шару. Труды ГГО, вып. 170.

D'iachenko, L. N., and Kondrat'ev, K. Ia. (1965). The global distribution of the budget of long-wave radiation of the atmosphere. *Tr. Gl. Geofiz. Observ.* **170**, 192–201. MGA 17.7-263.

Ефимова Н. А. (1962). Радиационный баланс поверхности суши земного шара. Труды ВНМС, т. IV. Гидрометеоиздат, Л.

Efimova, N. A. (1962). The radiation budget of the land surface of the globe. *Tr. Vses. Nauch. Meteorol. Soveshch. 1st, Leningrad, 1961*, **4**, pp. 186–195. Gidrometeoizdat, Leningrad.

Ефимова Н. А., Строкина Л. А. (1963). Распределение эффективного излучения на поверхности земного шара. Труды ГГО, вып. 139.

Efimova, N. A., and Strokina, L. A. (1963). Distribution of net longwave radiation at the surface of the earth. *Tr. Gl. Geofiz. Observ.* **139**, 16–26.

Зайцев Г. Н. (1960). Тепловой баланс Норвежского и Гренландского морей и факторы его образующие. Сб. «Советские рыбохозяйственные исследования в морях Европейского Севера». Пищепромиздат, М.

Zaitsev, G. N. (1960). Heat balance of the Norwegian and Greenland Seas and factors in its formation. *In* "Sovetskie Rybokhoziaistvennye Issledovaniia v Moriakh Evropeiskogo Severa." Pishchepromizdat, Moscow.

Зубенок Л. И. (1949). Опыт расчета радиационного баланса косвенным методом. Труды ГГО, вып. 18.

Zubenok, L. I. (1949). An experiment at calculating the radiation budget by an indirect method. *Tr. Gl. Geofiz. Observ.* **18**.

Зубенок Л. И. (1962). Тепловой баланс континентов. Труды ВНМС, т. IV. Гидрометеоиздат, Л.

Zubenok, L. I. (1962). Heat balance of the continents. *Tr. Vses. Nauch. Meteorol. Soveshch.*, *1st*, Leningrad *1961*, **4**, 173–186. Gidrometeoizdat, Leningrad.

Зубенок Л. И., Строкина Л. А. (1963). Испарение с поверхности земного шара. Труды ГГО, вып. 139.

Zubenok, L. I., and Strokina, L. A. (1963). Evaporation from the surface of the earth. *Tr. Gl. Geofiz. Observ.* **139**, 93–107; *Sov. Hydrol.* **1963**, No. 6, 597–611 [1964].

Кастров В. Г. (1928). К вопросу об основной актинометрической формуле. Метеорол. вестн., № 7.

Kastrov, V. G. (1928). The problem of the basic actinometric formula. *Meteorolog. Vestn.* No. 7.

Кондратьев К. Я. (1965). Актинометрия. Гидрометеоиздат, Л.

Kondrat'ev, K. Ia. (1965). "Aktinometriia." Gidrometeoizdat, Leningrad; Actinometry. *NASA Tech. Transl.* **TT F-9712** (1965). MGA 17.8-2.

Константинов А. Р. [и др.]. (1966). Тепловой и водный режим Украины. Гидрометеоиздат, Л.

Konstantinov, A. R., Sakali, L. I., Goisa, N. I., and Oleinik, R. N. (1966). "Teplovoi i Vodnyi Rezhim Ukrainy (Heat and Water Regimes of the Ukraine)." Gidrometeoizdat, Leningrad.

Макеров Ю. В. (1961). Тепловой баланс Черного моря. Труды ГОИН, вып. 61.

Makerov, Iu. V. (1961). Heat balance of the Black Sea. *Tr. Gos. Okeanogr. Inst.* **61**.

Маршунова **М. С.** и Черниговскии Н. Т. (1965). Климат советскои Арктики (радиационный режим). Гидрометеоиздат, Л.

Marshunova, M. S., and Chernigovskii, N. T. (1965). "Klimat Sovetskoi Arktiki (Radiatsionnyi Rezhim) (Climate of the Soviet Arctic—Radiation Regime)." Gidrometeorizdat, Leningrad.

Махоткин Л. Г. (1957). Прямая радиация и прозрачность атмосферы. Изв. АН СССР, сер. геогр., № 5.

Makhotkin, L. G. (1957). Direct radiation and the transparency of the atmosphere. *Izv. Akad. Nauk SSSR Ser. Geogr.* No. 5.

Мезенцев В. С. (1959). Годовые характеристики теплообеспеченностн Западно-Сибирской равнины. Изв. Омского отдела Геогр. об-ва СССР, вып. 3(10).

Mezentsev, V. S. (1959). Annual characteristics of heat expectancies in the West-Siberian plain. *Izv. Omsk. Otd. Geogr. Obshchest. SSSR* **3** (10).

Мухенберг В. В. (1967). Альбедо поверхности суши земного шара. Труды ГГО, вып. 193.

Mukhenberg, V. V. (1967). Albedo of the land surface of the earth. *Tr. Gl. Geofiz. Observ.* **193**, 24–36.

Мухенберг В. В., Строкина Л. А. (1967). Распределение поглощенной радиации на материках и океанах. Труды ГГО, вып. 193.

Mukhenberg, V. V., and Strokina, L. A. (1967). Distribution of absorbed short-wave radiation on the continents and oceans. *Tr. Gl. Geofiz. Observ.* **193**, 37–43.

Огнева Т. А. (1955). Некоторые особенности теплового баланса деятельной поверхности. Гидрометеоиздат, Л.

Ogneva, T. A. (1955). "Nekotorye Osobennosti Teplovogo Balansa Deiatel'noi Poverkhnosti. (Some Characteristics of the Heat Balance of the Active Surface)." Gidrometeoizdat, Leningrad. MGA 8.7-21.

Огнева Т. А. (1968). О соотношении составляющих теплового баланса на территории Советского Союза. Труды ГГО, вып. 233.

Ogneva, T. A. (1968). On the relation between components of the heat balance in the USSR. *Tr. Gl. Geofiz. Observ.* **233**, 110–117.

Пивоварова З. И. (1960). Основные характеристики радиационного режима Европейской территории СССР. Труды ГГО, вып. 115.

Pivovarova, Z. I. (1960). The chief characteristics of the radiation regime of the European territory of the USSR. *Tr. Gl. Geofiz. Observ.* **115**, 77–94; U.S. Weather Bur., WB/T 58. U.S. Weather Bur., Washington, D.C., 1961.

Пивоварова З. И. (1963). Прямая солнечная радиация на территории СССР. Труды ГГО, вып. 139.

Pivovarova, Z. I. (1963). Direct solar radiation in the USSR. *Tr. Gl. Geofiz. Observ.* **139**, 27–42.

Пивоварова З. И. (1966). Изучение режима солнечной радиацни в СССР. Сб. «Современные проблемы климатологии». Гидрометеоиздат, Л.

Pivovarova, Z. I. (1966). Study of the regime of solar radiation in the USSR. *In* "Sovremennye Problemy Klimatologii (Contemporary Problems of Climatology)" (M. I. Budyko, ed.), 41–56. Gidrometeoizdat, Leningrad.

Пивоварова З. И., Плешкова Т. Т. (1962). О радиационном режиме СССР по материалам наблюдений сети станций. Труды ВНМС, т. IV. Гидрометеоиздат Л.

Pivovarova, Z. I., and Pleshkova, T. T. (1962). On the radiation regime of the USSR from observational data at network stations. *Tr. Vses. Nauch. Meteorol. Soveshch. 1st, Leningrad, 1961,* **4**, pp. 195–205. Gidrometeoizdat, Leningrad. MGA 14:2321.

Померанец К. С. (1964). Тепловой баланс Балтийского моря. Труды ГОИН, вып. 82.

Pomeranets, K. S. (1964). The heat balance of the Baltic Sea. *Tr. Gos. Okeanogr. Inst.* **82.**

Раунер Ю. Л. (1961). Тепловой баланс леса и его роль в формировании микроклимата лесных и безлесных ландшафтов. Материалы к V Всесоюзному совещанию по вопросам ландшафтоведения, М.

Rauner, Iu. L. (1961). The heat balance of forest and its role in the formation of the microclimate of wooded and treeless landscapes. *Vop. Landshaftoved., Vses. Soveshch., 5th Moscow, 1961*; Translated in *Sov. Geog.* 3, No. 6, 40–47 (1962).

Русин Н. П. (1961). Метеорологический и радиационный режим Антарктиды. Гидрометеоиздат, Л.

Rusin, N. P. (1961). "Meteorologicheskii i Radiatsionnyi Rezhim Antarktidy." Gidrometeoizdat, Leningrad. MGA 15.5-6; "Meteorological and Radiational Regime of Antarctica." OTS 64-11097. Isr. Program Sci. Transl., Jerusalem 1964. MGA 16.8-5.

Русин Н. П., Строкина Л. А., Брагинская Л. Л. (1966). Суммарная солнечная радиация. Радиационный баланс. Атлас Антарктики, т. 1, стр. 73—75.

Rusin, N. P., Strokina L. A. and Braginskaia L. L. (1966). Summarnaia Solnechnaia Radiatsiia. Radiatsionnyi Balans (Total solar radiation; radiation budget). *Atlas Antarktiki* **1,** 73–75.

Самойленко В. С. (1966). Теплооборот и влагооборот в Тихом океане. В кн. «Тихий океан», т. I. Метеорологические условия над Тихим океаном. Изд. «Наука» М.

Samoilenko, V. S. (1966). Heat- and water-turnover in the Pacific Ocean. *In* Akademiia Nauk SSSR Institut Okeanologii, "Tikhii Okean" (V. G. Kort, ed.), Vol. 1, "Meteorologicheskie Usloviia nad Tikhim Okeanom," (V. S. Samoilenko, ed.), Izdat. Nauka, Moscow. MGA 18.8-7.

Сапожникова С. А. (1948). Тепловой баланс деятельной поверхности в основных климатических зонах СССР. Труды второго всесоюзного географического съезда т. II. Географгиз, Л.

Sapozhnikova, S. A. (1948). The heat balance of the active surface in the principal climatic zones of the USSR. *Tr. Vses. Geograf. S"ezd, 2d, Leningrad, 1947,* **2.** Geografgiz, Leningrad.

Серяков Е. И. (1959). Тепловой баланс поверхности южной части Баренцева моря. Сб. «Материалы конференции по проблеме «Взаимодействис атмосферы и гидросферы в северной части Атлантического океана» вып. 5. Гидрометеоиздат Л.

Seriakov, E. I. (1959). The heat balance of the surface of the southern part of the Barents Sea. *Mater. Konf. Probl. Vzaimodeistvie Atmos. Gidrosfery v Severnoi Chasti Atl. Okeana* Leningrad, 1958, **5.** Gidrometeoizdat, Leningrad. MGA 13E-190.

Сметанникова А. В. (1963). Расчет аномалий потерь тепла осенью в Карском море по аномалиям гидрометеорологических элементов. Труды ААНИИ т. 264.

Smetannikova, A. V. (1963). Calculation of anomalies of heat fluxes in autumn from the Caspian Sea from anomalies of hydrometeorologic elements. *Tr. Arkt. Antarkt. Nauchn Issled. Inst.* **264.** MGA 15.5-183.

Солянкин Е. В. 1963. Радиационный баланс поверхностного слоя Черного моря. Труды ИОАН, т. 72.

Soliankin, E. V. (1963). The radiation budget of the surface layer of the Black Sea. *Tr. Inst. Okeanol. Akad. Nauk SSSR* **72.**

Строкина Л. А. (1959). Новый расчет среднего многолетнего теплового баланса деятельной поверхности северной части Атлантического океана. Сб. «Материалы конференции по проблеме «Взаимодействие атмосферы и гидросферы в северной части Атлантического океана» вып. 5. Гидрометеоиздэт Л.

Strokina, L. A. (1959). A new calculation of the mean long-term heat balance of the active surface of the northern part of the Atlantic Ocean. *Mater. Konf. Probl. Vzai-*

modeistvie Atmos. Gidrosfery v Severnoi Chasti Atl. Okeana Leningrad, 1958, **5**. Gidro-meteoizdat, Leningrad. MGA 13E-190.

Строкина Л. А. (1962). Тепловой баланс в различных климатических зонах океанов. Труды ВНМС т. IV. Гидрометеоиздат Л.

Strokina, L. A. (1962). The heat balance in different climatic zones of the oceans. *Tr. Vses. Nauch. Meteorolog. Soveshch. 1st, Leningrad, 1961*, **4**, 205–215. Gidrometeoizdat, Leningrad.

Стыро Б. И., Грицюте Л. П. (1955). Радиационный баланс территории Литовской ССР. Труды АН ЛитССР, сер. Б, № 2.

Styro, B. I., and Gritsiute, L. P. (1955). Radiation budget of the Lithuanian SSR. *Liet. TSR Mokslu Akad. Darb. Ser. B* **No. 2**.

Тверской П. Н. (1934). Курс геофизики. Гостехиздат, Л.—М.

Tverskoi, P. N. (1934). "Kurs Geofiziki (Geophysics)." Gostekhizdat, Leningrad and Moscow.

Тролле Г. Г. (1938). Опыт расчета баланса тепловой энергии во всем столбе атмо-сферы и почвы в данной географической точке. Труды ГГО, вып. 21.

Trolle, G. G. (1938). An experiment in calculating the balance of thermal energy in the entire column of atmosphere and soil at a specific geographical point. *Tr. Gl. Geofiz. Observ.* **21**.

Цуцкиридзе Я. А. (1964). Радиационный баланс территории Закавказья. Труды ЗакНИГМИ, вып. 15.

Tsutskiridze, Ia. A. (1964). Radiatsionnyi Balans Territorii Zakavkaz'ia (Radiation Budget of the Caucasus). *Tr. Zakavkaz. Nauch. Issled. Gidrometeorol. Inst.* **21**.

Шихлинский Э. М. (1963). Тепловой баланс Азербайджанской ССР. Изв. АН АзССР, сер. геол.-геогр., № 3.

Shikhlinskii, E. M. (1963). Heat balance of the Azerbaidzhan SSR. *Izv. Akad. Nauk Azerb. SSR Ser. Nauk Zemle*, No. 3.

Шулейкин В. В. (1935). Элементы теплового режима Карского моря. Труды Таймыр-ской гидрографической экспедиции, ч. 2.

Shuleikin, V. V. (1935). Elements of the thermal regime of the Kara Sea. *Tr. Taimyrskii Gidrograf. Ekspeditsiia* Pt. 2.

Шулейкин В. В. (1941). Физика моря. Изд. АН СССР, Л.—М.

Shuleikin, V. V. (1941). "Fizika Moria (Physics of the Sea)." Akad. Nauk SSSR, Leningrad and Moscow. MGA 13E-289.

Albrecht, F. (1940). Untersuchungen über den Wärmehaushalt der Erdoberfläche in verschiedenen Klimagebieten. *Wiss. Abh. Reichsamt. Wetterdienst*, **8**, No. 2.

Albrecht, F. (1949). Über die Wärme- und Wasserbilanz der Erde. *Ann. Meteorol.* H. 5/6.

Albrecht, F. (1951). Monatskarten der Verdunstung und des Wasserhaushaltes des Indischen und Stillen Ozean. *Ber. Deuts. Wetterdienstes* U.S. Zone, No. 29.

Albrecht, F. (1952). Strahlung- und Wärmehaushaltsuntersuchungen während einer Seereise durch den Indischen Ozean im Juni 1949. *Ber. Deut. Wetterdienstres* U.S. Zone, Band 7, No. 42, pp. 5–10.

Albrecht, F. (1960). Jahreskarten des Wärme- und Wasserhaushaltes der Ozeane. *Ber. Deut. Wetterdienstes* **9**, No. 66.

Albrecht, F. (1965). Untersuchungen des Wärme- und Wasserhaushaltes der Südlichen Kontinente. *Ber. Deut. Wetterdienstes* **14**, No. 99.

Allen, C. W. (1958). Solar radiation. *Quart. J. Roy. Meteorol. Soc.* **84**, No. 362.

Angot A. (1883). Recherches théoriques sur la distribution de la chaleur à la surface du globe. *Ann. Bur. Central Météorol. Paris*, vol. 1.

"Atlas balanzu promienowania w Polsce. Pod red. Journ Paszyńskiego, (Atlas of the Radiation Balance in Poland)" (1966). Dokumentacia geograficzna zeszyt 4. Inst. geogr. Pol. Akad. Nauk Warsaw.

Baur, F., und Philipps, H. (1934). Der Wärmehaushalt der Lufthülle der Nordhalbkugel. *Gerlands Beitr. Geophys.* **42**, 160–207.

Baur, F., und Philipps H. (1935). Der Wärmehaushalt der Lufthülle der Nordhalbkugel. *Gerlands Beitr. Geophys.* **45**, 82–132.

Bernhard, F., und Philipps, H. (1958). Die räumliche und zeitliche Verteilung der Einstrahlung, der Ausstrahlung und der Strahlungsbilanz im Meeresniveau Pt. 1. Teil I, *Abh. Meteorol. Hydrogr. Dienstes DDR*, No. 45.

Bernhard, F., und Philipps, H. (1966). Die räumliche und zeitliche Verteilung der Einstrahlung, der Ausstrahlung und der Strahlungsbilanz im Meeresniveau Pt. 2 and 3, *Abh. Meteorol. Dienstes DDR* No. 77.

Drummond, A. J., and Hickey, J. R. (1968). The Eppley—JPL solar constant measurement program. *Sol. Energy* **12**.

Fletcher, J. O. (1965). The heat budget of the Arctic Basin and its relation to climate. *Rep.* R-444-PR. Rand Corp., Santa Monica, California.

Houghton, H. G. (1954). On the annual heat balance of the Northern Hemisphere. *J. Meteorol.* **11**, No. 1.

Jacobs, W. C. (1943). Sources of atmospheric heat and moisture over the North Pacific and North Atlantic Oceans. *Ann. N.Y. Acad. Sci.* **44**.

Kondrat'ev, K. Ya., and Nikolskii, G. A. (1968). Direct solar radiation and aerosol structure of the atmosphere from balloon measurements in the period IQSY. *Comm. Sver. Meteorol. Hydrol. Inst. Ser. B*, No. 28.

Landsberg, H. E., Lippman, H., Paffen, K.-H., and Troll, C. (1965). Global distribution of solar and sky radiation. *In* "World maps of climatology" (E. Rodenwaldt and H. J. Jusatz, eds.). Springer, Berlin and New York.

Löf, G. O. G., Duffie, J. A., and Smith, C. O. (1966). World distribution of solar radiation. *Sol. Energy* **10**, No. 1.

London, J. (1957). A study of the atmospheric heat balance. Final Rep., Contract No. AF 19(122)—165. New York Univ., New York.

Mani, A., Chacko, O., Krishnamurthy, V., and Desikan, V. (1967). Distribution of global and net radiation over the Indian Ocean and its environments, *Arch. Meteorol. Geophys. Bioklimatol. Ser. B*, **15**, Pt. 1–2, pp. 82–98.

Milankovich, M. (1930). "Mathematische Klimalehre und astronomische Theorie der Klimaschwankungen." (Hdbuch. Klimatologie, **1**, Teil A), Gebrüder Borntraeger, Berlin (Русский перевод: М. Миланкович Математическая климатология и астрономическая теория колебаний климата. ОМТИ, М., 1938).

Miller, D. H. (1965). The heat and water budget of the Earth's surface. *Advan. Geophys.* **11**.

Möller, F. (1960). Der Strahlungshaushalt der Troposphäre. *Meteorol. Rundsch.* **13**, Pt. 3.

Pouillet, C.-S.-M. (1838). Mémoire sur la chaleur solaire, sur les pouvoirs rayonnants et absorbants de l'air atmosphérique, et sur la température de l'espace. Acad. des Sci., Paris, *Comptes Rendus* **7**, 24–65.

Privett, D. W. (1960). The exchange of energy between the atmosphere and the oceans of the Southern Hemisphere. *Geophys. Mem.* **13**, No. 104.

Radiation instruments and measurements (1958). *Ann. Int. Geophys. Year* **5**, Pt. VI.

Raschke, E., Möller, F., Bandeen, W. (1968). The radiation balance of the earth-atmosphere system over both polar regions obtained from radiation measurements of the Nimbus II meteorological satellite. *Comm. Sver. Meteorol. Hydrol. Inst. Ser. B*, No. 28.

Sauberer, F., und Dirmhirn, I. (1954). Über den Strahlungshaushalt der Ozeane auf der Nordhalbkugel. *Arch. Meteorol., Geophys., Bioklimatol Ser. B* 6, Pt. 1–2.

Schmidt, W. (1915). Strahlung und Verdunstung an freien Wasserflächen; ein Beitrag zum Wärmehaushalt des Weltmeers und zum Wasserhaushalt der Erde. *Ann. Hydrol. Marit. Meteorol.* 43, Pt. 3 and 4.

Sellers, W. D. (1965). "Physical Climatology." Univ. Chicago Press, Chicago, Illinois.

Simpson, G. (1929). The distribution of terrestrial radiation. *Mem. Roy. Meteorol. Soc.* 4, No. 23.

Sverdrup, H. U. (1945). "Oceanography for Meteorologists." Prentice-Hall, New York.

Tomlain, J. (1964). Geograficke rozloženie globálneho ziarenia na území CSSR. *Meteorol. Zpr.* 17, No. 6.

Vonder Haar, T. H., and Suomi, V. E. (1969). Satellite observations of the Earth's radiation budget. *Science* 163, 667–669.

Vowinkel, E., and Orvig, S. (1964). Energy balance of the Arctic. *Arch. Meteorol. Geophys. Bioklimatol. Ser. B*, 13, Pt. 3–4.

Wyrtki, K. (1965). The average annual heat balance of the North Pacific Ocean and its relation to ocean circulation. *J. Geophys. Res.* 70, No. 18.

Ångström, A. (1920). Application of heat radiation measurements to the problems of evaporation from lakes and the heat convection at their surfaces. *Geograf. Ann.* 2, 237–252.

Ångström, A. (1925). On radiation and climate. *Geograf. Ann.* 7, 122–142.

II

Methods for Determining
the Components of the Heat Balance

1. The Radiation Balance at the Earth's Surface

Actinometric observations

When studying the radiation balance at the earth's surface, it is important to use data of actinometric observations.

At present, the number of stations making actinometric observations in various countries is close to one thousand. About 200 of them are situated in the territory of the USSR.

It must be indicated that the world actinometric network has an uneven density. There is a significant number of such stations in the USSR, the USA, and Japan, but very few in the vast lands of the developing countries (such as, for example, in South America). On the oceans, systematic actinometric observations are carried out on board ships designed for meteorological observations (weather ships).

At most actinometric stations, only the fluxes of short-wave solar radiation are observed. In recent years, a wider coverage of measurements of the radiation balance at the earth's surface has been made. Such observations are being carried out now in the USSR, at approximately 100 actinometric stations.

Systematic measurements of radiation balance were organized at several dozen stations throughout the world during the International Geophysical Year.

For actinometric observations in various countries, a multitude of instruments is applied, descriptions of which can be found in a number of publications (Radiation Instruments and Measurements, 1958; Kondrat'ev, 1965; and others). All these instruments measure the elements of the radiation regime with errors that are not easily estimated beforehand. For this reason, systematic comparison is very important for clarifying the accuracy of actinometric instruments.

Investigation of errors of actinometric instruments and the results of international comparisons have shown that the accuracy of measurements of short-wave radiation is sufficient for studying radiation regimes both for short and for long periods of time. Measuring the fluxes of long-wave radiation and the radiation balance by means of available instruments is associated with somewhat larger errors. These errors, however, do not prevent study of the regime of these elements, at all events over long averaging periods.

In many countries, the data of actinometric observations are published in special yearbooks or issued together with the data of basic meteorological observations.

Data of actinometric observations made in the Soviet Union are published in "Актинометрический ежегодник (Actinometric Yearbook)". The results of Soviet observations during the period of the International Geophysical Year and the International Geophysical Cooperation have been published in a special edition.

Beginning in 1964, at the request of the World Meteorological Organization, the Main Geophysical Observatory has been publishing an international actinometric monthly, including data on solar radiation and radiation balance. Observational data of a large number of actinometric stations situated in the territory of sixty countries are published in this monthly, "Солнечная радиация и радиационный ьаланс (мировая сеть) (Solar Radiation and Radiation Balance Data (The World Network))".

Along with periodical publications, the data of actinometric observations are published in various handbooks and reference books, such as the summary of short-wave observational data in foreign countries prepared by T. G. Berliand and including data from 570 actinometric stations, "Актинометрический справочник, зарубежные страны (Actinometric Handbook, Foreign Countries)", (1964).

Methods for calculation of total short-wave radiation

It has been already mentioned that available data from direct measurements of elements of the radiation regime are limited and often insufficient for extended climatological generalizations. Therefore, great importance for studies of spatial distributions of the radiation balance at the earth's surface and its components attaches to indirect methods of calculation, using observational data of the basic meteorological elements—temperature and humidity of the air, cloudiness, soil and water temperature, and so on.

The procedure of climatological calculations of the elements of the radiation regime can be more or less detailed, depending on the choice of meteorological data to be used for the calculation (for example, what kind of data are available—cloudiness in different layers or total cloudiness only, and so on). At the same time, the degree of detail of the procedure being used should depend on the object of the calculation. Thus, for example, the calculation of schematic maps of mean values of radiation balance for continents and oceans can be accomplished by a less differentiated procedure than calculations for small regions in microclimatic investigations, or for individual short periods of time.

It should be borne in mind that at present, climatological methods for calculating elements of the radiation regime for considerable averaging periods (mean long-term annual and monthly values) are better developed. The problem of procedures for calculating radiation values for short periods of time is not yet completely solved.

In climatological calculations of radiation balance at the earth's surface, its value is usually determined as the difference between absorbed radiation $Q(1 - \alpha)$ (where Q is the total short-wave radiation, α the albedo) and the net long-wave radiation I. Using such a calculation method for deriving the radiation balance, one must first find the value of the total short-wave radiation Q.

The first investigations devoted to calculation of the values of short-wave radiation incident on the earth's surface were restricted to determining direct-beam solar radiation. In the above-cited paper by Angot (1883) and in subsequent investigations by Savinov (1925, 1928), Milankovich (1930 and elsewhere), Kastrov (1928), Gal'perin (1949a, 1956), Averkiev (1956, 1958), and other authors, methods were elaborated for calculation of the quantity of direct radiation reaching the earth's surface, in relation to conditions of transparency of the atmosphere.

In subsequent papers, attempts were made to calculate the amount of incoming scattered short-wave radiation and to evaluate the effect of cloudiness on total short-wave radiation.

Most of the results of these investigations have not found application in calculations of total radiation because of the cumbersome formulas derived, and the necessity to consider in the computations parameters having considerable variability and not thoroughly investigated.

Both a simple and a sufficient method for determination of total radiation is offered in the works of Ångström (1922), Kimball (1928), and Savinov (1933).

In studies published in 1922, Ångström offered the following formula for determining total short-wave radiation:

$$Q = Q_0[\eta + (1 - \eta)]\frac{s}{s_0}, \qquad (2.1)$$

where Q and Q_0 are the total radiation under actual conditions and without cloudiness, respectively; s/s_0 is the ratio between the duration of sunshine according to the heliograph s and the possible duration s_0 for the given period; and η is a coefficient determining the fraction of the possible radiation actually received under conditions of complete cloudiness.

Ångström found that the last coefficient, according to data of observations in Stockholm, is equal to 0.235.

In Kimball's paper, based on the data of observations at several American stations, a similar dependence was derived:

$$Q = Q_0[0.29 + 0.71(1 - n)] \qquad (2.2)$$

where n is the mean cloudiness in fractions of a unit.

Savinov studied the relationship between the values s/s_0 and $(1 - n)$, according to data of observations at Pavlovsk, and found that these values differ markedly from each other. He came to the conclusion that the true value of the ratio of the actual sum of solar radiation to the possible sum is in best agreement with the arithmetic mean of s/s_0 and $(1 - n)$.

On this basis, for calculation of direct and total solar radiation, Savinov offered the following formulas:

$$S = S_0(1 - \bar{n}), \qquad (2.3)$$

$$Q = Q_0(1 - c\bar{n}), \qquad (2.4)$$

where S is the direct radiation, S_0 is the direct radiation with cloudless skies, c is the coefficient defining the effect of cloudiness on radiation, and

$$1 - \bar{n} = \frac{1 - n + (s/s_0)}{2}.$$

According to the conclusions by Savinov and by Gal'perin (1949a) and other authors, application of the $\bar{n}$ coefficient for calculations of total radiation gives better results than the application of values of total cloudiness or duration of sunshine. However, in many regions there are no reliable data of sunshine, which makes it necessary to limit oneself to the use of the data of general cloudiness when determining total short-wave radiation.

The works of Savinov have contributed much to a wide use of the formulas given here in climatological calculations of short-wave radiation. Of great importance has been the fact that the possible radiation Q_0 included in

Eqs. (2.1), (2.2), and (2.4) has proved comparatively stable, depending basically on latitude and season. Such regularity makes it much easier to use these formulas for calculations of total radiation.

In investigations by scientists of the Main Geophysical Observatory, associated with preparation of the first edition of "Атлас теплового баланса (Atlas of the Heat Balance)" (1955), the following formula was used for calculation of total radiation:

$$Q = Q_0[1 - (1 - \eta')n]. \tag{2.5}$$

In contemporary literature, it is usually called the formula of Savinov–Ångström (η' is an empirical coefficient).

The parameters occurring in this formula were determined by T. G. Berliand on the basis of the then available data of actinometric observations.

Later, as a result of generalizing numerous new observational data, it was established that somewhat more accurate results in calculating total radiation could be obtained by use of the following formula (Berliand, 1960):

$$Q = Q_0[1 - (a + bn)n] \tag{2.6}$$

where a and b are dimensionless coefficients. The use of the quadratic dependence in this formula permits us to take into account the correlations between the amount of clouds and their form. With an increase in cloudiness, the frequency of low clouds, which reduce solar radiation the most, is usually increased. Thus, as cloudiness increases, the reduction of radiation occurs slowly at first and then more rapidly.

We should point out that though Eq. (2.6) is somewhat more accurate than Eq. (2.5), in many cases calculation of the mean monthly values of radiation according to these formulas gives similar results.

For calculating mean monthly values of possible radiation Q_0, corresponding to different latitudes and months of the year, T. G. Berliand used a method proposed by Ukraintsev (1939). In accordance with Ukraintsev's method, graphs have been constructed for a number of stations situated in various latitudinal zones, the abscissas of which correspond to days of the year and the ordinates to daily values of the total short-wave radiation from several years' observations. The points on the graphs fall within areas having a distinct upper boundary. As the upper points probably relate to clear days, then by drawing a smooth curve through these points, one can obtain the annual cycle of daily values of total radiation with cloudless skies.

The dependence on latitude of the values of possible radiation thus obtained in various months is shown in Table 3.

It must be indicated that the values of possible radiation in this table are somewhat greater than the corresponding values determined in most previous papers. This difference is probably connected to some extent with the fact

TABLE 3

Total Radiation with Cloudless Sky (kcal cm^{-2} month^{-1})[a]

Latitude (degrees)	Jan.	Feb.	Mar.	Apr.	May	June	July	Aug.	Sept.	Oct.	Nov.	Dec.
90 N	0	0	0.1	10.0	21.9	26.0	23.8	12.9	2.4	0	0	0
85	0	0	0.7	10.2	21.8	25.8	23.4	13.1	3.0	0	0	0
80	0	0	2.4	10.8	21.4	25.2	23.0	13.4	4.3	0.5	0	0
75	0	0.5	4.0	11.7	21.0	24.5	22.2	13.8	5.8	1.3	0	0
70	0	1.6	6.0	13.1	20.5	23.6	21.2	14.6	7.5	2.7	0.5	0
65	0.7	2.8	8.0	14.5	20.1	22.8	21.0	15.6	9.5	4.3	1.4	0.2
60	1.8	4.3	9.9	16.0	20.8	22.9	21.4	16.7	11.3	6.1	2.6	1.1
55	3.1	6.2	11.7	17.3	21.4	23.4	21.9	17.9	12.9	7.8	4.0	2.3
50	4.8	8.2	13.3	18.5	22.2	23.7	22.6	19.1	14.4	9.7	5.8	3.9
45	6.7	10.3	14.8	19.5	22.6	23.9	23.2	20.1	15.8	11.5	7.8	5.9
40	8.8	12.2	16.4	20.3	23.0	24.0	23.4	20.9	17.0	13.2	9.7	7.7
35	10.7	14.0	17.6	21.0	23.0	24.0	23.6	21.6	18.1	14.7	11.4	9.7
30	12.5	15.5	18.6	21.4	23.0	23.8	23.4	21.8	19.1	16.1	13.1	11.5
25	14.1	16.8	19.5	21.6	23.0	23.4	23.1	21.8	19.8	17.4	14.6	13.1
20	15.5	17.9	20.2	21.6	22.5	22.8	22.6	21.6	20.4	18.5	16.1	14.7
15	16.9	19.0	20.8	21.4	21.9	22.0	21.9	21.2	20.9	19.3	17.4	16.1

10	18.1	19.8	21.1	21.2	21.2	21.0	21.1	20.6	21.2	20.1	18.5	17.5
5 N	19.3	20.4	21.4	21.0	20.2	19.9	20.0	20.0	21.3	20.6	19.5	18.8
0	20.2	20.9	21.5	20.4	19.3	18.8	19.1	19.3	21.2	21.2	20.4	19.2
5 S	21.0	21.4	21.4	19.9	18.3	17.6	17.9	18.3	20.8	21.4	21.8	21.0
10	22.0	21.8	21.1	19.2	17.7	16.	16.3	17.3	20.4	21.4	21.8	22.0
15	22.6	22.0	20.6	18.3	16.0	14.9	15.4	16.1	19.7	21.3	22.4	22.9
20	23.2	22.0	20.0	17.2	14.7	13.4	13.8	14.9	18.9	21.0	22.6	23.6
25	23.6	22.0	19.4	16.0	13.0	12.0	12.6	13.6	18.0	20.6	23.0	24.1
30	23.9	21.8	18.6	14.9	11.9	10.6	11.1	12.1	17.0	20.1	23.0	24.6
35	24.0	21.3	17.6	13.6	10.4	9.0	9.6	10.6	15.9	19.5	23.0	25.0
40	24.0	20.6	16.4	12.2	8.7	7.3	8.1	9.0	14.3	18.7	22.8	25.2
45	24.0	19.9	15.2	10.7	7.1	5.5	6.3	7.3	13.4	17.7	22.4	25.2
50	23.6	18.9	13.8	9.2	5.4	3.8	4.6	5.5	12.0	16.6	21.8	25.0
55	23.2	17.8	12.3	7.5	3.8	2.3	3.0	3.8	10.3	15.4	21.2	24.6
60	22.6	16.6	10.8	5.6	2.4	1.0	1.6	2.3	8.5	14.1	21.0	24.4
65	22.4	15.3	9.1	3.9	1.1	0.1	0.4	1.0	6.7	12.6	20.8	24.5
70	22.6	14.2	7.3	2.2	0.1	0	0	0	5.0	11.4	21.0	24.9
75	23.2	13.4	5.7	0.9	0	0	0	0	3.5	10.4	21.2	25.4
80	24.0	12.8	4.3	0	0	0	0	0	2.1	9.7	21.9	26.0
85	24.6	12.4	2.9	0	0	0	0	0	0.9	9.2	22.4	26.6
90 S	24.9	12.3	1.7	0	0	0	0	0	0	9.0	22.6	27.0

[a] Computed for the mean duration of each month, 30.4 days.

47

that in the previous calculations of possible radiation, comparatively limited observational material was used. Furthermore, such material often included measurements of radiation performed with old instruments, underestimating scattered radiation. In addition, the peculiarity of Ukraintsev's method (which provides the possible radiation for a high transparency of the atmosphere rather than for mean transparency) could lead to the values of possible radiation in Table 3 being somewhat high. Besides, when determining possible radiation by Ukraintsev's method, values might in some cases be over-estimated because of the effect of scattered cloudiness (the amount of clouds reaching 2–3 tenths), which sometimes does not only not reduce but even increases the total radiation in comparison with cloudless conditions. However, this fact, as will be explained below, should not lead to any noticeable systematic error in calculations of total short-wave radiation by Eqs. (2.5) or (2.6).

For determination of coefficients η', a, and b, permitting us to take into account the effect of cloudiness on total radiation, observational data of different latitudinal zones were used in the works of T. G. Berliand.

The coefficient η', which represents the ratio of actual radiation with complete cloudiness to the possible must depend on the mean altitude of the sun, the properties of the cloudiness, and the conditions of reflection of short-wave radiation (the value of albedo).

As a result, mean values of the coefficient η' would probably be different in different regions; this coefficient also varies slightly in the diurnal and annual cycles.

The mean annual values of the coefficient η', averaged for different latitudes, are given in Table 4.

Investigation of the parameters in Eq. (2.6) has shown that the coefficient b is comparatively stable, and therefore its mean value for various latitudes, which equals 0.38, can be used in calculations.

TABLE 4

LATITUDINAL MEANS OF THE COEFFICIENTS η' AND a

ϕ	85°	80°	75°	70°	65°	60°	55°	50°	45°
η'	—	—	0.55	0.50	0.45	0.40	0.38	0.36	0.34
a	0.14	0.15	0.16	0.18	0.25	0.36	0.41	0.40	0.38

ϕ	40°	35°	30°	25°	20°	15°	10°	5°	0°
η'	0.33	0.32	0.32	0.32	0.33	0.33	0.34	0.34	0.35
a	0.38	0.38	0.36	0.35	0.37	0.39	0.40	0.40	0.38

Mean annual values of coefficient a for various latitudes are also presented in Table 4.

Since the coefficients η' and a presented in this table have been computed directly by Eqs. (2.5) and (2.6), taking into account the means of actually observed values of Q, then it is clear that a small systematic error in the values of Q_0 must change the values of these coefficients accordingly. In this case, some compensation of the effect of errors in determining the parameters of Eqs. (2.5) and (2.6) on the calculations of the total short-wave radiation is assured.

When determining total radiation by these formulas and Tables 3 and 4, the effect of variations in transparency of the atmosphere and in the height and form of the clouds is taken into account just as is the mean latitudinal factor (through latitudinal variations of the values Q_0 and η' or a). Besides, in such calculations, variation in the values of η' and a in the annual cycle, which according to data of several papers might take place, are not considered.

As a consequence, the procedure of calculating the total short-wave radiation must be considered rather schematic, and applicable mainly for calculations of radiation distribution over large expanses of global and continental scale. This procedure has the important advantage of using the more accessible data of total cloudiness. (Climatological data of the frequency of various forms of cloud for many territories and for a portion of the oceans are either absent or not reliable enough.)

Besides the method cited here, other formulas taking into account the effect of cloudiness on total solar radiation have been offered (Black, 1956; Ångström, 1957; Bernhardt and Philipps, 1958; and others). In a number of cases, total radiation has been assumed to be proportional to the radiation incident on the outer boundary of the atmosphere, the coefficient of proportionality being considered a function of cloudiness. Comparisons have shown that such an approach does not improve on the accuracy of calculations by the method cited above.

A more differentiated procedure for calculation of total solar radiation should take into account the effect of the form and altitude of the clouds on radiation and also the effect of variations in the transparency of the atmosphere.

The effect of changes in the properties of cloudiness on radiation during the annual cycle could be taken into account, approximately, by changing the values of the coefficient η'. The problem of the annual cycle of appropriate coefficients for the formulas of Savinov and Ångström was considered in a paper of Gal'perin (1949b). It was indicated in this investigation that the coefficient c in Savinov's formula, Eq. (2.4), changes noticeably in some regions during the annual cycle.

Another method for calculating the effect of the properties of cloudiness on total short-wave radiation consists of introducing into the calculation formulas data on the amounts of clouds in different layers. Thus, for example, in the paper of Kuz'min (1950), the ratio of the actual radiation to the possible is assumed to be equal to

$$1 - c_1(n - n_\mathrm{H}) - c_2 n_\mathrm{H},$$

where n is total cloudiness, n_H is lower cloudiness, and c_1 snd c_2 are numerical coefficients. This calculation method might be applied when data on the quantity of lower cloudiness are available.

In the studies of Braslavskii (Braslavskii and Vikulina, 1954), special attention was paid to the problem of taking into account the effect of additional factors in determining total radiation. Braslavskii pointed out that when calculating possible radiation by a theoretical method, it is necessary to take into account in a direct form the effect of surface albedo on scattered (and, consequently, total) radiation. Using for calculations the values of possible radiation found from observational data for the actual state of the surface, the effect of albedo on the total radiation is, to some extent, taken into account automatically.

The calculations of Braslavskii have shown that variations of transparency of the atmosphere associated with variations of humidity and of altitude of the terrain up to several kilometers have relatively little influence on total short-wave radiation.

The problem of climatological calculation of the diurnal cycle of total radiation was examined by Biriukova (1956a). For this purpose she used Eq. (2.5) and determined its parameters from the data of actual observations.

The values of possible radiation in the diurnal cycle were calculated by Biriukova by taking into account Ukraintsev's idea. Graphs of the diurnal cycle were drawn for all months and for seven points of the USSR: Pavlovsk, Riga, Sverdlovsk, Irkutsk, Odessa, Vladivostok, and Tbilisi. The calculations showed that values of possible radiation depend mainly on the latitude, season, and hour of day. The results obtained from these calculations of possible radiation (i.e., total radiation with cloudless skies) in various latitudes are presented in Table 5.

Having data on the diurnal cycle of possible radiation and comparing them to data from observations of total radiation, it is easy to calculate by Eq. (2.5) the diurnal cycle of the coefficient η' and to determine its mean dependence on the altitude of the sun.

This relation, derived from the data of calculations for several points in the territory of the USSR, is presented in Fig. 8. It is seen from this graph that the value of coefficient η' diminishes with a decrease of the sun's altitude $h_\odot$. The cause of such change probably lies in the fact that when cloudiness is present, the increase of length of the path of the solar ray in the atmosphere greatly reduces the amount of radiation reaching the earth's surface, in comparison with cloudless conditions.

Using Eq. (2.5), Table 5, and Fig. 8, one might calculate the diurnal cycle of total radiation for mean long-term conditions. The question of the possibility of applying this procedure to calculate total radiation for short calendar periods is not quite clear yet.

Along with the data of total short-wave radiation, the data of direct and scattered radiation incident on a horizontal surface are often of importance.

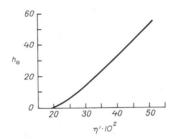

Fig. 8 Dependence of coefficient η' on the sun's altitude.

There are different methods for determining the values of direct and scattered radiation. For calculation of their mean monthly values, one could use a procedure set forth in a paper of T. G. Berliand (1961). In this investigation, a relationship was established between the ratio of scattered to total radiation, and the relative duration of sunshine. Using this relationship and taking into account available data on total radiation, one could determine monthly mean values of scattered and direct radiation.

Absorbed radiation

For determining the value of that fraction of total solar radiation absorbed by the earth's surface, it is necessary to estimate the albedo of the underlying surface for short-wave radiation.

At present, there is a great deal of observational material on mean values of albedo for various natural underlying surfaces. Mukhenberg (1963) made great efforts to generalize observational data of albedo obtained at meteorological stations.

Summaries of the results of albedo measurements at different types of surfaces have been presented in a number of works (Budyko, 1948; Berliand, 1948; Gaevskii, 1961; Kondrat'ev, 1965; and others). Mean values of albedo

TABLE 5

Total Radiation with Cloudless Sky[a] Q_0 (cal cm^{-2} hr^{-1})

North latitude	Month	Hours									
		21 3	20 4	19 5	18 6	17 7	16 8	15 9	14 10	13 11	12
	Jan.	—	—	—	—	—	—	2	6	10	12
	Feb.	—	—	—	—	1	5	13	19	24	29
	Mar.	—	—	—	2	6	15	25	31	49	37
	Apr.	—	1	3	10	21	31	40	49	53	56
	May	—	4	10	19	29	39	47	55	58	60
60°	June	2	5	13	22	31	40	48	55	60	62
	July	1	5	12	19	29	40	47	55	59	61
	Aug.	—	2	7	14	24	34	40	47	51	53
	Sept.	—	—	1	4	12	21	30	39	43	44
	Oct.	—	—	—	—	3	11	19	27	31	34
	Nov.	—	—	—	—	—	2	5	10	15	18
	Dec.	—	—	—	—	—	—	2	3	6	8
	Jan.	—	—	—	—	—	2	7	13	18	20
	Feb.	—	—	—	—	2	8	18	28	33	36
	Mar.	—	—	—	3	13	21	33	42	46	49
	Apr.	—	—	3	10	20	31	42	50	56	58
	May	—	2	6	17	28	39	50	57	60	62
55°	June	1	4	11	20	30	41	50	58	62	66
	July	—	3	8	15	27	37	47	56	62	63
	Aug.	—	2	5	13	24	34	42	50	55	58
	Sept.	—	—	1	6	14	24	36	45	50	53
	Oct.	—	—	—	1	5	13	23	32	39	40
	Nov.	—	—	—	—	—	3	10	18	24	27
	Dec.	—	—	—	—	—	—	2	6	11	13

[a] According to data of observations in the territory of the USSR.

according to the most reliable measurements made under different geographical conditions are given in Table 6.

For comparatively schematized climatological calculations of absorbed radiation, it is convenient to use the more broadly averaged values of albedo presented in Table 7 [refer to Budyko *et al.* (1961)]. The data from this table were used in preparing the "Атлас теплового баланса земного шара (Atlas of the Heat Balance of the Earth)" (1963). Monthly mean values of albedo of different geographical regions have been determined with respect to the areas occupied by different types of underlying surfaces in each region (Mukhenberg, 1962, 1963).

As has been pointed out, the albedo of the earth's surface frequently changes in the course of the year. As an example, we give here a graph de-

TABLE 5 (Continued)

TOTAL RADIATION WITH CLOUDLESS SKY[a] Q_0 (cal cm^{-2} hr^{-1})

North latitude	Month	21 3	20 4	19 5	18 6	17 7	16 8	15 9	14 10	13 11	12
										Hours	
	Jan.	—	—	—	—	—	3	11	19	25	27
	Feb.	—	—	—	1	4	11	21	34	42	45
	Mar.	—	—	1	4	12	24	38	48	52	54
	Apr.	—	—	3	10	21	33	44	54	61	63
	May	—	—	5	15	28	41	53	60	65	68
50°	June	—	2	9	19	30	44	54	62	68	70
	Jule	—	2	6	14	27	40	52	61	66	68
	Aug.	—	1	4	12	25	36	46	54	61	63
	Sept.	—	—	—	6	15	27	40	51	57	59
	Oct.	—	—	—	2	7	16	26	36	43	46
	Nov.	—	—	—	—	1	5	13	23	29	31
	Dec.	—	—	—	—	—	1	6	12	18	20
	Jan.	—	—	—	—	1	5	15	24	32	35
	Feb.	-	—	—	1	4	14	25	39	46	50
	Mar.	—	—	—	4	13	25	42	53	59	61
	Apr.	—	—	2	9	21	35	48	59	66	68
	May	—	—	4	14	30	45	58	66	70	73
45°	June	—	2	7	19	31	46	58	69	75	77
	July	—	1	5	15	30	45	58	66	71	74
	Aug.	—	—	3	11	26	39	50	61	67	70
	Sept.	—	—	—	5	16	30	45	57	64	66
	Oct.	—	—	—	2	9	19	30	43	49	51
	Nov.	—	—	—	—	2	5	17	28	34	37
	Dec.	—	—	—	—	—	3	10	20	26	29

[a] According to data of observations in the territory of the USSR.

fining the mean annual cycle of albedo from data of observations conducted at an open site in the Leningrad region (Fig. 9). It is seen from this figure that the albedo reaches its maximum in winter, when there is snow cover.

Investigations of Iaroslavtsev (1952), Kondrat'ev and Ter-Markariants (Kondrat'ev, 1954), Tooming (1961), Goisa (1962), and other authors show that the values of albedo of a land surface often vary during the diurnal cycle. When the sun's altitude is low (in morning and evening hours), albedo usually increases. The cause of the albedo increase in this case is associated with the change in reflectivity of a rough underlying surface for different angles of incidence of the sun's rays. (With a high position of the sun, the flux of direct-beam radiation penetrates deep into the vegetation cover and is absorbed there, while at a low altitude of the sun this flux penetrates the vegetation less and is reflected from its surface to a greater extent.)

TABLE 6

ALBEDO OF NATURAL SURFACES

Type of surface	Albedo
Snow and ice	
Fresh, dry snow	0.80–0.95
Clean, moist snow	0.60–0.70
Dirty snow	0.40–0.50
Sea ice	0.30–0.40
Bare soil	
Dark soils	0.05–0.15
Moist, grey soils	0.10–0.20
Dry loam or grey soils	0.20–0.35
Dry light sandy soils	0.35–0.45
Fields, meadows, tundra	
Rye and wheat fields	0.10–0.25
Potato fields	0.15–0.25
Cotton fields	0.20–0.25
Meadows	0.15–0.25
Dry steppe	0.20–0.30
Tundra	0.15–0.20
Arboreal vegetation	
Coniferous forest	0.10–0.15
Deciduous forest	0.15–0.20

Furthermore, the variation of albedo during the diurnal cycle is influenced by the change in spectral composition of short-wave radiation at different altitudes of the sun.

In climatological calculations of the diurnal cycle of absorbed radiation, the dependence of albedo on the altitude of the sun, found by Biriukova (1956b) by generalizing observational data, can be utilized. Biriukova indi-

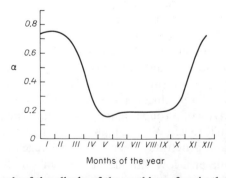

Months of the year

Fig. 9   Annual march of the albedo of the earth's surface in the Leningrad region.

TABLE 7

MEAN VALUES OF ALBEDO

Type of surface	Albedo
Stable snow cover in high latitudes (more than 60°)	0.80
Stable snow cover in middle latitudes (less than 60°)	0.70
Forest with stable snow cover	0.45
Unstable snow cover in spring	0.38
Forest with unstable snow cover in spring	0.25
Unstable snow cover in autumn	0.50
Forest with unstable snow cover in autumn	0.30
Steppe and forest during the transition period after snow cover disappears and before the mean daily temperature of the air reaches 10°	0.13
Tundra without snow cover	0.18
Steppe or deciduous forest during the period after the temperature goes above 10° in spring and before snow cover appears in autumn	0.18
Needleleaf forest during the period after the temperature goes above 10° in spring and before snow cover appears in autumn	0.14
Forest dropping leaves during a dry season, savanna and semidesert {During the dry season	0.24
{During the wet season	0.18
Desert	0.28

cated that in the snowless period albedo changes during the diurnal cycle depend mainly on sun altitude and cloudiness. Increasing cloudiness in this situation reduces the dependence of albedo on the sun's altitude for a well-understood reason—the increase of cloudiness reduces the direct and increases the scattered radiation, and the absorption of scattered radiation depends little on the altitude of the sun.

The relationship between the value $\Delta\alpha$ (the difference between the albedo at a given hour of the day and its value at noon) and the sun's altitude is presented in Fig. 10 for mean conditions of cloudiness (according to data

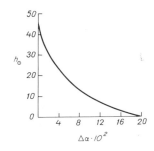

Fig. 10 Dependence of the albedo of a snow-free land surface on the sun's altitude.

from middle latitudes). This graph can be used for estimating the diurnal cycle of absorbed radiation in snow-free periods. With snow cover present, taking account of albedo changes in the determination of absorbed radiation is not necessary, according to Biriukova.

When determining the albedo of water surfaces, it is necessary to take into account the fact that reflection of direct-beam radiation depends on the altitude of the sun. As is seen from Fig. 3, the albedo for direct radiation in such conditions has a very wide variation.

The albedo of a water surface for scattered radiation varies much less and is on the average equal to 0.08–0.10. Accounting for the variations in albedo for scattered radiation that depend on cloudiness and other factors might be of some importance when calculating the amount of radiation reflected from a water surface. However, for the calculations under consideration of the amount of absorbed radiation (which usually is much greater than the reflected), the possible variations in the albedo for scattered radiation produce a relatively small effect.

As a consequence of the large dependence of the albedo of water bodies on the sun's altitude, the albedo for total incoming short-wave radiation has annual and diurnal cycles (Kirillova, 1970; and elsewhere).

For determining the mean albedo of water bodies, we used in our work (Budyko *et al.*, 1954a,b) the data of Sivkov (1952), who, by generalizing available experimental data and the conclusions drawn from theoretical calculations, established the relation of water-surface albedo in direct-beam radiation to the altitude of the sun. Considering that the albedo for scattered radiation is equal, on the average, to 0.10, and taking into account the mean fractions of direct and scattered radiation in different latitudes, we determined values of water-surface albedo for total radiation. These are presented in Table 8. The data from this table can also be used for calculations for the

TABLE 8

ALBEDO OF A WATER SURFACE FOR TOTAL SHORT-WAVE RADIATION

North lati- tude	Jan.	Feb.	Mar.	Apr.	May	June	July	Aug.	Sept.	Oct.	Nov.	Dec.
70°	—	0.23	0.16	0.11	0.09	0.09	0.09	0.10	0.13	0.15	—	—
60°	0.20	0.16	0.11	0.08	0.08	0.07	0.08	0.09	0.10	0.14	0.19	0.21
50°	0.16	0.12	0.09	0.07	0.07	0.06	0.07	0.07	0.08	0.11	0.14	0.16
40°	0.11	0.09	0.08	0.07	0.06	0.06	0.06	0.06	0.07	0.08	0.11	0.12
30°	0.09	0.08	0.07	0.06	0.06	0.06	0.06	0.06	0.06	0.07	0.08	0.09
20°	0.07	0.07	0.06	0.06	0.06	0.06	0.06	0.06	0.06	0.06	0.07	0.07
10°	0.06	0.06	0.06	0.06	0.06	0.06	0.06	0.06	0.06	0.06	0.06	0.07
0°	0.06	0.06	0.06	0.06	0.06	0.06	0.06	0.06	0.06	0.06	0.06	0.06

Southern Hemisphere, taking into account the corresponding change of seasons.

When making climatological calculations of solar radiation absorbed in water bodies, it must be borne in mind that a change in the state of the water surface by waves definitely affects the albedo. It must be noted, however, that these changes cannot substantially influence the values of absorbed radiation. As mean albedo values for water surfaces do not usually exceed 0.10, it is clear that comparatively large variations of this value change the value of absorbed radiation relatively little. This permits us to neglect the effect of wave disturbance on the albedo when calculating the sums of absorbed radiation for such periods as months, ten-day periods, and so on.

Net long-wave radiation

Besides the loss of a portion of incoming short-wave radiation due to reflection, it is necessary to calculate the outgo of radiative energy by the net exchange of long-wave radiation when computing the radiation balance. In the investigations that have been made, it has been established (Kondrat'ev, 1956; and others) that the value of net long-wave radiation depends on air temperature, humidity, cloudiness, and the vertical gradients of temperature and moisture in the atmosphere.

As a result of these investigations, formulas were found that relate the value of net long-wave radiation under cloudless skies to the temperature and humidity of the air. These formulas have the following form:

$$I_0 = \delta\sigma T^4(a_1 + b_1 \cdot 10^{-c_1 e}) \tag{2.7}$$

and

$$I_0 = \delta\sigma T^4(a_2 - b_2\sqrt{e}), \tag{2.8}$$

where I_0 is the net long-wave radiation; δ is the coefficient of emissivity, relating the properties of the radiating surfaces to those of a black body; T is the air temperature; e is the pressure of water vapor; and a_1, b_1, c_1, a_2, and b_2 are coefficients.

The first of these formulas was offered by Ångström (1916) and the second by Brunt (1932). The coefficients of the formulas have been determined in a number of studies of observational data.

In climatological calculations of net long-wave radiation, Ångström's formula with the coefficients given in Linke's reference book (Linke, 1934), $a_1 = 0.194$, $b_1 = 0.236$, $c_1 = 0.069$, has often been used (vapor pressure is expressed in millimeters of mercury).

In the investigations of a number of authors, theoretical methods for determining net long-wave radiation have been worked out. Of much importance in the development of these investigations have been the works of

Kondrat'ev, who has used for radiation calculations a model of differential accounting of the spectrum of the coefficients of absorption of long-wave radiation in the atmosphere.

Using results obtained by Kondrat'ev, M. E. Berliand established a theoretical dependence of net long-wave radiation under cloudless skies upon the temperature and humidity of the air (Berliand and Berliand, 1952).

The dependence found by M. E. Berliand can be approximately expressed in the analytical form

$$I_0 = \delta\sigma T^4(0.39 - 0.058\sqrt{e}),\qquad(2.9)$$

where e is in millimeters of mercury. The coefficient δ in this formula varies relatively little for different natural surfaces. Therefore, its mean value, which equals 0.95, is commonly used in calculations.

For checking the available formulas, Efimova processed a great many observational data of net long-wave radiation, obtained during the period of the International Geophysical Year at actinometric stations in the USSR (Efimova, 1961). It was established in her work that Berliand's formula is corroborated well by the data of observations made at average and high humidities. At a small absolute humidity, which, for example, corresponds to winter conditions in regions with a continental climate, Berliand's formula gives results that are too high. Therefore, the dependence of net long-wave radiation on humidity should be used in a somewhat modified form:

$$I_0 = \delta\sigma T^4(0.254 - 0.0066e).\qquad(2.10)$$

Besides the temperature and humidity of the air, net long-wave radiation is considerably influenced by cloudiness and by the difference between temperatures of the surface and the air. The effect of cloudiness on net long-wave radiation is usually accounted for by the formula

$$I = I_0(1 - c'n),\qquad(2.11)$$

where I is the net long-wave radiation with actual cloudiness, I_0 is the net long-wave radiation with cloudless skies, n is the cloudiness in fractions of unity, and c' is a coefficient.

Ångström found the value of c' to be equal, on the average, to 0.75. Asklöf (1920), Dorno, and other authors established the fact that the value of c' is different for clouds of different layers, being much smaller for high clouds than for low. Taking this fact into account, Evfimov (1939) suggested that net long-wave radiation be calculated in relation to cloudiness by the formula

$$I = I_0[1 - (c_B'n_B + c_C'n_C + c_H'n_H)]\qquad(2.12)$$

where n_H, n_C, and n_B represent the cloudiness of the lower, middle, and upper layers; c_H', c_C', and c_B' are the corresponding coefficients.

Evfimov found these coefficients to be $c_B' = 0.15$ to 0.20; $c_C' = 0.50$ to 0.60; $c_H' = 0.70$ to 0.80.

In some investigations, there are indications that observational data show that the decrease of net long-wave radiation with an increase of cloudiness is not linear, but more rapid. Therefore, this formula for determining it has been offered:

$$I = I_0(1 - c'n^\tau), \tag{2.13}$$

where τ is assumed equal to 1.5–2.0.

A theoretical calculation of the mean values of the coefficient c' for different latitudes has been made by M. E. Berliand. In this calculation, the mean frequency of clouds of different layers at each latitude is taken into account. The values obtained for the coefficient c' are given in Table 9. The reduction of values of this coefficient in low latitudes is explained mainly by the higher mean altitude of clouds in these regions.

TABLE 9

MEAN LATITUDINAL VALUES OF THE COEFFICIENT c'

ϕ	75°	70°	65°	60°	55°	50°	45°	40°	35°	30°	25°	20°	15°	10°	5°	0°
c'	0.82	0.80	0.78	0.76	0.74	0.72	0.70	0.68	0.65	0.63	0.61	0.59	0.57	0.55	0.52	0.50

In some works (Kuz'min, 1948; Bolz, 1949; Kirillova, 1952; and others), the effect of cloudiness on long-wave radiation is assumed to be taken into account by introducing a correction, not to net long-wave radiation, but to the counterradiation from the atmosphere. Kondrat'ev indicated that such a method for calculating the effect of clouds on long-wave radiation does not have any substantial advantage over using Eq. (2.11) or (2.13).

In climatological calculations made in the Main Geophysical Observatory in connection with the preparation of the first edition of the "Атлас теплового баланса (Atlas of Heat Balance)" (1955), Eq. (2.13) with $\tau = 2$ was used.

In the investigations of Efimova (1961), generalizing many observational data, it was found that the form of the dependence of the monthly mean values of net long-wave radiation on cloudiness varies appreciably in different climatic regions and in different seasons. Therefore, in Eq. (2.13) the value τ is actually variable, changing roughly from 1.0 to 1.5.

In addition, Efimova confirmed the variability of the coefficient c' during the annual cycle, which had been noted earlier by several authors.

Thus, for accurate determination of the total net long-wave radiation by Eq. (2.13), one should use detailed information on the values of the coefficients in this formula for different geographical regions in different periods of the year.

At the same time, for approximate computations of the radiation balance, it is possible to limit consideration to schematized values of the parameters mentioned. Thus, for example, in work done in the Main Geophysical Observatory for constructing world maps of radiation balance in "Атлас теплового баланса земного шара (Atlas of the Heat Balance of the Earth)" (1963) and other works, it was assumed that $\tau = 1$, and mean latitudinal values of the coefficient c' from Table 9 were used.

The above formulas for calculation of net long-wave radiation relate to cases when the temperature of the earth's surface is close to that of the lower layer of air. If these temperatures differ substantially, then the formulas must be modified to account for the effect of their difference on radiation, since the true radiation of the earth's surface is defined by its own temperature T_w and not by the temperature of the air. The complete formula for calculating net long-wave radiation then becomes

$$I = I_0(1 - c'n) + 4\delta\sigma T^3(T_w - T). \qquad (2.14)$$

The second term of the right side of this formula permits us to take into account the effect on radiation of the difference between the temperatures of the underlying surface and the air. In the presence of such a difference between temperatures, net long-wave radiation changes by the quantity $\delta\sigma T_w^4 - \delta\sigma T^4$, which might be considered to be approximately equal to $4\delta\sigma T^3(T_w - T)$, as the difference between the values T_w and T is always small in comparison to their values in the absolute temperature scale.

The question of accounting for the effect of this correction has been discussed in several papers (Kondrat'ev, 1951; Berliand and Berliand, 1952; and others). In the investigation of Efimova (1961), it was established that the indicated way of taking the effect of temperature difference on radiation into account is corroborated by observational data. This conclusion requires an additional check for large differences of temperatures of the earth's surface and the air.

When calculating net long-wave radiation for water bodies by Eq. (2.14), the temperature T_w can usually be determined from observational data.

Since for land conditions there are not, as a rule, reliable data on the temperature of the underlying surface, it is often better to use an indirect method in computing the correction $4\delta\sigma T^3(T_w - T)$ when calculating a radiation balance. This method is based on the following considerations. Let us write the equation of the radiation balance in the following form:

$$R = Q(1 - \alpha) - I_0(1 - c'n) - 4\delta\sigma T^3(T_w - T). \qquad (2.15)$$

We shall use the heat-balance equation

$$R = LE + P + A, \qquad (2.16)$$

and the formula for determining the turbulent flux of sensible heat from the earth's surface into the atmosphere (refer to Section 2 of this chapter)

$$P = \rho c_p D(T_w - T), \qquad (2.17)$$

where ρ is air density, c_p is the specific heat of air, and D is the integral coefficient of turbulent diffusion.

From Eqs. (2.15–2.17), it follows that

$$R = [Q(1 - \alpha) - I_0(1 - c'n)]\frac{1}{1 + G'} + (LE + A)\frac{G'}{1 + G'}, \qquad (2.18)$$

where

$$G' = \frac{4\delta\sigma T^3}{\rho c_p D}.$$

This formula can be used for calculation of the radiation balance when there are no data on the temperature of the underlying surface.

When using this formula for determination of average values of the radiation balance, one can use mean values of the ratio G' since the variation of this value does not greatly influence the calculation results. As available data have shown, G' in the warm season is, on an average, equal to 0.7. In desert regions, where turbulent exchange is more intense, this value reduces, on an average, to 0.4–0.5. In the cold season in middle and high latitudes, when turbulent mixing diminishes, the mean value of G' increases slightly and can be assumed to be close to 1.0. All the given values of the ratio G' are diurnal means.

The methods for calculating the values of the latent-heat flux LE and the heat flow A into the soil, included in Eq. (2.18), will be discussed later.

The stated procedure for climatological calculation of net long-wave radiation permits us to determine its value using only the data of standard meteorological observations of air temperature and humidity, total cloudiness, and (for water bodies) the temperature of the water surface with information on the heights and forms of clouds and also on the vertical distributions of temperature and humidity in the troposphere, it is possible to use more detailed methods for determining net long-wave radiation. Thus, for example, in the study of Berliand and Berliand (1952) and other investigations, the mean values of coefficients c_B', c_C', and c_H' for different forms of clouds are given. Application of these coefficients with information on cloud types can make the calculations of net long-wave radiation more accurate.

The necessity of taking into account the vertical distributions of temperature and humidity when calculating radiation has been discussed in a number of papers. Calculations by Mukhenberg and Efimova (1961) show that in determining long-term mean values of net long-wave radiation in single months, accounting for vertical gradients actually observed does not introduce any substantial change in the values of net long-wave radiation found on the basis of the above-mentioned model and the use only of data of near-surface meteorological observations.

However, it may be assumed that in climatic regions where strong inversions of temperature are observed, the vertical structure of the troposphere has an appreciable influence on net long-wave radiation.

It is also probable that for calculating net long-wave radiation over short calendar periods, it is important to take into account the vertical gradients of temperature and humidity. For such calculations, the methods worked out in the investigations of Shekhter (1950), Kirillova and Kovaleva (1951), Elsasser and Culbertson (1960), Kondrat'ev and Niilisk (1960), and other authors are useful.

2. The Turbulent Flux of Sensible Heat from the Earth's Surface into the Atmosphere

Turbulent exchange in the layer of air near the ground

The temperature of the earth's surface for both land and water bodies usually is not equal to that of the layers of air lying above it. As a consequence, there appears a vertical flux of heat between the underlying surface and the atmosphere, conditioned by the eddy or turbulent heat conductivity of the air.

The value of the turbulent sensible-heat flux depends essentially on the intensity of turbulent exchange in the lower layer of the atmosphere. A quantitative relationship between the turbulent sensible-heat flux at ground level and the characteristic intensity of turbulent mixing (the coefficient of exchange) can be obtained from the following considerations.

Considering, according to the idea of Taylor (1915) and Schmidt (1917), the process of turbulent diffusion to be similar to that of molecular diffusion, it is possible to use the following equation to describe the turbulent heat exchange in the lower layer of the atmosphere:

$$\frac{dT}{dt} = \frac{\partial}{\partial z}\left(k\,\frac{\partial T}{\partial z}\right),$$ (2.19)

where t is time, z is the vertical coordinate, k is the coefficient of turbulent exchange, and T is the temperature.

Designating an individual time-derivative of temperature by a partial derivative, we obtain

$$\frac{\partial T}{\partial t} + u\,\frac{\partial T}{\partial x} = \frac{\partial}{\partial z}\left(k\,\frac{\partial T}{\partial z}\right),$$ (2.20)

where x is the horizontal coordinate measured along an axis, the direction of which coincides with that of the vector of wind velocity u.

After integrating Eq. (2.20) with respect to z from 0 to z, we obtain the relation

$$\int_0^z \left(\frac{\partial T}{\partial t} + u \frac{\partial T}{\partial x} \right) dz = k \frac{\partial T}{\partial z} + \frac{P}{\rho c_p}, \tag{2.21}$$

where $P/\rho c_p$ is the constant of integration, which is equal to the ratio of the turbulent heat flux P at ground level to the product of air density ρ by heat capacity of the air at constant pressure c_p.

Evaluating the order of magnitude of the term

$$\int_0^z \left(\frac{\partial T}{\partial t} + u \frac{\partial T}{\partial x} \right) dz,$$

one can easily establish that for the lowest layer of air it will always be small in comparison with the other two members of Eq. (2.21).

As has been found in appropriate calculations, the height of this layer is usually of the order of several meters at night and several tens of meters in the daytime. Within the limits of this layer [which we have called a quasi-stationary sublayer—Budyko (1946d)], the turbulent sensible-heat flux changes little together with height. Its value is equal to

$$P = -\rho c_p k \frac{\partial T}{\partial z}. \tag{2.22}$$

In a number of investigations for calculating the vertical turbulent heat flux in the higher layers of the air, an assumption has been used that the turbulent heat flux at certain levels in the free atmosphere is proportional to the product of the turbulent exchange coefficient by the vertical gradient of temperature; that is, a formula similar to Eq. (2.22) has been applied. In this case, the vertical gradient of absolute temperature is replaced by the gradient of potential temperature. It is evident that with such an assumption the turbulent heat flux becomes zero when the vertical gradient of temperature becomes equal to the adiabatic gradient, i.e., to approximately 1° per 100 m. Such a method of using Eq. (2.22) is not quite accurate.

In papers of Budyko and Iudin (1946, 1948), Budyko (1967), Iudin (1967 and elsewhere), it has been pointed out that transport of heat by means of turbulent diffusion in the vertical direction differs slightly from turbulent diffusion of so-called "passive admixtures", which do not themselves influence the process of mixing. In these investigations, the hypothesis has been expressed that there is a definite correlation between the deviation of temperature of a turbulent eddy at a given level from the mean temperature of the level and the direction of eddy movement (warmer eddies more often ascend and colder ones descend). As a result of analyzing observational data, it has been found that for this reason the turbulent heat flux becomes zero at a vertical gradient of temperature less than the adiabatic gradient and approximately equal to 0.6° per 100 m. This temperature gradient has been called the equilibrium gradient.

The concept of the equilibrium gradient is very important for explanation of the so-called "Schmidt paradox", which will be discussed below (refer to Chapter III, Section 3). At the same time, in using Eq. (2.22) for the surface air layer, there is no necessity to consider the value of the equilibrium gradient, since the temperature gradients observed in the surface layer usually exceed the values of the equilibrium gradient by a factor of 10–100 times.

As pointed out above, the turbulent heat flux is proportional to the value of the turbulent exchange coefficient. In its physical meaning, this coefficient is similar to the corresponding coefficient for the conditions of molecular diffusion. However, unlike the latter, the coefficient of turbulent exchange in the lower layers of the atmosphere changes considerably in space and in time, depending on a number of meteorological factors.

Information available on the coefficient of exchange in the surface air layer has been obtained mainly from experimental investigations and semi-empirical theories.

In the papers of Rossby (1932) and Rossby and Montgomery (1935), for determining the characteristic of turbulent mixing in the lower layer of the atmosphere, a semiempirical theory of the boundary turbulent layer was used.

In accordance with the point of view of Prandtl (1932), Rossby and Montgomery assumed that with an adiabatic temperature distribution the mixing length in the lower layer of air increases linearly with altitude, turning, at the level where the wind velocity is equal to zero (at $z = 0$), into a value proportional to the roughness of the underlying surface, that is,

$$l = \kappa(z + z_0) \tag{2.23}$$

where l is the mixing length, z_0 is the roughness, and κ is a dimensionless constant, approximately equal (according to experiments in pipes) to 0.38–0.40 (von Kármán constant).

According to Prandtl, the value of the turbulent friction stress τ, equal to $\rho\kappa(\partial u/\partial z)$, can be determined by the formula

$$\tau = \rho l^2 \left(\frac{\partial u}{\partial z}\right)^2 = \rho\kappa^2(z + z_0)^2\left(\frac{\partial u}{\partial z}\right)^2, \tag{2.24}$$

where $\partial u/\partial z$ is the vertical gradient of wind speed.

Having accepted the assumption that in the lower layer of air the value τ

is constant with height, we can derive, after having integrated Eq. (2.24) with respect to z, the equation for the wind profile,

$$u = \frac{1}{\kappa} \left(\frac{\tau}{\rho}\right)^{1/2} \ln \frac{z + z_0}{z_0}, \tag{2.25}$$

and for the coefficient of turbulent exchange,

$$k = l^2 \left(\frac{\partial u}{\partial z}\right) = \kappa^2(z + z_0) \frac{u_1}{\ln[(z_1 + z_0)/z_0]}, \tag{2.26}$$

where u_1 is the wind speed at height z_1.

It follows from Eq. (2.26) that in the lower layer of air the exchange coefficient is proportional to height z and wind speed u.

Experimental investigations have shown that application of these formulas gives satisfactory results in the absence of any substantial vertical gradient of temperature in the surface air layer up to a height of several tens of meters. In this situation, the exchange coefficient can be calculated from data on wind speed at a single level and roughness of the earth's surface.

For determination of the roughness parameter, which defines the effect of the uneven surface on wind speed, it is necessary to have data on wind speed at two or more different levels. It is then possible to exclude the value of turbulent friction from Eq. (2.25) and calculate the value of z_0, which depends on the ratio of wind speeds at the two levels.

Without any such observational data available, the value of roughness can be approximated from the kind of underlying surface. For a smooth surface of ice or snow, roughness is usually of the order of 10^{-3}–10^{-2} cm. For a smooth meadow covered with low grass, the value of roughness is usually equal to 10^{-1}–10^{0} cm. With high grass or such agricultural plants as potatoes, roughness increases to 1–10 cm. Over shrub vegetation and forest, the values of roughness may be equal to 10–100 cm [refer to Sutton (1953), Priestley (1959), and others].

It should, however, be borne in mind that application of Eq. (2.26) is possible only in comparatively rare cases, because a simple dependence of wind-speed gradient on speed itself, corresponding to this formula, is realized only at small vertical gradients of temperature.

Numerous observations of wind profile in the lower layers of air have shown that in real conditions the value of vertical gradient of wind speed over a given underlying surface depends materially on both the wind speed and the vertical distribution of temperature.

Thus, in our works (Budyko, 1945, 1946b), there was established from experimental data a relation of the ratio of wind speeds at heights of 5 m and 1 m to the wind speed at 2 m and the difference of temperature between 0.2 and 1.5 m. The relation, given in Fig. 11, shows the important influence that thermal stratification produces in the wind profile in the surface layer of air. With temperature decreasing with height (which in the figure corresponds to positive values of ΔT), the ratio of wind speed at the two heights decreases considerably in comparison to the ratio under inversion conditions.

In connection with this conclusion, the necessity of considering the effect of vertical temperature distribution when determining the exchange coefficient becomes evident.

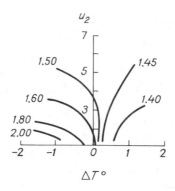

Fig. 11   Dependence of the ratio of wind speeds at heights of 5 and 1 m to speed at the height of 2 m (u_2) and the temperature difference between heights of 20 and 150 cm (ΔT), from observational data.

The question of the effect of the vertical profile of temperature on turbulent exchange in the surface layer has been discussed in many papers, both experimental and theoretical. Even in the first works in this direction, it was established that the values of the exchange coefficient in the surface air layer in daytime considerably exceed those determined by Eq. (2.26) for isothermal stratification. For night conditions, the reverse dependence was established. In light of this fact, it has turned out that utilization of Eq. (2.26) for determination of the turbulent exchange coefficient must lead to substantial errors in calculations of the turbulent heat flux.

This conclusion has been corroborated by the results of checking the calculations of evaporation made by Thornthwaite and Holzman (1942), who used the formula for the exchange coefficient without considering the influence of thermal stratification. Such calculation of components of the heat and water balances has shown (Budyko, 1946c) that the equations of balance in this case do not close. From this, it follows that not considering the effect of stability on exchange leads to a significant error in determining evaporation and turbulent exchange of sensible heat.

In our works (Budyko, 1946b, 1948), the following relation was offered for the accounting of the effect of stability on turbulent exchange:

$$k = k_p \Phi \tag{2.27}$$

where k_p is the exchange coefficient at the equilibrium state, and Φ is a function depending on the Richardson number in the surface layer of air.

The Richardson number [refer to Sutton (1953), Iudin (1948), and others] is a dimensionless criterion, defining the effect of thermal stratification on turbulent exchange. It is derived from the formula

$$\mathrm{Ri} = \frac{g(\partial T/\partial z)}{T(\partial u/\partial z)^2}, \tag{2.28}$$

where g is the acceleration of gravity, and T is temperature in the absolute scale.

It is easy to demonstrate that in the surface air layer, the Richardson number is approximately proportional to the ratio $\Delta T/(\Delta u)^2$ or $\Delta T/u^2$, where ΔT is the difference between temperatures at two heights, and Δu is the difference between wind speeds at two heights.

In accordance with this, we offered the formulas (Budyko, 1946b)

$$k = k_p \left[1 + \zeta_1 \frac{\Delta T}{(\Delta u)^2} \right] \tag{2.29}$$

and

$$k = k_p \left[1 + \zeta_2 \frac{\Delta T}{u^2} \right], \tag{2.30}$$

where ζ_1 and ζ_2 are coefficients to be derived from semiempirical considerations and depending on the levels at which temperature and wind speed are measured.

After the first papers of Rossby and Montgomery (1935), Sverdrup (1936b), Holzman (1943), Obukhov (1946), and others, the problem of the influence of thermal stratification on turbulent exchange was discussed in other investigations, in which different methods for determination of the Φ function in Eq. (2.27) were used.

To verify the formulas that permit the calculation of the values of the turbulent exchange coefficient, data were used in our work from experiments in which the values of the exchange coefficient were determined by different independent methods. Some of these methods are based on measurements of vertical fluxes of heat and moisture. They include, for example, a method for determining the exchange coefficient from the measurements of evaporation (Budyko, 1946a; and others). The gist of this method reduces to the following:

By analogy with Eq. (2.22) for conditions of the layer of air near the surface, it is possible to use the formula

$$E = -\rho k \frac{\partial q}{\partial z},\qquad(2.31)$$

where E is the rate of evaporation, and $\partial q/\partial z$ is the vertical gradient of specific humidity.

We take into account the fact that the turbulent exchange coefficient in the surface layer of air increases with height, according to the law approximated by the relation

$$k = k_1 z\qquad(2.32)$$

(where k_1 is a coefficient of proportionality). After having integrated the right side of Eq. (2.31) with respect to z, considering Eq. (2.32), we obtain the relation

$$E = \rho k_1 \frac{q_1 - q_2}{\ln(z_2/z_1)},\qquad(2.33)$$

where q_1 and q_2 are the specific humidities at heights z_1 and z_2.

It follows from this that the value k_1 can be calculated by the formula

$$k_1 = \frac{E \ln(z_2/z_1)}{\rho(q_1 - q_2)}.\qquad(2.34)$$

In some determinations of the exchange coefficient, a more general formula has been used

$$k_1 = -\frac{E}{\rho(\partial q/\partial \ln z)}.\qquad(2.35)$$

These formulas have been repeatedly used for determination of the exchange coefficient in experimental investigations with measurements of evaporation and the vertical gradient of humidity.

The results of calculating the exchange coefficient at a height of 1 m by this method, using observational data obtained in the region of Leningrad, are presented in Fig. 12, in relation to wind speed. It is seen from this figure that the values of the exchange coefficient observed in daytime on the average noticeably exceed the values corresponding to Eq. (2.26), which are represented by the straight line. The difference confirms the marked effect of stability on turbulent exchange in the surface layer of air.

Another method to determine the exchange coefficient (the so-called heat-balance method) is based on the use of a formula obtained from Eq. (2.22) by integrating it with respect to z, taking into account condition (2.32). This formula has the following form:

$$P = \rho c_p k_1 \frac{T_1 - T_2}{\ln(z_2/z_1)}.\qquad(2.36)$$

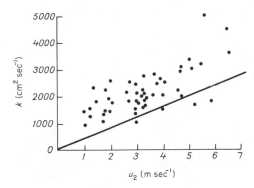

Fig. 12 Dependence of the coefficient of turbulent exchange on wind speed.

From Eqs. (2.33) and (2.36) and from heat-balance equation (2.16), we derive the formula

$$k_1 = \frac{(R - A) \ln (z_2/z_1)}{\rho[c_p(T_1 - T_2) + L(q_1 - q_2)]}. \tag{2.37}$$

Utilization of this formula implies the acceptance of the assumption that the exchange coefficients for heat transfer and water-vapor transfer are equal.

This problem has been discussed in a number of investigations. Considering the results, it is possible to assume that if differences between the exchange coefficients for heat and moisture do exist, then at any rate in the lowest layer of air they are relatively small.

Among other methods for experimental determination of the exchange coefficient, it is worth mentioning the one based on the measurements of the eddy fluctuations of wind speed and temperature. Application of this method involves the use of rather complicated apparatus and requires comparatively difficult processing of observational data. However, the method permits the obtaining of data that are very important for understanding the mechanism of turbulent exchange in the atmosphere.

As a result of applying experimental and semiempirical methods for determination of coefficients of turbulent exchange in the surface layer of air, it is found possible to draw the following general conclusions:

1. The exchange coefficient in the surface layer of air increases with height and is approximately proportional to height up to the level of several tens of meters. In the daytime (with temperature decreasing with height), the exchange coefficient usually increases with height somewhat faster than linearly. During the night (with inversions), the increase of the exchange coefficient with height is slower than linear. Deviations of the vertical profile

of the exchange coefficient from linearity are noticeable mainly at levels higher than several meters.

Thus, in climatological calculations of the variation of the exchange coefficient with height for the lowest layer of air, one can use the formula $k = k_1 z$ with sufficient accuracy. In this case, the vertical distributions of wind speed, temperature, and humidity following from the above formula would have the form of the well-known logarithmic laws.

2. Mean values of the exchange coefficient at a level of 1 m in the daytime period in the warm season on land are of the order of 1500–2000 cm^2 sec^{-1}. During the diurnal cycle of the warm period on land, the exchange coefficient varies significantly, reaching its maximum in the afternoon hours and its minimum at night and in the early hours of the morning. In conditions of clear weather, the exchange coefficient may change by one to two orders during the diurnal cycle. In overcast weather and at high wind speeds, the diurnal cycle of the exchange coefficient diminishes.

During the annual cycle in middle latitudes, the exchange coefficient reaches its greatest values in summer because of the increase of roughness and the large daytime temperature gradients. In winter, the exchange coefficient decreases because of the small roughness of the snow surface and the high frequency of daytime inversions.

3. Over large water bodies (especially the oceans), the exchange coefficient in the lower layer of air depends mainly on wind speed, since under these conditions the vertical gradients of temperature are usually small. Besides wind speed, the exchange coefficient is here influenced by the form of the water surface (waves), but this influence is comparatively limited.

4. Significant changes in the exchange coefficient because of the effect of variable factors make it difficult to use the mean values of the exchange coefficient in calculation of the turbulent heat flux by Eq. (2.36), especially for short periods of averaging with respect to time.

Turbulent diffusion between the earth's surface and the atmosphere

It was pointed out that the vertical turbulent flux of sensible heat is the consequence of the presence of a difference between the temperatures of the earth's surface and of the layers of air above it. As a result, the value of the heat flux depends not only on the intensity of exchange in the surface layer of air at some distance from the earth's surface, but also on the conditions of heat conductivity in the thin air layer immediately adjacent to the earth's surface.

Because turbulent exchange near the earth's surface is substantially weakened, the intensity of exchange in the lowest levels produces a considerable influence on the rates of the heat fluxes. Therefore, the problem of the regularities of turbulent exchange between the earth's surface and the atmosphere becomes of great importance when studying the vertical fluxes of heat and water vapor.

To establish the relations between the turbulent heat flux and the difference between the temperatures of the earth's surface and the atmosphere, Eq. (2.22) must be integrated with respect to z from 0 to z. Then we obtain

$$P = \frac{\rho c_p (T_w - T)}{\int_0^z dz/k},$$ (2.38)

where T_w is the temperature of the earth's surface, and T is the temperature at the level z.

This formula can be rewritten as

$$P = \rho c_p D(T_w - T),$$ (2.39)

where

$$D = \frac{1}{\int_0^z dz/k}.$$ (2.40)

The value D, widely used in modern investigations of heat balance, is usually called the integral coefficient of turbulent diffusion (Budyko, 1956). In terms of properties, this coefficient is considerably different from that of turbulent exchange in the surface air layer.

Thus, for example, unlike the coefficient k, the value D depends relatively little on height. Elementary estimates show that beginning at heights of the order of 1 m, a change in the level z by several times changes the coefficient D by only several per cent.

In determining the coefficient D for land conditions, it is possible to use two basic methods. The first is based on Eq. (2.40), that is, on the use of the relationship between the integral coefficient of diffusion and the exchange coefficient. When integrating the denominator in Eq. (2.40), one should bear in mind that the regularities of turbulent exchange near the underlying surface, that is, at very small z, are rather complicated.

In many theoretical investigations of heat exchange and evaporation for determination of the integral $\int_0^z dz/k$, authors have used various hypotheses concerning the form of the function $k(z)$ at small z without any substantiation of their feasibility.

For solving the problem of the conditions of diffusion near a natural rough surface, we carried out an experimental investigation (Budyko, 1947). In these experiments, the temperature of the underlying surface devoid of vegetation and the temperature of the air at several levels were measured with thin resistance thermometers.

The relationship between the measured values of temperature difference at the surface and at a height of 150 cm ($T_w - T_{150}$) for daytime conditions and the difference in temperatures between the heights of 55 cm and 150 cm ($T_{55} - T_{150}$) is presented in Fig. 13 as a group of points. In this figure, the relation between the values ($T_w - T_{150}$) and ($T_{55} - T_{150}$) shown as line 1 corresponds to the height relation of the exchange coefficient

$$k = k_1(z + z_0).\tag{2.41}$$

Line 2 defines a dependence derived under the condition

$$k = k_1 z + k_0,\tag{2.42}$$

where k_0 is the coefficient of molecular diffusion.

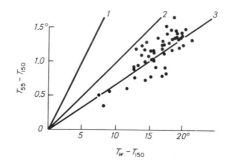

Fig. 13   Results of investigations of boundary conditions for heat and water exchange (see text).

It is seen from the figure that neither Eq. (2.42) nor Eq. (2.41) is satisfied, because the discontinuities in temperature between the underlying surface and the air that are predicted by these models turn out to be much underestimated. The location of points in Fig. 13 can be described on the average by line 3, corresponding to values of the ratio

$$\frac{T_w - T_{150}}{T_{55} - T_{150}} = 15.\tag{2.43}$$

The data in Fig. 13 indicate that the conditions of heat conductivity in the thin air layer near the ground have a very great effect on the turbulent sensible-heat flux. The differences between lines 1, 2, and 3 correspond to relative differences between the values of the heat flux that occur in relation to exchange conditions in this thin layer.

Taking into account that Eqs. (2.36) and (2.39) lead to the ratio

$$D = \frac{T_1 - T_2}{T_w - T_2} \frac{k_1}{\ln(z_2/z_1)}\tag{2.44}$$

(T_1 and T_2 are air temperatures at heights z_1 and z_2), we assume that

$$D = \vartheta k_1, \qquad (2.45)$$

where ϑ is a coefficient dependent on the boundary conditions of heat exchange at the underlying surface.

It follows from the given experimental data that for the above-indicated levels of temperature measurement the value ϑ is equal to $\frac{1}{15}$. Other experimental material relating to daytime hours and conditions of various bare surfaces usually give mean values of ϑ within the range from $\frac{1}{10}$ to $\frac{1}{20}$. For the night period with temperature inversions in the surface layer, the coefficient ϑ increases greatly in comparison to the daytime value—on an average, 3–5 times.

Although a precise determination of the coefficient ϑ is difficult to obtain in each individual case, Eq. (2.45) can nevertheless be used for estimating mean values of the coefficient D.

Other methods for determining the integral coefficient of diffusion by analogy with those for calculation of the exchange coefficient are based on measurements of the fluxes of heat and moisture. Thus, for example, with the availability of data on measurements of evaporation rate, one can use the following formula for determining the coefficient D:

$$D = \frac{E(T_1 - T_2)}{\rho(T_w - T_2)} \frac{1}{(q_1 - q_2)}, \qquad (2.46)$$

and with the availability of data from measurements of radiation balance R and heat exchange in the soil A, the formula

$$D = \frac{R - A}{\rho c_p(T_w - T)\left[1 + \dfrac{L(q_1 - q_2)}{c_p(T_1 - T_2)}\right]}. \qquad (2.47)$$

Application of these relations permitted us to obtain series of data on the integral coefficient of diffusion for land conditions.

As an example, we can mention the results of a special investigation done in the Leningrad region on a site covered with grass (Budyko et al., 1956). In this work observations of the earth's surface temperature were made by a radiation thermometer, which made it possible to provide the accuracy of measurements necessary for calculations. The mean value of coefficient D was found by Eq. (2.47) for several dozen series of observations conducted in daytime and proved to be equal to 1.02 cm sec^{-1}. Simultaneously, it was established that in daytime the coefficient D does not have a significant diurnal cycle.

A detailed climatological analysis of the coefficient D was carried out in the works of Broido (1957, 1958). In these investigations, the values of the coefficient were calculated for numerous points, and maps of its monthly means for the European part of the USSR were constructed.

It was established in Broido's papers that the mean value of the coefficient D does not vary much in time and space. Taking into account this fact and the insufficient accuracy of existing methods for climatological calculations of the coefficient D, one might consider that the information now available on the space–time distribution of this coefficient to a large extent has qualitative and not quantitative significance.

On the basis of available data, one can draw the following general conclusions concerning the basic properties of the integral coefficient of diffusion.

1. The integral coefficient of diffusion varies little in relation to the level at which the temperature (or humidity) of the air is measured, if this level is higher than 1 m.

2. Mean values of the integral coefficient of diffusion in the daytime for land conditions are of the order of 1.0–1.5 cm sec^{-1}. With inversions, the integral coefficient of diffusion decreases in comparison with its values at superadiabatic gradients of temperature; however, the dependence of the integral coefficient of diffusion on temperature stratification is noticeably less than the dependence of the exchange coefficient. (This is associated with changes in the conditions of heat exchange near the earth's surface that result in corresponding changes in the coefficient ϑ.)

The mean values of the coefficient D for mean daily conditions are noticeably less than those for daytime. In the warm season on land, they are approximately equal to 0.6–0.7 cm sec^{-1}.

3. In arid regions, the integral coefficient of diffusion is larger than in humid regions. On extensive water bodies, the integral coefficient of diffusion changes significantly with variations in wind speed. Under land conditions, the dependence of mean values of this coefficient on wind speed is less, since, first, the variability of mean wind speeds over a large part of the land surface is comparatively small, and, second, a decrease in wind speed at superadiabatic gradients leads to an increase of the thermal influence on turbulent exchange—this influence compensating the reduction of the integral coefficient of diffusion [refer to Budyko (1947, 1948), and elsewhere].

A smaller variability of the integral coefficient of diffusion for land conditions, in comparison with the variability of the exchange coefficient, facilitates the use of its mean values in climatological calculations. In addition, for conditions of water bodies, it is usually necessary, even in calculations of heat exchange for a long period of time, to take into account the dependence of the coefficient D on wind speed. This problem will be discussed in detail below.

Determination of the turbulent sensible-heat flux

Determination of the vertical turbulent flux of sensible heat both by means of direct measurements and on the basis of indirect climatological calculations has a number of difficulties.

Let us first consider some methods for determination of this heat flux from data of special observations. Among these methods, the gradient method is most generally used, associated with measurements of the vertical gradient of temperature in the surface layer of air.

In this case, calculation of the turbulent sensible-heat flux is done by Eq. (2.36), which includes two variables—the difference in temperature at two heights and the coefficient of turbulent exchange (k) at a single height. To determine the exchange coefficient, one uses Eq. (2.30) or (2.37). In the first case, for the determination of the exchange coefficient, it is necessary to have additional data on wind speed (and also on the roughness of the observational site); in the second case, one must have data on the radiation balance, the flow of heat into the soil, and the difference in specific humidity at two heights.

Experience has shown that determination of the turbulent sensible-heat flux by gradient observations requires thorough preparation. An especially difficult task is the choice of a site for gradient observations. This site ought to be open and absolutely homogeneous in terms of the state of the underlying surface within a radius of not less than several hundred meters. Even comparatively small obstacles not far from the observational site may distort the gradients observed. Considerable distortion of measured values may appear even at a seemingly quite homogeneous surface in case different parts are not equally moist.

Because the indicated requirements as to the choice of observational site are often not easy to meet, the data of mass gradient observations are not always of sufficiently high quality. On the other hand, data of gradient observations obtained under favorable conditions often give valuable material for investigating the regularities of turbulent heat exchange between the earth's surface and the atmosphere.

Special difficulties arise in conducting gradient observations at the surface of water bodies. In this case, observations on the masts of ships often give unsatisfactory results, since the hull of the ship significantly distorts the fields of temperature, humidity, and wind. Best results can be obtained by mounting the instruments on special devices extending out on the windward side of the ship to some distance from its hull. In some investigations, masts installed on floating buoys are used for this purpose.

When determining the turbulent sensible-heat flux with the aid of data of gradient observations on land, one should bear in mind that this flux often displays a pronounced diurnal cycle. Because of the substantial increase of the turbulent exchange coefficient when temperature decreases with height, in comparison with inversion conditions, the turbulent sensible-heat flux directed from the earth's surface to the atmosphere is usually much greater than the flux directed to the earth's surface. This regularity, which is some-times called the valve effect (Budyko, 1948), should be taken into account when determining the sums of turbulent heat fluxes over observational periods of greater or smaller length. Thus, for example, for calculation of the diurnal sums of the turbulent sensible-heat flux during the warm season, it is of great importance to determine the values of this flux for the daytime period, when they are usually much greater than those at night. Thus, calcu-lation of the turbulent flux from diurnal mean values of the turbulent ex-change coefficient and vertical gradient of temperature may lead to large errors.

For large water bodies, at the surface of which the diurnal cycle of the turbulent sensible-heat flux is insignificant, the valve effect does not occur.

Determination of the turbulent sensible-heat flux by methods other than the method of gradient observations is associated with the use of special instruments. Among these are methods for calculation of the heat flux on the basis of measurements of pulsations of air temperature and vertical wind speed. There are also instruments for measuring turbulent heat flux that are based on the compensation principle (Aizenshtat, 1951; and others). These instruments are suitable for the measurement of the turbulent heat flux under conditions of bare soil.

These methods are not yet widespread and are used only in individual experimental investigations. A partial exception to this is the method of gradient observations, now being used at several dozen Soviet meteorological stations.

Since data of specific observations of turbulent sensible-heat exchange now available are comparatively few, much importance for climatological research attaches to the use of calculation methods for determination of this component of the heat balance.

Equation (2.39), permitting the connection of the turbulent sensible-heat flux with the difference between temperatures of the earth's surface and atmosphere, is often used for this purpose. When using this formula for calculating the value of the turbulent heat flux at land surfaces, much diffi-culty is encountered in determining the temperature of the earth's surface T_w.

A comparatively reliable method for determination of the temperature of the land surface is the method of the radiation thermometer, i.e., the method for calculating temperature on the basis of measurements of the flux of long-wave radiation. This method has been successfully used in a number of studies.

Among other methods for measuring the value T_w, the use of thin resistance thermometers may in some cases give satisfactory results. These thermometers are laid on the more or less even surface of bare soil.

Less accurate results in measuring the temperature of the underlying surface are given by mercury thermometers laid on the soil surface. Some studies [for example, Zubenok (1947)] have shown that even for conditions of bare soil, the utilization of mercury thermometers may give noticeable errors in measuring the temperature of the underlying surface. It should be noted, however, that the errors appearing with application of mercury thermometers are to some degree of a systematic character, which facilitates taking them into account when determining the sensible-heat flux.

One of the papers on climatology of the heat balance (Budyko, 1947) proposed an approximate method for calculation of sums of the turbulent sensible-heat flux, according to data of mass meteorological observations with the use of materials from measurements of the temperature of the soil surface with mercury thermometers.

Such a method for calculating total turbulent sensible-heat flux was used in drawing the maps of this heat-balance component over the southern part of the European territory of the USSR. The values of the heat flux found in this way were confirmed by the heat-balance equation, with satisfactory results.

Most often, in climatological calculations of the turbulent sensible-heat flux for land conditions, its values are determined from the heat-balance equation. In this case, the simplest way is to determine the turbulent sensible-heat flux as the residual component of the balance by the formula

$$P = R - LE - A. \tag{2.48}$$

This method, used in a whole series of papers, provides satisfactory results in those cases when the value P is not very small compared to other heat-balance components (mainly, as compared to the radiation balance). In those cases in which the turbulent flux is much less than the radiation balance, the "residual components" method may lead to large relative errors in calculation. There is even the possibility of an error in sign (that is, in direction) of the turbulent sensible-heat flux.

Let us turn now to the problem of the turbulent sensible-heat exchange between a water surface and the atmosphere.

Climatological calculations of the turbulent heat flux at water bodies are, as a rule, simplified in comparison with those for land, because of the possibility of using data of mass measurements of water-surface temperature. Here the diffusion method for calculation of the turbulent heat flux, based on application of Eq. (2.39), can be used for determining the values of the heat flux by data of mass observations. This requires only the evaluation of the diffusion coefficient D in relation to meteorological factors.

The problem of calculating this coefficient for water surfaces was discussed in a study by Sverdrup (1936a) aimed at determining evaporation from a water surface. Sverdrup assumed that over the sea surface there is a thin sublayer of height h, in which the exchange coefficient is equal to that of molecular diffusion ($k = k_0$). Sverdrup considered that above this sublayer the turbulent exchange coefficient depends on height according to Eq. (2.41), namely,

$$k = k_1(z + z_0).$$

After having integrated Eq. (2.31) by z from 0 to z in the layer of turbulent diffusion, we can derive the ratio

$$E = \frac{\rho k_1(q_0 - q)}{\ln[(z_1 + z_0)/z_0]} \tag{2.49}$$

(q is the specific humidity at height z_1, q_0 is the specific humidity at the upper boundary of the sublayer of molecular diffusion).

Integrating Eq. (2.31) with respect to z within the limits of the sublayer of molecular diffusion, we find

$$E = \frac{\rho k_0(q_s - q_0)}{h} \tag{2.50}$$

(q_s is the saturation specific humidity at the temperature of the evaporating surface).

Excluding q_0 from Eqs. (2.49) and (2.50) and inserting the value of k_1 from Eq. (2.26), Sverdrup obtained an equation for evaporation from the ocean surface:

$$E = \frac{\rho k_0 u(q_s - q)}{uh + (k_0/\kappa^2) \ln^2[(z_1 + z_0)/z_0]}, \tag{2.51}$$

where u is the wind speed at height z_1.

One can obtain from these formulas the following equations for determination of D and P:

$$D = \frac{k_0 u}{uh + (k_0/\kappa^2) \ln^2[(z_1 + z_0)/z_0]}, \tag{2.52}$$

and

$$P = \frac{\rho c_p k_0 u(T_w - T)}{uh + (k_0/\kappa^2) \ln^2[(z_1 + z_0)/z_0]}, \tag{2.53}$$

where T is temperature at height z_1. This formula was first derived by Kuz'min (1938).

In using Eqs. (2.51) and (2.53), one must determine two parameters: the roughness of the sea surface z_0 and the thickness of the sublayer of molecular diffusion h.

Sverdrup postulated that in accordance with the known aerodynamic relation derived for rough pipes, the value of sea-surface roughness was equal to $\frac{1}{30}$ of mean wave height. To estimate the value h, Sverdrup used the data of his observations in Spitsbergen and the data of observations made above the sea surface by Wüst. On the basis of these materials, he assumed a mean value of h equal to 0.10 to 0.15 cm.

Rossby (1936) showed that roughness of the sea surface depends little on wave height and as a consequence can be considered constant for different wind speeds.

Further investigations led to the conclusion that, although wind speed influences the roughness of the sea surface, this influence usually does not remain the same, due to the frequent lack of correspondence between the nonstationary regimes of wind and waves. When this correspondence is present, the roughness of the sea surface probably decreases with an increase in wind speed at comparatively low speeds, and increases with rising wind speed at high speeds (Wu, 1969).

In a number of further papers (Sverdrup, 1937; and others), the Sverdrup formula received various improvements, but the relations found in these papers have not come into general use for calculations of evaporation and turbulent sensible-heat flux from water bodies. This might be associated with the fact that the models of diffusion in the lowest layer of air, used by Sverdrup as well as subsequent authors, have been difficult to confirm by reliable experiments.

For this reason, most subsequent investigators, when studying the turbulent heat exchange at water bodies, preferred to use a simple hypothesis, according to which

$$\frac{1}{\int_0^z dz/k} = \chi u, \tag{2.54}$$

where u is wind speed, and χ is a dimensionless coefficient, which, at the given heights of measuring air temperature and wind speed, is considered to be constant. In this case, for calculation of the turbulent sensible-heat flux, they use the formula

$$P = \chi \rho c_p u (T_w - T), \tag{2.55}$$

by which averaged values of the turbulent flux are determined, averaged values of temperature and wind speed being generally used as initial data.

The first such formula for evaporation was obtained in experimental studies of Shuleikin (1935), who applied it to studying the heat balance of the

Kara Sea. A little later, similar formulas for both the turbulent fluxes were proposed by Sverdrup (1937). Later, the Shuleikin–Sverdrup formulas became generally used for determination of the mean values of the turbulent heat fluxes on seas and oceans.

We should make some comment on the physical meaning of hypothesis (2.54).

With an assumption that the turbulent sensible-heat flux is constant with height, it is easy to derive the relation

$$\frac{1}{\int_0^z dz/k} = \frac{T_2 - T_3}{T_w - T} \frac{1}{\int_{z_2}^{z_3} dz/k},$$
(2.56)

where T_2 and T_3 are air temperatures at levels z_2 and z_3.

It is known that in the absence of a vertical gradient of temperature, the value of $1/\int_{z_2}^{z_3} dz/k$ is equal to $\kappa^2 u_1/[\ln(z_3/z_2) \ln(z_1/z_0)]$, where u_1 is wind speed at height z_1, and κ is von Kármán's constant; that is, the value is proportional to wind speed. The value of the ratio $(T_2 - T_3)/(T_w - T)$ defines, in this case, the conditions of turbulent diffusion in the air layer near the underlying surface. This value has been studied in a number of experimental investigations, which have shown that it depends relatively little on wind speed [refer to Budyko and Gandin (1966), and others]. Therefore, hypothesis (2.54) can be considered natural for small gradients of temperature. The question to what extent it is possible to use hypothesis (2.54) for calculations of turbulent fluxes when there is a substantial vertical temperature gradient requires special consideration.

As pointed out above, it was long ago established that thermal stratification substantially influences the turbulent fluxes of heat and moisture in the near-surface layer of the atmosphere above the land. It has been found that in the lower layer of air, there is the so-called valve effect, according to which the turbulent sensible-heat fluxes directed downward are usually small in comparison to the fluxes directed upward. Hence, the conclusion was reached that the mean values of the fluxes above the land surface are mainly determined by their values in daytime (Budyko, 1946c).

It follows from general considerations that the effect of vertical gradients of temperature on variations in intensity of the turbulent exchange above the ocean is less than the effect above land.

Let us take into account the fact that the variation in intensity of turbulent exchange that occurs under the influence of thermal stratification depends on the Richardson number, which is proportional to the ratio

$$\frac{T_2 - T_3}{u_1^2} = \text{Ri}_z,$$
(2.57)

where $T_2 = T(z_2)$, $T_3 = T(z_3)$, and $u_1 = u(z_1)$ are values of temperature and wind speed at certain fixed levels in the lower layer of the atmosphere, with $z_3 > z_2$.

The wind speed u_1 above a water surface is, on the average, noticeably larger than above land, and the temperature difference $T_2 - T_3$ is considerably less. Therefore, the typical significant values of Ri_z above the sea are comparatively small, which defines the smallness of the effect of stratification on the exchange above the sea. The first quantitative estimates of this effect showed that at moderate and high wind speeds, stratification changes the turbulent heat flux above the sea very little. Only at low wind speeds might these changes become substantial (Budyko, 1948).

Budyko and Gandin (1966) found mean values of ratio (2.57) for conditions on the land and oceans. It follows from these data that the value of the ratio for the North Atlantic is $\frac{1}{15}$ to $\frac{1}{30}$ as large as its mean value in summer daytime conditions in the European territory of the USSR. Using these data, it has been possible to calculate the effect of thermal stratification on the intensity of turbulent fluxes in the northern part of the Atlantic Ocean. This calculation shows that the effect of stratification increases turbulent exchange above the sea, on the average, by 5% in winter and 2% in summer. It is evident that these values are unimportant and lie within the range of the probable error of determination of the coefficient of turbulent exchange.

It must be indicated that the above-mentioned evaluation characterizes the effect of stratification on the turbulent exchange at the height of 1 m. Let us take into account the fact that the Richardson number increases with altitude according to the same law as the turbulent-exchange coefficient. (This follows from the inverse proportionality of the vertical gradients of temperature and wind speed to the exchange coefficient.) Therefore, the influence of stratification on the intensity of turbulent exchange that occurs immediately at the sea surface is unimportant. At the same time, the value of the integral coefficient of turbulent diffusion fundamentally depends on the intensity of exchange at the lowest levels, where the values of the local exchange coefficient are minimal. For this reason, as calculations show, the effect of temperature stratification on the integral coefficient of diffusion and on the vertical turbulent fluxes of heat and moisture turns out to be smaller than the effect of stratification on the exchange coefficient that relates to the 1 m level.

Thus, it appears that for estimation of the mean values of turbulent heat fluxes on the oceans, one could use formulas of the type of Eq. (2.55) with a constant value of the coefficient χ, though for individual values of the fluxes over comparatively short periods, this is not always permissible.

An analogous conclusion can be drawn concerning the necessity of taking into account the dependence of the coefficient χ on wind speed. Some authors, beginning with the above-mentioned investigations of Sverdrup, have considered this coefficient to be dependent on wind speed. This was the consequence of taking into account the influence of the sublayer of molecular diffusion, and also the hypotheses on the relationship between roughness and wind speed or other hypotheses. Since this dependence in the class interval of most frequent wind speeds usually is weak, its effect on the results of calculations of mean long-term values of the turbulent sensible-heat fluxes has been small. At the same time, it might be substantial in determinations of instantaneous values of the turbulent fluxes.

Let us now turn to the problem of the possibility of using such formulas as Eq. (2.55) for determining monthly sums of the corresponding fluxes, not according to the data of individual observations, but according to the mean monthly values of the meteorological elements.

When studying the geographical distribution of the turbulent heat fluxes at ocean surfaces, it is often difficult to use data of individual observations. Therefore, the question arises: to what extent would the calculation results be distorted if the monthly mean values of turbulent heat fluxes were determined from such formulas as Eq. (2.55) by substituting in them the monthly mean values of wind, temperature, and humidity?

It was long ago indicated (Budyko, 1948) that for conditions at the land surface, such a method will often not do. Substitution of the daily mean values of temperature differences along the vertical into the formula for determining the turbulent flux not only reduces the value of this flux considerably but also is capable of misrepresenting its sign. It might be thought, however, that above the sea, due to the small diurnal variability of changes in temperature and humidity, calculation by means of formulas of the type of Eq. (2.55) with mean monthly values should not lead to substantial errors. This supposition was confirmed by calculations of Strokina (1963), done during the preparation of maps of the heat balance of the oceans. Similar results have been obtained by Malkus (1962). According to her evaluations, the error in the values P and E, when calculated from monthly mean values, amounts to only 7%, the ratio P/E turning out practically free of error.

These conclusions were subsequently confirmed in a paper of Budyko and Gandin (1966), based on the materials of observations at weather ships in the North Atlantic, which were worked up in the study of Kraus and Morrison (1966). These authors, using Eq. (2.55) and the analogous formula for evaporation, made calculations of the mean monthly values of the fluxes P_K and LE_K from routine data of observations at nine weather ships. For the same weather ships, Budyko and Gandin made similar calculations from the monthly mean values (P_r and LE_r). Figures 14 and 15 present the comparison of these results with the data of Kraus and Morrison. The coincidence proved very close, which confirms the possibility of using monthly mean

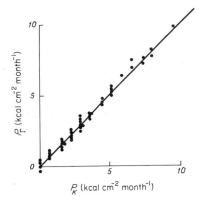

Fig. 14 Monthly means of the flux of sensible heat found by averaged (P_r) and nonaveraged (P_K) values of the meteorological elements.

values of wind, temperature, and humidity when calculating turbulent fluxes at sea.

It should be stressed that in Figs. 14 and 15, there is no systematic discrepancy of any kind between the data of calculations made by the author and Gandin and the data of Kraus and Morrison. This is explained by the small difference between the coefficient χ applied in the calculations by Budyko and Gandin and the value used by Kraus and Morrison. Such difference is quite natural, since in our calculations the value χ was deter-

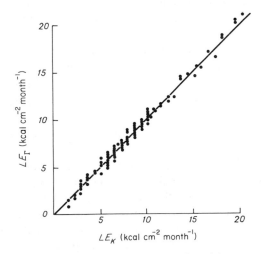

Fig. 15 Monthly means of the flux of latent heat found by averaged (LE_r) and non-averaged (LE_K) values of the meteorological elements.

mined by closing the heat-balance equation using just the monthly mean values and not the original data for the hours of observation.

The problem of the possibility of utilizing averaged values of meteorological elements in calculations of the turbulent heat fluxes from the oceans was also discussed by Garstang (1965). To determine the turbulent sensible-heat flux, he used Eq. (2.55) and the similar one for calculation of heat conversion in evaporation. Assuming that the parameter χ is a function of wind speed and the Richardson number, Garstang calculated values of turbulent fluxes characteristic of various synoptic situations during two short periods at a weather ship on station in one of the regions of the Atlantic Ocean.

Then, having estimated the frequency of occurrence of these situations under conditions of different tropical regions, Garstang constructed maps of the long-term means of the turbulent fluxes for the low latitudes of the Atlantic Ocean. These maps turned out appreciably different from those of the "Атлас теплового баланса земного шара", and Garstang explained this difference by the use of nonaveraged data of the meteorological elements in his calculations.

This explanation is, however, wrong. Comparing Garstang's formulas with those used for the construction of the maps for the "Атлас теплового баланса земного шара," one can easily see that they are but little different. For the interval of values of meteorological parameters used in the work of Garstang, the coefficient χ in his formulas is, on the average, equal to 2.1×10^{-3}, with the average deviation in individual cases being equal only to 10% of this value, which is sufficiently close to the value of the coefficient applied by the authors of the maps for the "Атлас теплового баланса земного шара" (2.0×10^{-3}).

Thus, in order to check the magnitude of the effect of using nonaveraged original data in calculations of the turbulent sensible-heat flux, it will suffice to compare the products $\bar{u}\,\overline{(T_w - T)}$ and $\overline{u(T_w - T)}$ using the data of observations used by Garstang. Such comparison shows that the products differ by 2.4%, a very small amount.

A similar analysis of the calculation of the latent-heat flux gives a still smaller difference, amounting only to 0.3%.

Thus, the materials of Garstang's work not only do not demonstrate the presence of substantial errors resulting from using averaged parameters when calculating the turbulent heat fluxes, but, on the contrary, confirm once more the possibility of such simplification of calculations.

We must indicate that, indeed, the maps of turbulent fluxes drawn up by Garstang differ considerably from the corresponding sections of maps comprised in "Атлас теплового баланса земного шара (Atlas of the Heat Balance of the Earth)." However, such differences are explicable by the impossibility of ascertaining the long-term mean regime of the turbulent fluxes in different seasons on the vast expanses of the Atlantic Ocean from the data of two short periods of observations conducted in one region.

Thus, the above data confirm the possibility of applying such formulas as Eq. (2.55) to the calculation of the turbulent fluxes of heat and moisture above the sea by use of averaged original data.

Among other problems associated with the determination of turbulent sensible-heat fluxes, we would mention the role of the surface film of water with a lowered temperature and the effect of spray formed by waves, problems set forth in the works of Montgomery (1940, 1947). The first of these problems was investigated by Timofeev (1963), who established that a thin surface film of water is slightly colder than the underlying layers. Such an effect can noticeably influence the oceanic heat exchange with the atmosphere, especially at low wind speeds. The problem of a possible effect of the cooled water film on the monthly mean values of the turbulent heat fluxes on the oceans does not seem quite clear, because of the insufficient amount of data concerning the existence of such film at appreciable wind speeds and in the presence of more or less significant wave disturbance.

The analysis of this problem by Malevskii-Malevich (1970) deserves special attention. It follows from his observational and computational data that the presence of the cooled water film at low and moderate wind speeds may somewhat influence the turbulent sensible-heat flux directed from the water surface to the atmosphere. In middle latitudes, such an influence is unimportant in the winter months (when strong winds prevail), but becomes more noticeable in the warm season. In the summer months, the influence of the film could reduce the transport of heat from the ocean's surface by 7–10%. This, however, does not substantially change the annual sums of turbulent heat flux, due to the smallness of its absolute values in summer.

The second problem was studied in the papers of Grabovskii (1956), who has shown, as a result of measuring the concentration of salt particles above the oceans, that spray formation influences the mean values of evaporation but little. This conclusion does not mean, however, that during short periods of time the heat exchange of spray with the surrounding air might not be considered comparable with the total heat exchange of the ocean with the atmosphere.

It follows from the above that for the determination of the turbulent heat fluxes between the ocean and the atmosphere for a more or less long period, it is advisable at present to use the well-known formulas of Shuleikin-Sverdrup. In this method, it is possible to use in calculations the time-averaged original meteorological observations.

The value of the coefficient χ in these formulas has been determined by many scientists [refer to Robinson (1966) and elsewhere]. In research work carried out in GGO during the preparation of "Атлас теплового баланса (Atlas of the Heat Balance)" (1955), the value of $\rho\chi$, found by closing the heat-balance equations for the world ocean, proved equal to 2.4×10^{-6} g cm^{-3} (under conditions of measuring wind speed and air temperature at the heights usual in ship observations).

In subsequent research, carried out in work on the "Атлас теплового баланса земного шара (Atlas of the Heat Balance of the Earth)" (1963), a slightly larger value of $\rho\chi$, equal to 2.5×10^{-6} g cm^{-3}, was found. Other data on this coefficient will be given in the following chapter in connection with the discussion of problems of the water balance of the oceans.

We shall only point out here that for individual regions of the world ocean and for different bodies of water, the mean values of the coefficient χ may be slightly different. There are, for example, data indicating that this coefficient for inland seas (the Caspian Sea and the Aral Sea) is somewhat less than its mean values for the world ocean.

It should be noted that, whereas mean values of the coefficient χ relating to individual seas and oceans and to long periods of time vary comparatively little, the values of this coefficient over short periods of time may vary much more.

For calculations of turbulent fluxes at water bodies for short periods of time, it may become necessary to take into account factors that are not very important when determining the long-term means of fluxes. In such cases, it is advisable to use more detailed formulas, such as those obtained in the works of Bortkovskii and Biutner (1969, 1970). Taking into account the limited available materials for checking these formulas by experimental data, it is possible to consider that they permit us to determine the values of the turbulent fluxes for short periods of time more accurately than the schematized formulas of Shuleikin–Sverdrup.

At the same time, the errors in calculating instantaneous values of the turbulent fluxes with such formulas are probably large, particularly for the reason that the wave regime is often nonstationary and does not correspond to the wind observed at the given moment of time. In this connection, the roughness of the water surface varies within wide limits, which possibly affects the instantaneous values of the coefficient χ. Formation of spray and other factors may also influence this coefficient.

For determination of the turbulent sensible-heat flux at water bodies, formulas based on the so-called "Bowen ratio" are often employed. These can be derived as follows.

Integrating Eq. (2.31) by z, we find a relation analogous to Eq. (2.39),

$$E = \rho D(q_s - q), \tag{2.58}$$

where q_s is the saturation specific humidity at the temperature of the water surface.

It follows from Eqs. (2.39) and (2.58) that

$$\frac{P}{LE} = \frac{c_p(T_w - T)}{L(q_s - q)}.$$ (2.59)

This formula permits the calculation of values of the turbulent sensible-heat flux when data on evaporation are available. In cases when there are no data on evaporation, but there are data on the radiation balance R and internal heat exchange in the water body A, one can use for calculation of the sensible-heat flux the relation

$$P = \frac{R - A}{1 + \dfrac{L(q_s - q)}{c_p(T_w - T)}},$$ (2.60)

derived from the heat-balance equation (2.16) and Eq. (2.59).

The turbulent heat flux above water bodies can be determined also by Eq. (2.48). However, its application in this case is often complicated by the difficulty of making a sufficiently accurate calculation of the value of A for more or less extensive water bodies (or portions of them).

Summing up, we should indicate that for climatological calculations of the turbulent sensible-heat flux from water bodies, it is best to use Eq. (2.55), which permits determination of the value of this flux from data only on water-surface temperature, air temperature, and wind speed.

For determination of annual means of the turbulent sensible-heat flux at land surfaces, the heat-balance equation is often used in climatological calculations—the turbulent heat flux being calculated as a residual component of the balance. The annual and monthly means of the turbulent heat flux on land can also be calculated by means of jointly solving the equations of the heat and water balances, with calculation of the annual cycle of evaporation and soil moisture. This method will be discussed below.

3. The Flux of Latent Heat

Evaporation from the land surface

The conversion of energy in evaporation [latent-heat flux] is equal to the product of the latent heat of evaporation by the amount of evaporation. The latent heat of evaporation under natural conditions varies slightly in accordance with the change in temperature of the evaporating surface. The dependence has the form

$$L = 597 - 0.6T \text{ cal g}^{-1},$$ (2.61)

where T is the temperature in degrees Celsius. In many climatological calculations, one can use a constant value of the latent heat of evaporation, which is approximately equal to 0.6 kcal g^{-1}.

There are many different methods for determining evaporation under natural conditions. In discussing these methods, we shall take up first the relatively more complicated problem of determining evaporation from the land surface.

As mentioned above, one of the oldest methods for determining evaporation is based on using evaporation meters [or lysimeters], the various constructions of which for land conditions are based on measurements of the change in moisture in an isolated monolith of soil.

It is known that because of complete or partial isolation of the soil monolith in the lysimeter from surrounding layers of soil, substantial distortions of evaporation conditions appear. Distortion of water-exchange conditions in the isolated monolith may lead to errors in determination of evaporation; however, it must be borne in mind that weighed lysimeters can give errors in evaporation measurement even if such distortions are absent. This conclusion follows from the elementary theory of weighed lysimeters (Budyko and Timofeev, 1952).

Weighed lysimeters of the generally used types of construction cannot be considered absolute instruments, that is, instruments directly measuring evaporation. It is easy to understand that with the use of the weighed lysimeter, only the moisture content of the monolith contained in the lysimeter can be measured. Therefore, when using the lysimeter at a frequency of weighing equal to once in several days, it is necessary to have data on precipitation and on surface and below-ground run-off. With respect to periods when the values of deep percolation and run-off are small compared to total precipitation (particularly in the warm season under conditions of insufficient moisture), it is generally considered that evaporation for this period of time is equal to

$$E' = r + \Delta w', \qquad (2.62)$$

where r is total precipitation, and $\Delta w'$ is the change in moisture content in the soil monolith contained in the lysimeter.

Actually, the value of evaporation in these conditions must be considered equal to

$$E = r + \Delta w, \qquad (2.63)$$

where Δw is the change in moisture content in the whole layer of active water exchange in the soil.

As a consequence, the relative error of determination of evaporation when using the weighed lysimeter is equal to

$$\frac{E - E'}{E} = \frac{\Delta w - \Delta w'}{r + \Delta w}, \qquad (2.64)$$

and, in a period without precipitation,

$$\frac{E - E'}{E} = \frac{\Delta w - \Delta w'}{\Delta w}. \tag{2.65}$$

Thus, in order to estimate the error involved in using a weighed lysimeter, it is necessary to calculate the ratio of the change in moisture content in the soil layer, the thickness of which corresponds to the depth of the lysimeter, to the change in moisture content in the whole layer of active water exchange.

If the condition

$$\Delta w \neq \Delta w' \tag{2.66}$$

is encountered, then in measuring evaporation an error appears that is not associated with disturbance in the conditions of water exchange in the isolated monolith and which takes place with any frequent substitution of a monolith in the lysimeter.

We shall illustrate this statement by the following example. Suppose that we utilize the lysimeter in a rainless period under soil conditions in which the upper layer has dried out to a depth equal to the depth of the lysimeter. In this situation, further flux of moisture originates from the deeper layers of soil. It is evident that in this case the weighed lysimeter would give wrong results (zero evaporation) with either frequent or infrequent change of monoliths.

A similar situation will always appear if a noticeable flux of moisture in the evaporation process originates from layers of soil that are deep in comparison with the depth of the lysimeter.

Using available observational data on soil moisture, one can estimate with the aid of Eq. (2.64) the results of utilization of lysimeters of 500-mm depth under different climatic conditions.

It follows from these data that under conditions of the steppe and forest–steppe zones, and also in the forest zone during the second half of summer, a change in the amount of moisture in the 500–1000-mm layer is fully comparable with that in the 0–500-mm layer, and often exceeds it.

We can draw the conclusion that utilization of weighed lysimeters of 500-mm depth under conditions of insufficient moisture is associated with definite errors in evaporation measurements. These errors, mainly relating to underestimation of the evaporation in rainless periods, may reach sizes comparable to the measured value itself. For periods of more or less abundant precipitation, the relative error in evaporation measurements will be appreciably reduced, as is seen from the above formulas.

Thus, the weighed lysimeter of a limited depth (for example, 500 mm) cannot be considered a universal instrument that permits measurement of total evaporation under different climatic conditions. These lysimeters might, perhaps, give more or less reliable results with sufficiently damp soil and in the absence of massive root systems of transpiring plants.

Evaluating the observational material on soil lysimeters, we should indicate that at present some conclusions of a climatological character can be drawn, mainly on the basis of data obtained with the aid of the weighed lysimeters used in the network of stations in the USSR. However, taking into account the limited volume and not always sufficient accuracy of these data, we must recognize that for climatological calculations of the evaporative heat flux, data from lysimeters have essentially a supplementary value.

Among other methods for determining evaporation [evapotranspiration], associated with the utilization of special observational data, it is necessary to note the gradient methods. These are analogous to the corresponding modes of determining the turbulent sensible-heat exchange (refer to Section 2 of this chapter).

The most reliable method for determining evaporation from the data of gradient observations is the heat-balance method. It follows from the heat-balance equation (2.16) and Eqs. (2.22) and (2.31) that

$$R = -L\rho k \frac{\partial q}{\partial z} - \rho c_p k \frac{\partial T}{\partial z} + A. \tag{2.67}$$

From Eqs. (2.31) and (2.67) we obtain

$$E = \frac{R - A}{L + c_p \dfrac{\partial T/\partial z}{\partial q/\partial z}}, \tag{2.68}$$

or, after having integrated by z,

$$E = \frac{R - A}{L + c_p \dfrac{T_1 - T_2}{q_1 - q_2}}, \tag{2.69}$$

where $T_1 - T_2$ and $q_1 - q_2$ are the differences of temperature and specific humidity at two heights.

The last formula, similar to Eq. (2.60), permits us to determine the value of evaporation in periods of time with not very small values of the principal components of the heat balance, that is, mainly daytime conditions in the warm season.

In this case, one must remember that in making calculations by this formula, one often can either neglect the value A or approximate it, since for a more or less long averaging period it is, as a rule, considerably smaller than the value R. This simplifies the determination of evaporation appreciably.

We should note that some investigators, when performing calculations of evaporation on land by Eq. (2.69), made errors when they utilized the diurnal mean or monthly mean of the differences $T_1 - T_2$ and $q_1 - q_2$. Since both these values have a considerable diurnal cycle, such averaging may lead, because of the relationship between them, to large errors in the determination of evaporation.

To test this supposition, we compared the results of evaporation calculations at an observation point over a year by Eq. (2.69), using values of $T_1 - T_2$ and $q_1 - q_2$ from hourly observations and by use of the annual means (Budyko, 1946c, 1948). In the second case, the value of evaporation turned out twice as great as in the first case, which confirmed the impossibility of employing the mean characteristics of temperature and humidity gradients in evaporation calculations by Eq. (2.69).

At present, Eq. (2.69) is generally used for determining evaporation according to data of expedition and special-station observations. This method is applied to determine evaporation at the heat-balance stations in the USSR. [Refer to "Руководство по градиентным наблюдениям и определению составляющих теплового баланса (Manual for Gradient Observations and Determination of Components of the Heat Balance)," 1964, and "Руководство по производству наблюдений за испарением с сельскохозяйственных полей (Manual for Observing Evaporation from Agricultural Lands)," 1957.]

The limited amount of available data of gradient observations make it difficult to use the method more generally in investigations of the evaporation regime.

The same thing applies to the diffusion method for the determination of evaporation. This method, based on the utilization of Eq. (2.33), has been used in a number of investigations. Thus, for example, Thornthwaite and Holzman (1939, 1942, and elsewhere) developed the idea of Schmidt, who had suggested that evaporation be determined with reference to the vertical turbulent flux of water vapor [refer to Schmidt (1917, 1925, 1935)], and applied it to determining evaporation by Eq. (2.33) and the Rossby–Montgomery formula for the turbulent-exchange coefficient. In this case, to determine the difference in specific humidities $q_1 - q_2$, Thornthwaite and Holzman constructed special instruments with which detailed observations of evaporation over about a year were carried out.

As mentioned above, it was subsequently established (Budyko, 1946c, 1948), that the calculations made by Thornthwaite and Holzman gave estimates of evaporation that were too low, in consequence of the fact that the Rossby–Montgomery formula did not take into account the effect of thermal stratification on turbulent exchange.

As has been shown in these papers, utilization of such formulas as Eq.

(2.30) for determination of the exchange coefficient provides more accurate results in calculating evaporation by the diffusion method.

Not dwelling on the more detailed features of the diffusion method, we shall indicate only that at present it is, with the heat-balance method, used mainly when generalizing the data of special-station and expedition observations.

The pulsation or eddy method, based on the determination of evaporation by the fluctuations of humidity and the vertical component of wind speed, has also not yet become widespread.

Let us turn now to the problem of determining evaporation from the land surface by calculation methods that utilize the data of mass hydrometeorological observations.

Evaporation in the mean annual period according to the water-balance equation can be determined by the formula

$$E = r - f, \tag{2.70}$$

that is, as the difference between precipitation and run-off.

This method for determining mean annual evaporation has been widely used in many investigations. Calculations of evaporation by the water balance have permitted the construction of a number of maps of evaporation and latent-heat flux (Kuzin, 1940, 1950; Budyko, 1947; Troitskii, 1948; "Водные ресурсы и водный баланс территории СССР [Water Resources and Water Balance in the USSR]," 1967; and others) and have provided considerable material on evaporation means for the year.

It must be kept in view that calculations of evaporation by Eq. (2.70) give more reliable results for relatively large areas, of the order of thousands or tens of thousands of square kilometers. For more limited areas, calculations made by Eq. (2.70) may lead to noticeable errors because of the difficulty of keeping accurate account of the redistribution of moisture by ground-water flow.

For shorter averaging periods—for calculations of the annual march of evaporation, for determination of evaporation in individual years and months, and so on—one must, instead of Eq. (2.70), use the more general equation

$$E = r - f - \Delta w. \tag{2.71}$$

Since the value of change of moisture content in the upper layers of the lithosphere Δw is hard to determine accurately, its value often being comparable with evaporation in the indicated periods, calculations of evaporation by Eq. (2.71) do not always provide sufficiently reliable results.

It is easiest to use Eq. (2.71) for determination of evaporation in the warm season under conditions of insufficient moisture, when the changes in moisture content are mainly determined by the dynamics of moisture in the upper layers of the soil.

Because the moisture of the upper layers of the soil is measured in the USSR at numerous agrometeorological stations, it is possible to calculate evaporation for these conditions by Eq. (2.71) with the use of the data of mass hydrometeorological observations. In this case, the great spatial heterogeneity of the field of soil moisture should also be taken into consideration. This requires considerable averaging of the basic data in carrying out climatological calculations of evaporation.

Since considerable areas of land are without run-off data, the utilization of Eq. (2.71) without any additional relationships cannot be considered a universal means of determining evaporation from land, even for mean annual conditions.

For this reason, a number of investigations are directed toward working out methods for determining evaporation from land surfaces by use only of data of mass observations of the principal meteorological elements: precipitation, air temperature, and humidity.

In one of the first pieces of research of this orientation (Wundt, 1937), by generalizing calculated evaporation data by the water balance, an empirical relationship between annual evaporation and precipitation with the annual mean temperature was established. Wundt's nomogram, constructed on the basis of this relationship, has been used in some hydrological research, for example, by L'vovich (1945) when he calculated the norms of run-off on the different continents.

Checking Wundt's nomogram shows (Budyko, 1951) that it gives rather noticeable errors in calculated evaporation. These errors are presumably associated to some extent with the fact that Wundt was not quite successful in selecting annual mean temperature as an index of the influence of the thermal regime on evaporation. (It is known that mean annual temperatures in middle and high latitudes depend substantially on conditions of the cold season, while evaporation in these latitudes is almost completely determined by conditions of the warm season.)

Another approach to the task of determining annual mean evaporation was offered by Ol'dekop (1911), in whose work the dependence of evaporation on precipitation and potential evaporation was found. In our papers (Budyko, 1948, and others), on the basis of combined analysis of the equations of the heat and water balances of the land surface, we obtained the relationship equation—the dependence of evaporation upon precipitation and the radiation balance, which is a generalization of Ol'dekop's formula.

This equation establishes the relationship between the ratio of annual mean evaporation to precipitation E/r, and the ratio of the radiation balance to the amount of heat required for evaporation of the annual precipitation R/Lr, that is,

$$\frac{E}{r} = \Phi\left(\frac{R}{Lr}\right),\tag{2.72}$$

where Φ is a function determined from semiempirical considerations.

The development of the relationship equation will be provided in Chapter VI. We give here a table constructed on the basis of this equation and permitting the calculation of annual evaporation (Table 10).

TABLE 10

RELATION BETWEEN PRECIPITATION, EVAPORATION,
AND RADIATION BALANCE

R/Lr	E/r	R/Lr	E/r
0.10	0.10	1.20	0.76
0.20	0.20	1.40	0.82
0.30	0.28	1.60	0.86
0.40	0.35	1.80	0.88
0.50	0.44	2.00	0.90
0.60	0.50	2.50	0.94
0.70	0.56	3.00	0.97
0.80	0.62		
0.90	0.66		
1.00	0.70		

Compared to the problem of determining annual evaporation, the task of calculating evaporation from data of mass meteorological observations for such periods as months and ten-day periods is much more difficult.

In one of the first studies of this task, Kuzin suggested that land evaporation under the conditions of surplus moisture be determined by a method similar to the mode of calculation of evaporation from water surfaces. In his papers (1934, 1938), Kuzin used for determination of evaporation the formula

$$E = \Omega d,\tag{2.73}$$

where d is the humidity deficit, and Ω is a dimensional coefficient.

In one of these studies Kuzin (1938) also offered an empirical formula for determination of evaporation in individual months under conditions of insufficient moisture.

Poliakov (1946, 1947) was the first to use routine material on changes in moisture of the upper soil layers for determination of evaporation. This enabled him to find the empirical relations of evaporation with meteorological factors for the condition both of surplus and of insufficient moisture.

Albrecht (1951) offered several methods for calculation of the annual march of evaporation from land. Some of these methods are based on utilization of the formula

$$E = (e_s\phi - e)\, Y(u), \tag{2.74}$$

where e_s is the absolute saturation humidity at the temperature of the earth's surface, e is the absolute humidity, $Y(u)$ is a function depending on wind speed, and ϕ is a parameter defining the influence of properties of the underlying surface on the reduction of evaporation. (Albrecht calls it "the portion of the surface covered with water.")

In this formula, with a completely wet surface, $\phi = 1$ (and the formula converts into the well-known relationship for evaporation from a water surface); with a partially dried soil, $\phi < 1$.

Equation (2.74) does not seem satisfactory enough, since it plainly gives the wrong dependence of evaporation on humidity. Indeed, if a soil is partly dry and evaporation is reduced in comparison with that from a water surface, ϕ must be less than unity. Let us assume, for example, that $\phi = 0.7$. Then, according to Albrecht, evaporation (under the conditions of isothermal stratification in the air layer near the surface) must equal zero when relative humidity is equal to 70%, and when relative humidity exceeds 70% condensation must begin. The observational data of humidity gradients in the air near the surface show that nothing of this kind is observed under natural conditions.

It is typical that Albrecht did not succeed (as he admits) in establishing the relationship between the parameter ϕ and the humidity of the upper layer of the soil, though, according to the implication of the problem, this parameter must primarily represent the changes in soil moisture.

Among other methods for climatological calculation of evaporation recommended by Albrecht, we shall mention the heat-balance method, based on utilization of the following equations:

$$E = \frac{1}{L}(R - P - A), \tag{2.75}$$

and

$$P = (T_w - T)\, Y'(u), \tag{2.76}$$

where $Y'(u)$ is a function depending on wind speed.

Application of this method (similar to the method used in our paper of 1947) is made difficult by the complicated interpretation of available data from network observations of soil-surface temperature. Besides, in calculating evaporation by Eq. (2.75), we often get a rather large relative error, because the difference between the values R and $(P + A)$ is, in some cases, not very great relative to the value of R.

There are a number of investigations, in which various empirical and semi-empirical formulas have been offered for determining evaporation from land for limited periods of time (Turc, 1955; Konstantinov, 1968; Mezentsev and Karnatsevich, 1969; and others). Not dwelling on their contents, which have been discussed in a number of published monographs, we will turn to the question of determining evaporation by means of calculation of components of the water balance.

Determination of evaporation from land according to the water balance

The water-balance method, based on utilization of Eqs. (2.70) and (2.71) has, from our point of view, the best prospects for determining evaporation from land over limited periods of time. Since the values of run-off and changes in moisture content included in these equations are often unknown, then for calculating evaporation it is necessary to take into account the relation of these water-balance components with the observed hydrometeorological elements. The first scheme of evaporation calculation based on this idea (Budyko, 1950) involved the employment of relatively complicated calculations. Later on, it turned out to be possible to simplify the developed model of evaporation calculations, and at the same time make it more detailed.

We shall set forth here the concept of this method for calculating the annual cycle of evaporation.

At the beginning of this century, it was known that the process of evaporation from the soil surface is defined by several different phases. In the first phase of evaporation, with the availability of a considerable amount of moisture in the soil, the evaporation rate depends little on soil moisture and is determined, in general, by external meteorological factors. This statement was corroborated in the papers of Alpat'ev (1950, 1954), who showed that for fields covered with agricultural vegetation, the first phase of evaporation is observed over a comparatively wide range of soil moistures.

In this case, evaporation is equal to the value of potential evaporation, which is defined by meteorological conditions and to a limited extent depends on the properties of the evaporating surface. It can be shown that potential evaporation is closely connected with the balance of radiant energy at the earth's surface (refer to Chapter VI of this book).

As the soil becomes dry, beginning at its critical moisture the evaporation passes into a second phase, in which the evaporation rate rapidly decreases with the decrease of soil moisture. There are many experimental data showing that, in this case, the relation of the rate of evaporation from soil to the soil moisture can be considered close to linear.

On the basis of these considerations, and taking into account the relations of river run-off with other components of the water balance of the land, we can construct a quantitative model permitting the calculation of evaporation for individual periods dependent on meteorological elements observed in the network of stations [refer to Budyko, (1950, 1955), Budyko and Zubenok (1961)].

Let us assume that, with the moisture of the upper soil layer w being equal to or more than a certain critical value w_0, evaporation E is equal to potential evaporation E_0. At $w < w_0$, evaporation reduces in correspondence with the decrease in moisture by the formula

$$E \doteq E_0 \frac{w}{w_0}, \tag{2.77}$$

the values w and w_0 characterizing the amount of available water in the soil (that is, accessible to plants).

In determining the values of critical soil moisture w_0, it has been established that for the upper soil layer of 1 m depth, the value of w_0 is usually equal to a layer of available moisture of 10–20 cm, these values varying slightly, depending on geographical conditions and season. As a result of analysis of data on the water balance of the soil, Zubenok (1968) obtained the following rounded values of the parameter w_0 for various climatic conditions in the territory of the USSR.

In the forest zone, the value of w_0 varies from 20 cm at a monthly mean air temperature below 10° in spring, to 15 cm in summer. In the forest–steppe, steppe, and semidesert zones, w_0 in spring amounts to 17 cm. In summer, the values of w_0 reduce to 12 cm in the forest–steppe zone and to 10 cm in the steppe and semidesert zones. With an autumn decrease in monthly mean temperature below 3° in all zones, a certain increase of w_0 is typical. Under desert conditions, w_0 is about 15 cm, increasing to 30 cm in summer in those months when the potential evaporation exceeds 20 cm month^{-1}. Absence of any noticeable annual cycle of critical humidity is characteristic of the zone of permafrost. In this zone, the monthly means of w_0 are approximately equal to 20 cm.

Variations of the value of w_0 are associated with changes in the state of vegetation and to some extent show the activity of the root system of plants. The more developed the root system and the more efficiently it extracts water from soil, the smaller is the value of w_0.

Since the value of soil moisture w in most regions cannot be obtained from observational data, then in order to calculate evaporation in single months, one could use the water-balance equation in addition. This equation has the following form (see Eq. 2.71):

$$r = E + \Delta w + f, \tag{2.78}$$

where r is the precipitation; Δw is the variation of the amount of water in the active layer of the soil, where, in general, water exchange occurs; and f is the horizontal flow, equal to the sum of surface and ground run-off.

It must be noted that the value f by no means coincides with the value of stream run-off in the given period, since the formation of stream run-off is a rather long process. The horizontal flow included in Eq. (2.78) approaches the value of stream run-off only in the mean annual period.

Calculation of evaporation by Eqs. (2.77) and (2.78) becomes noticeably simplified under conditions of a climate with insufficient moisture, when horizontal flow is absent. For this reason, we shall first set forth the calculation scheme for this simpler case.

Under conditions of extreme insufficiency of moisture, the water-balance equation has the form

$$r = E + \Delta w. \tag{2.79}$$

If we designate the mean moisture of the active soil layer at the beginning of a month by w_1, and that at the end of it by w_2, then Eq. (2.79) can be rewritten as

$$r = E + (w_2 - w_1). \tag{2.80}$$

In this case,

$$E = E_0 \frac{w_1 + w_2}{2w_0} \qquad \text{at } 0 < \frac{w_1 + w_2}{2} < w_0, \tag{2.81}$$

$$E = E_0 \qquad \text{at } \frac{w_1 + w_2}{2} \geqslant w_0. \tag{2.82}$$

To calculate the evaporation in each month, it is possible to use the method of successive approximation.

Choosing at random a value for soil moisture at the beginning of the first month, we can calculate, with the aid of Eq. (2.80), the moisture at the end of this month w_2 and determine the evaporation by Eq. (2.81) or (2.82). Then a similar calculation can be carried out for the next month, assuming that for this month the value w_1 is equal to the value w_2 in the first month, and so on. After summing up all the calculated monthly values of evaporation, the result should be compared with the annual sum of precipitation. If the annual sum of precipitation is more than the computed evaporation, it means that the value of w_1 chosen for the first month was underestimated, and if it is less, then the chosen value was overestimated. Changing the value of w_1 in the appropriate direction and repeating the calculation, one can use the method of successive approximation to find such a value of w_1 in the first month for which the annual sums of precipitation and evaporation will coincide. The obtained monthly values of evaporation represent the desired result.

Such a calculation method can be applied to conditions of insufficient humidification, when in each month precipitation is much less than potential evaporation. Such conditions are observed in many regions of desert, savanna, and dry steppe in low latitudes.

It must be indicated that this simplified scheme can be used for determination of evaporation both if run-off is present, in case it appears chiefly as a result of spring snow melting, and if its annual mean is known from observational data. Calculation of evaporation and soil moisture in this case is carried out for the warm season with the mean temperature in each month above zero. Determining evaporation for the first month with a positive temperature, one must add to the total precipitation in this month the sum of precipitation in the cold season with temperatures below zero and subtract from this sum the annual run-off. In determining the water-balance equation by the method of successive approximation, one must compare evaporation over the year with the difference between the annual sums of precipitation and run-off. This method can be used, for example, for many regions of the USSR with a climate of insufficient and moderately surplus moisture.

The above models for calculation of monthly values of evaporation do not solve the problem of determining evaporation in those cases in which the annual sums of precipitation are close to the values of potential evaporation and when run-off is formed in different seasons.

To determine evaporation under different conditions of moisture, one can use a more general model, in which the formula of the water balance for each month is taken into account in the form of the full Eq. (2.78).

Since the value of horizontal flow in each month, as a rule, cannot be determined from observational data, we must calculate it from other hydrometeorological elements. This task is complicated by the fact that horizontal flow is, to a considerable extent, associated with extreme values of the elements of the hydrometeorological regime and depends to a lesser degree on the monthly means used in our calculations.

However, taking into account the availability of certain relations between mean and extreme values of the elements, it is possible to offer an approximate scheme for keeping an account of run-off values, which is based on the following considerations.

For each month the run-off coefficient f/r has values from 0 to 1. (When calculating the run-off coefficient during a period of snow melting, one must add to the sum of precipitation for this period the sum of solid precipitation during the cold season.)

It is evident that the run-off coefficient depends on the soil moisture. It can be considered that for a completely dry soil at $w/w_k = 0$, run-off is also equal to zero. (w_k designates the greatest supply of available moisture that can remain in the upper layers of soil in the absence of any connection with ground water.) With an increase in moisture, the run-off coefficient grows, reaching its maximum at $w/w_k = 1$. This relation can be presented in the form

$$\frac{f}{r} = \mu \frac{w}{w_k}, \tag{2.83}$$

where μ is a dimensionless coefficient of proportionality. It is evident that the value of μ will depend on intensity of precipitation and will increase in the regions of frequent convective rains.

Equation (2.83) can be used for estimating run-off under conditions of insufficient humidification, when the monthly value of potential evaporation is greater than precipitation ($E_0 > r$). Under conditions of plentiful moisture, when precipitation is greater than potential evaporation, run-off is immediately influenced by the value of the difference $r - E_0$. With complete humidification of the soil, when $w/w_k = 1$, the value of run-off will approach as a limit $r - E_0$, that is, in this case the run-off coefficient will be close to the value $1 - E_0/r$. At $w/w_k < 1$ and $r > E_0$, the run-off coefficient will be less than the indicated value, its value being dependent both on the parameter $\xi = 1 - E_0/r$ and also on the intensity of the rains.

We present this dependence in the form

$$\frac{f}{r} = [\mu^2(1 - \xi^2) + \xi^2]^{1/2} \frac{w}{w_k}. \tag{2.84}$$

Thus we obtain an equation for calculation of horizontal flow:

$$f = r \frac{w}{w_k} \left\{ \mu^2 \left[1 - \left(1 - \frac{E_0}{r} \right)^2 \right] + \left(1 - \frac{E_0}{r} \right)^2 \right\}^{1/2} \qquad \text{at } r > E_0, \tag{2.85}$$

$$f = \mu r \frac{w}{w_k} \qquad \text{at } r < E_0. \tag{2.86}$$

We must mention that in these equations, the presence of two forms of run-off having different physical meanings is taken into account. The first, having taken place at $r < E_0$, is a consequence of short falls of heavy precipitation that create a brief over-saturation of the soil and are to a known degree disposed of as run-off. The sum of this form of run-off is equal to $\mu r(w/w_k)$. In cases when $r > E_0$, to the first form of run-off is added the second, which appears as a result of surplus moisture being available all through the month. Such run-off does not depend on the character of the rains and with high soil moisture approximates the difference between the precipitation and the potential evaporation.

It must be indicated that Eqs. (2.83–2.86) are interpolative and their accuracy is limited. Application of such formulas to calculations of evaporation is justified in those sufficiently frequent cases when changes in run-off have relatively little effect on the value of evaporation.

The practical accuracy of calculations of the annual march of run-off by Eqs. (2.85) and (2.86) can be increased if there are reliable materials on the annual norm of run-off in the given region, obtained from observations. In such a case, the annual mean of the coefficient μ can be calculated from the comparison of the annual sum of calculated run-off with observational data.

If there are no observational data on run-off, the parameter μ can be calculated from data on the annual sum of run-off obtained by climatological calculation methods, or approximate values of this parameter can be used for different geographical zones.

Calculations have shown that the coefficient μ has the smallest values in high and middle latitudes. In subtropical and tropical latitudes the coefficient μ increases, because of the frequent rain showers. In carrying out calculations for constructing world maps of evaporation, the mean value of $\mu = 0.2$ was used for regions northward from 45° N and southward from 45° S. For areas between 45° N and 45° S, the coefficient μ was assumed equal to 0.4–0.8, depending on the conditions of humidity.

Comparisons of the results of determining monthly means of evaporation according to the above models with data from the water balance are presented in the paper of Budyko and Zubenok (1961).

In the papers of Zubenok (1966a, 1968, and others), these models have been used for calculation of evaporation in individual months of different years. The data obtained were compared with evaporation values calculated according to data of gradient observations conducted at the stations in various regions of the USSR. This comparison shows that independent methods for determining evaporation provide sufficiently close results, which are in especially good conformity in regions of sufficient moisture. The models mentioned for calculation of evaporation have been applied in various investigations, including studies on the theory of climate (Manabe and Bryan, 1969, and elsewhere).

It must be indicated that application of the above method (as well as the application of all other methods for the calculation of evaporation that are based only upon climatic factors) provides better results when evaporation means are determined for large areas. For calculation of evaporation from limited areas, such a model must in many cases be made more detailed, taking into account the effect of peculiarities of the soil, vegetation cover, and relief on evaporation.

The task of determining evaporation from limited areas in terrain where the earth's surface has a heterogeneous structure may be very complicated. Difficulties associated with its solution are at present still not fully overcome.

Evaporation from the surface of water bodies

The task of determining evaporation from the surface of water bodies is simplified in comparison with land conditions, as a result of the fact that humidity at the level of the water surface is equal to the saturation humidity at the temperature of the water surface. At the same time, data on the water balance of small bodies of water permit us, in many cases, to determine evaporation in the annual cycle more reliably than for land conditions.

Let us look first on the question of applying evaporimeters to the measurement of evaporation from reservoirs.

Methods for determination of evaporation with the use of evaporimeters differ slightly between the cases of measuring evaporation from the surface of small water bodies and those of measuring evaporation from the seas and oceans. Most papers on the procedure of using evaporimeters are aimed at the solution of the first of these tasks, which has practical importance.

In early papers on measuring evaporation, it was supposed that the rate of evaporation from a small open vessel, filled with water and placed in the open air, is equal to that from a body of water. As a consequence, to determine evaporation from the water body, the value from the evaporimeter [or evaporation pan] was directly multiplied by the ratio of the water body area to the area of the pan. However, it was long ago noticed that such a calculation leads to considerably overestimated values of the evaporation rate from water bodies.

This phenomenon has been explained by differences in the physical conditions of evaporation from an isolated pan and from a water body. For this reason, investigators directed their efforts to the development of floating evaporation pans, for which it was supposed possible to reach a full identity of evaporation conditions with those of the body of water. As a result of numerous observations, however, it became clear that floating pans also do not always give accurate results, because even with complete preservation of the natural conditions of water-vapor diffusion, the evaporation rate varies because of the distortion of heat-exchange conditions in the upper layers of water. (The heat conductivity of water in the pan differs noticeably from that of the upper layers of a water body, which is determined by turbulent mixing.) At the same time, utilization of floating pans often involves considerable technical difficulties, especially at high wind speeds.

Measurement of the evaporation rate on seas and oceans by means of evaporimeters commenced in the middle of the last century with Ladly's observations. After the unsuccessful effort of Mohn to use floating evaporation pans at sea (they are easily flooded by waves), ship evaporimeters mounted on the deck were used for observations. Initially, the evaporation rate from ship evaporimeters was measured by the reduction in water volume, but, as a consequence of difficulty in overcoming errors due to overflow of water from the pans because of rolling and pitching, this method was replaced by calculating the evaporation rate from the change in concentration of salt contained in the evaporimeter water, proposed by Dieulafait (1883).

An original ship evaporimeter was constructed by Shuleikin (1941, 1953), who in order to measure evaporation used an open calorimeter filled with sea water, the heat exchange of which with the surrounding air takes place only through the water surface.

It is possible to determine from the reading of a thermometer inserted in the vessel the rate of change in heat content of the water in the calorimeter, which defines the evaporation rate in the case when the algebraic sum of the radiation balance at the evaporimeter surface and the value of the sensible-heat flux from the evaporating surface to the atmosphere is small relative to the sum of heat converted in evaporation over the given interval of time.

It has been pointed out repeatedly that ship evaporimeters do not measure the precise value of evaporation from the sea because of the difference in conditions of evaporation for an isolated instrument and from the sea surface.

More reliable results, in comparison to the method of evaporimeters, are commonly given by calculations of evaporation from water bodies made from their water balance. It follows from the water-balance equation that evaporation from water bodies can be determined from precipitation data, horizontal transport of water, and variation in water level. In some cases, it turns out to be necessary to take into account also the infiltration of water through the bottom of the water body, though usually this constitutes a small value compared to other components of the water balance.

The method for determination of evaporation by the water balance is applicable, mainly, to restricted bodies of water over more or less long periods of averaging. It is usually impossible to determine evaporation by water balance for a portion of a water body (for example, for a single oceanic region), since in this circumstance it is extremely difficult to evaluate the horizontal redistribution of water.

For comparatively short periods, the method of water balance is also difficult to use because the accuracy of determining water-balance components for short intervals often proves inadequate.

For more or less detailed calculations of evaporation from water bodies, the diffusion method and the method of the heat balance are most frequently used.

The diffusion method for determination of evaporation from water bodies is based on the application of Eq. (2.58), which has been long used as an empirical relation, often called Dalton's law.

Empirical formulas of this type usually have been applied in the form

$$E = (e_s - e) \ Y(u), \tag{2.87}$$

where e_s is the absolute humidity of air saturated with water vapor, calculated from the temperature of the evaporating surface; e is the absolute air humidity at some height; and $Y(u)$ is the "wind factor"—an empirically established function of the dependence of the evaporation rate on wind speed u.

For the function $Y(u)$ different authors have obtained a number of expressions, in most cases having the form $Y(u) = M + Ku$ (M and K are numerical coefficients), but sometimes the form of a power dependence of the type $Y(u) \approx u^m$, with numerical values of the coefficient m from 0.5 to 1.0.

It must be indicated that numerous experimental works carried out under diverse conditions confirm the direct proportionality of the evaporation rate to the humidity deficit calculated from the temperature of the water surface. The difference between the relations of evaporation to wind speed found in some investigations can be explained to a considerable extent by insufficient comparability of conditions of various evaporation pans, evaporimeters, and laboratory installations by means of which the relations were studied.

It is clear from a comparison of Eqs. (2.87) and (2.58) that the question of form of the "wind factor" function coincides with that of the dependence of the integral diffusion coefficient D on wind speed. Because over more or less large bodies of water the vertical gradients of temperature in the lowest layer of air are, as a rule, markedly smaller than the corresponding gradients above land, the dependence of the exchange coefficient on wind speed in this case is satisfactorily described by the Rossby–Montgomery formula.

This gives a basis for considering that the coefficient of integral diffusion on water bodies is proportional to wind speed, that is,

$$E = \chi \rho u (q_s - q). \tag{2.88}$$

This equation, as indicated above, was first obtained by Shuleikin and at present is generally used in calculations of evaporation and the latent-heat flux.

As was pointed out in the previous section, in determining evaporation, the value of the coefficient $\chi \rho$ can be assumed constant and approximately equal to 2.5×10^{-6} g cm^{-3} (when measuring wind speeds and air temperatures at the heights usually applicable for ship observations).

In those cases when the temperature of the surface on a large water body differs considerably from the air temperature, it might appear necessary, in determining evaporation, to take into account the effect of thermal stratification on turbulent exchange and evaporation.

It was noted in the previous section that the effect of thermal stratification on evaporation decreases with an increase of wind speed, when the value of the Richardson number decreases due to the growth of the vertical gradient of wind speed. This inference was corroborated by calculations [refer to Budyko (1948)]. As a result of these calculations, it was established that for moderate and high wind speeds (usually observed over large water bodies, including the main portion of the ocean), the effect of the difference between the temperatures of water and air on the turbulent heat exchange and evaporation is insignificant.

Not dwelling any longer on the problem of determining evaporation from extensive water areas, we shall point to some special features in the calculations of evaporation from the surface of comparatively small and restricted bodies of water.

In order to determine evaporation from restricted water bodies, lakes, and so forth, one must often use observational data of the principal meteorological elements at meteorological stations near the shore. It has been established in the works of several authors that above a water body of even a few hundred meters size, wind speed, humidity, and temperature of the air often vary appreciably, because of the transformation of air masses above the water. These variations commonly produce a rather large influence on evaporation. As a result, in determining evaporation it becomes necessary to cast a quantitative accounting of the transformation process.

In the papers of Jeffreys (1918), Giblett (1921), Sutton (1934), Laikhtman (1947), Iudin (in Budyko et al., 1952), Braslavskii and Vikulina (1954), Timofeev (1963), and other authors, various methods have been developed to determine evaporation from water bodies with consideration of the transformation of air streams. The results of these investigations permit us now to carry out calculations of evaporation from a variety of limited water bodies.

Along with the diffusion method for the determination of evaporation from water bodies, the heat-balance method is in general use for this purpose in modern investigations.

In 1915, Schmidt, who had calculated radiation balances of latitudinal zones of the oceans, made an attempt to determine the amounts of heat disposed of for evaporation in these zones. On the basis of very rough hypotheses, Schmidt assumed that the ratio of the latent-heat flux to the radiation balance in different latitudinal zones was equal to 0.4–0.8. Subsequent authors pointed out the inaccuracy of these estimates, and Schmidt later agreed with them.

Ångström calculated the heat balance of one of the Swedish lakes (1920) and came to the conclusion that the ratio of the amount of heat used in evaporation to the total amount disposed of in evaporation and the turbulent sensible-heat exchange with the atmosphere was equal to 0.9. This estimate was used by Mosby (1936), who determined the latitudinal distribution of evaporation from the oceans with an assumption that in all zones the heat outgo for evaporation corresponded to 91% of the radiation balance.

The possibilities of reliable determination of evaporation from water bodies by the heat balance have become much greater after the Bowen ratio, Eq. (2.59), came into general use.

With the aid of this ratio, it is possible to calculate from the heat-balance equation the evaporation (or the conversion of heat in it) on the basis of data on the radiation balance, temperature of the water surface, and humidity.

In this case, the following formula is commonly used:

$$LE = \frac{R - A}{1 + \dfrac{c_p(T_w - T)}{L(q_s - q)}},\qquad(2.89)$$

where T_w is the temperature of the water surface, and q_s is the specific humidity of saturated air at the temperature of the water surface.

Such a method for determination of evaporation gives, as numerous checks have shown, rather accurate results, especially in determining evaporation for long periods of time. Calculations of evaporation made by this method for short periods are, as a rule, less accurate, since in this case it is usually necessary to determine the values of the heat flux A, which is attended with much difficulty.

Summing up the discussion of various methods for determination of the heat disposal in evaporation, we point out that for land conditions, it is more rational for climatological calculations of the annual mean of evaporation to use the method of the water balance or the relationship equation. To determine evaporation in single months or 10-day periods, one can use the method of solving the equation of the water balance outlined above.

For climatological calculations of the outgo of heat for evaporation from water bodies, it is usually most convenient to use the simple equation (2.88), i.e., the Shuleikin–Sverdrup formula. At the same time, methods based on the equations of the water and heat balances can be successfully used for this purpose.

Determination of other components of the heat balance

In most cases, all other components of the heat balance equation are markedly less in value than its principal components—the radiation balance, the latent-heat flux from evaporation, and the sensible-heat flux. Therefore, in calculating these additional components, one may often use simplified methods that permit obtaining an approximation to their values.

Let us consider first the problem of determining the heat flux directed from the earth's surface to lower layers of the soil or water.

The heat flux directed from the earth's surface to the lower layers for land conditions can be calculated from the heat content of the upper layers of soil, the temperature of which varies over the corresponding period of time. Such calculation is easy to carry out if there are data on soil temperature at different depths through the whole layer of heat exchange, and the thermal capacity of the soil is known.

If, in the period of time under consideration, some soil moisture freezes or melts, the component A will equal the sum of the change in heat content and the gain (or loss) of heat when freezing (or melting) of soil water takes place. The latter value can be approximately determined by data on soil moisture and the difference in the levels of the 0° isotherm at the beginning and end of the period under examination.

When the annual cycle of heat exchange in the soil is calculated, observational data obtained by the use of soil thermometers do not usually embrace the whole depth of the layer of heat exchange. To determine the inflow of heat to the soil with the availability of data on the temperature regime only in a layer of limited depth, one can add the change in heat content in the upper layer of soil to the value of the vertical heat flux between this layer and the underlying ones. The value of this flux can be calculated as the product of the coefficient of soil heat conductivity and the vertical gradient of temperature relating to the corresponding level. An example of such calculations is given in the paper of Tseitin (1953).

Calculation of heat inflow into the soil is complicated in the presence of snow cover, since the heat capacity and heat conductivity of snow change within very wide limits, depending on its density. At the same time, there are usually no routine data on the vertical distribution of temperature in snow cover. At present, however, there is available a satisfactorily large amount of material on heat exchange in soil, both in the warm season and, partially, in the period of snow cover. Some conclusions drawn from this material can be used for approximate estimations of heat turnover in soil during the annual march.

It is clear from general physical considerations that the annual cycle of the heat flux in the soil is closely connected with the annual amplitude of variation of the temperature of the air. If the annual variation of temperature is insignificant, then, presumably, the monthly means of heat inflow into the soil must also be close to zero.

The results of calculation of this heat flux actually show that at an annual variation of temperature less than 10–15°, the monthly sums of the heat flux are comparatively small and can be neglected in most approximate calculations of the heat balance. This means that the heat flux in the soil is not of substantial importance in the monthly sums of the heat balance in most tropical regions and many regions of marine climate in middle latitudes.

According to calculations made by Mukhenberg for regions of the Northern Hemisphere with a significant annual variation of temperature, the annual march of the heat flux in the soil A_1 has, on the average, the form presented in Table 11. The values of the soil-heat flux A_1 in this table are expressed in the fractions of its maximum monthly value A_m.

TABLE 11

ANNUAL CYCLE OF RELATIVE VALUES OF THE SOIL-HEAT FLUX[a]

	Jan.	Feb.	Mar.	Apr.	May	June
A_1	-0.82	-0.64	0.03	1.00	1.00	0.91
A_2	-0.76	-0.59	-0.29	0.03	0.58	1.10

	July	Aug.	Sept.	Oct.	Nov.	Dec.
A_1	0.56	0.26	-0.15	-0.52	-0.78	-0.85
A_2	1.10	0.95	-0.14	-0.48	-0.72	-0.72

[a] Sign convention: + into the soil, − out of the soil.

The maximum monthly value of the heat flux, as calculations show, depends on the annual variation of air temperature. According to available data, this dependence can be expressed, on the average, by the values presented in Table 12.

For northern regions, where thawing of the soil begins at the end of spring or in summer, the relations presented in these tables vary slightly. In those

TABLE 12

RELATION BETWEEN ANNUAL VARIATIONS OF
AIR TEMPERATURE ΔT AND MONTHLY
MAXIMA OF SOIL-HEAT FLUX A_m

ΔT (degrees)	A_m (kcal cm^{-2} month^{-1})
10	0.35
15	0.52
20	0.68
25	0.82
30	0.97
40	1.25
50	1.50

cases when the disappearance of stable snow cover begins after the first of May, the magnitudes of the soil-heat flux can be determined from the values in line A_2 in Table 11 (also expressed as a fraction of A_m).

Using Tables 11 and 12, one can obtain from data only on the annual variation of temperature an approximate idea of the annual cycle of the soil-heat flux. In this case, the data obtained define mean conditions for a large region. (For specific points, the heat exchange in the soil possesses a large microclimatic variability, owing to differences in the thermal properties of the soil.

Calculation of heat exchange in water bodies is generally more complicated than that of heat exchange in the soil, because of the absence of any mass data from systematic measurements of water temperature at different depths in most water bodies, including the seas and oceans.

For individual parts of seas, oceans, or other water bodies one can determine the value of the heat flux A as the residual component of the heat-balance equation. The annual mean of these values thus defines the redistribution of heat owing to the activity of currents and horizontal heat conductivity.

For those water bodies for which there is a sufficient amount of data on temperature at different depths, it is possible to determine the value of the change in heat content. Such a calculation, compared to that for land conditions, on the one hand, becomes simpler because of the virtual stability of the heat constants of water; on the other hand, for small water bodies, it might become more complicated because of the necessity of taking into account the heat exchange of the water with the underlying ground, which is usually difficult to determine.

Because of the great importance of changes in heat content of the upper layers of ocean water in the heat balance of the oceans, it has been attempted many times to work out methods for determining this value without utilizing observational data on temperature at various depths. One of the first methods of the type was offered by Fritz (1958), who established a relation between mean variations of temperature of the ocean surface and changes in heat content of the upper 100-m layer of water during the annual cycle. Later this method was improved by Strokina (1963, 1967a), in whose papers many oceanographic observations were used for studying these relationships.

In Fig. 16, we give a graph of the relation between changes in water heat content from month to month in the 100-m layer (B) and the corresponding changes in water-surface temperature (ΔT), constructed by Strokina. The lines in this graph pertain to different seasons.

Strokina found that the dependence shown in Fig. 16 changes little in different regions of the world ocean.

Among other components of the heat balance, we should mention the accounting for the outgo (or release) of heat owing to melting (or freezing)

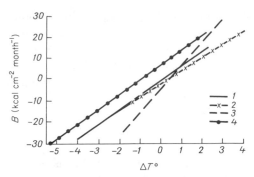

Fig. 16 Graph of the relationship between the changes in heat content of the 100-m oceanic layer and changes in water-surface temperature in the Northern Hemisphere. (1) Oct.–Nov., Nov.–Dec., Dec–Jan., Jan.–Feb., Feb.–Mar., Mar.–Apr.; (2) Apr.–May, May–June, June–July; (3) July–Aug.; (4) Aug.–Sept., Sept.–Oct.

of ice and snow, and the accounting of the redistribution of heat associated with falling atmospheric precipitation.

Transformation of water from the solid to the liquid phase at the earth's surface, as well as the reverse process, conditions a gain or loss of heat that is considerably smaller than the annual sums of the principal components of the heat balance. (An exception to this might be in regions of more or less stable snow or ice cover.) However, for monthly sums of the balance components in certain periods in many regions of middle and high latitudes, the accounting of this component is very important. The procedure of such calculations is based on the determination of the quantity of surface moisture being melted or frozen. This value is multiplied by the latent heat of freezing, which approximately equals 80 cal g^{-1}.

In those cases in which there are no data from direct observations of the quantity of water melted or frozen, one can use for its calculation a number of procedures, some of which are based on heat-balance equations. Statements of such procedures are contained, for example, in papers of Sverdrup (1936b), Kuz'min (1947, 1948, 1950), and other authors and also in Chapter IV of this book.

The transformation of more or less significant amounts of heat with falling precipitation is observed mainly in low-latitude regions, where, in the rainy season, the fall of large quantities of comparatively cold water may lead to a noticeable cooling of the earth's surface. The method for calculation of this component of the heat balance is very simple—its value is equal to the product of the quantity of fallen water by the difference between the temperatures of the water and the active surface. This method, however, is difficult to use, largely because of the absence of data of routine observations of the temperature of falling rain.

Some examples of calculations of this component for tropical regions are contained in the works of Albrecht (1940) and others.

Not dwelling on the problem of determining other components of the heat balance that are usually smaller in magnitude than the above-mentioned components, we shall only note that Chapter VIII will deal with the task of determining the conversion of energy in photosynthesis of plants. Although this heat-balance component is, as a rule, much smaller than the principal components of the balance, its determination is extremely important for a number of biologic and geographic problems.

4. The Heat Balance of the Atmosphere

Utilization of special observations for the determination of the components of the atmospheric heat balance is associated with greater technical difficulty, as compared with observations of the components of the balance at the level of the earth's surface.

The existing methods of observation permit the measurement of all the principal elements of the radiation regime of the atmosphere. The instruments used for such measurements are similar to those applied for actinometric observations near the ground. At the same time, it is necessary to make some changes in construction of these instruments in order to use them in airplanes or other airborne carriers.

To measure the elements of the radiation regime of the atmosphere as a whole, the instruments used should be placed beyond the atmosphere or, at any rate, at such great altitudes that the effect of higher atmospheric layers on the total characteristics of the radiation regime is small.

Such a condition is met in observations conducted from earth satellites or geophysical rockets. The available calculations show that for estimating the radiation balance of the atmosphere as a whole, one can limit himself to considering radiative processes that occur in the troposphere (Kondrat'ev, 1956, and elsewhere). In this connection, observations from planes ascending into the lower stratosphere might also provide valuable data on the atmospheric radiation balance.

In earlier studies, observations made in the higher layers of the atmosphere have been used for elucidating general regularities in the radiative process in the atmosphere. At the same time, because of the comparatively short duration and nonsystematic character of these observations, they have not provided sufficient material for study of the radiation regime of the atmosphere.

In this respect, observations of elements of the radiation regime from satellites possess great advantages. Actinometric instruments installed in long-lived satellites permit us to obtain a detailed characterization of the regime of atmospheric radiation along the trajectory of the satellite. Such observations have acquired great importance for the climatology of the heat balance of the atmosphere.

To measure such components of the atmospheric heat balance as the release of the heat of condensation (Lr) and the income (or outgo) of heat due to the action of advective processes (F_a), direct methods are lacking. The problem of measuring the turbulent transfer of sensible heat from the earth's surface into the atmosphere (P) has been considered in Section 2 of this chapter.

As in investigations of the heat balance at the earth's surface, the utilization of calculation methods for determination of the heat-balance components is of great importance in studies on the climatological regime of the atmospheric heat balance. Let us look at the basic methods for such calculations.

To calculate the atmospheric radiation balance, it is necessary to have information about the amount of solar radiation incident upon the outer boundary of the atmosphere. As pointed out above (refer to Section 2 of Chapter I), these data are obtained as a result of comparatively simple geometrical calculations, if the value of the solar constant is known. Using the accepted value of the solar constant and the above formulas, it is possible to determine with sufficient accuracy the amount of solar radiation incident on the outer boundary of the atmosphere at each latitude and any period of time.

The determination of the amount of radiation absorbed in the atmosphere is a more complicated task. To calculate this value, one must compute the amount of solar radiation absorbed by the earth–atmosphere system, and then subtract from this quantity the radiation absorbed at the earth's surface. The method for determination of the last value is stated above, in Section 1 of this chapter.

The value of the albedo of the earth–atmosphere system α_s can be calculated by the formula

$$\alpha_s = f(\alpha)\,(1 - n) + \alpha' n, \tag{2.90}$$

where the function $f(\alpha)$ designates the relation of α_s for a cloudless sky to the value α, which is the albedo of the earth's surface; α' is the mean albedo of the earth–atmosphere system with complete cloudiness; n is cloudiness in fractions of unity.

Mean values of the albedo characterizing the reflection of solar radiation resulting from scattering by molecules of air, water vapor, and dust particles are comparatively small. In approximations, an appropriate value can be assumed equal to 0.08–0.10 [refer to Kondrat'ev (1954)]. Considering this estimate, Vinnikov (1965a) suggested that the expression $f(\alpha) = 0.66\alpha + 0.10$ be used for average conditions.

Values of albedo of the earth's surface are comparatively well known from observations and corresponding calculations, and can be determined by the use of the tables included in Section 1 of this chapter.

The albedo of the earth–atmosphere system is substantially influenced by clouds. Numerous observations have shown that the albedo of clouds varies over a wide range, in which its value depends on the depth of the cloud layer. For thin clouds, albedo is small, but for layers amounting to several hundreds of meters and more in depth, albedo values usually vary within a range from 0.3 to 0.8. In addition, the value of the albedo of clouds depends on their structure. The highest albedo values are noted for altocumulus clouds, which contain ice particles that substantially intensify reflection.

Because of the great variability of cloud albedo, utilization of mean values may lead to noticeable inaccuracies in calculation of the radiation balance, especially for comparatively short periods of time.

More justifiable is the application of mean values of cloud albedo to the determination of long-term means of the atmospheric radiation balance.

In the paper by Fritz (1949), the mean albedo of clouds for the whole earth is appraised at 0.50–0.55. In climatological calculations of Fedoseeva (1953), a mean cloud albedo equal to 0.50 was used.

Observational data from satellites show that these evaluations are slightly high and that the mean albedo of clouds probably is about 0.45 (refer to Section 4 of Chapter III).

In earlier study of the planetary albedo of the earth, the value was calculated from the brightness of the ashy light of the moon. It is known that the part of the moon's surface not illuminated by the sun is illuminated by rays reflected from the earth's surface. This phenomenon, usually easily visible when a small part of the disc of the moon is illuminated by the sun, is called the earthshine. Measuring the brightness of this light, one can evaluate the albedo of the part of the earth that faces the moon. This albedo value relates to the visible part of the spectrum. As a result of approximate evaluations of the reflectivity of the earth for different wavelengths and on the basis of observations of the earthshine, calculations of the integrated albedo of the earth were carried out and provided values equal to 0.35–0.40 (Bagrov, 1954).

Observations from satellites gave smaller values of the planetary albedo, close to 0.30 (Raschke et al., 1968; and others).

When determining the components of the atmospheric radiation balance, the greatest difficulty arises in connection with calculation of the value of outgoing long-wave radiation emitted to space.

For this purpose, one can use various radiation nomograms, following the method offered by Kondrat'ev and Filippovich (1952).

In this study, it was suggested that the flux of outgoing emission is approximately equal to the value of the flux of long-wave radiation at the level of the tropopause. Evaluation of the error due to this assumption showed that it probably did not exceed 6%.

In T. G. Berliand's investigation (1956), the formula of M. E. Berliand, obtained as a result of working out a theoretical model of long-wave radiation transfer in the atmosphere, was used to calculate outgoing radiation. This formula has the following form:

$$I_s = \delta\sigma T^4\left\{\left(\frac{T_H}{T}\right)^4 - \frac{\gamma}{\beta T}\left(\frac{T_m}{T}\right)^3 \sum_{n=1}^{4}[Ei(-\theta_n m_0 e^{-\beta H}) - Ei(-\theta_n m_0)]\right\}. \quad (2.91)$$

In this equation, T is the temperature near the earth's surface; T_H is the temperature at the tropopause; T_m is the mean temperature of the troposphere, which is equal to the mean between T and T_H; γ is the temperature gradient in the troposphere; β is a coefficient equal to 4.5×10^{-6} cm^{-1}; Ei is an integral function [Euler's function]; θ_n is the coefficient of absorption ($\theta_1 = 0.166$; $\theta_2 = 2.6$; $\theta_3 = 36.2$; $\theta_4 = 189.0$ cm^2 g^{-1}); m_0 is the mass of water vapor (in g cm^{-2}) in the atmospheric column of cross section 1 cm^2; δ is a coefficient defining the difference between the properties of the radiating surface and those of a black body; σ is the Stefan–Boltzmann constant; and H is the height of the tropopause.

Equation (2.91) relates to a cloudless atmosphere, being derived with the assumption that the outgoing emission equals the flux of long-wave radiation at the tropopause level.

This formula could be also used for determining the outgoing emission with complete cloudiness. In this case, one should assume T equal to the temperature of the upper boundary of the clouds and use data on the vertical temperature gradient in the troposphere above the layer of clouds.

To determine outgoing emission under the conditions of broken cloudiness of different layers, T. G. Berliand used the formula

$$I_s = I_{s0}[1 - (n_H + n_C + 0.5n_B)] + I_H n_H + I_C n_C + 0.5I_B n_B, \quad (2.92)$$

where I_{s0} is the outgoing emission with a cloudless sky; n_H, n_C, and n_B are the amounts of clouds of lower, middle, and upper layers, respectively; and I_H, I_C, and I_B are the outgoing emission from the lower, middle, and upper layers of clouds.

The coefficient 0.5 in the last term of Eq. (2.92) is introduced to account for the fact that the emission from the surface of clouds of the upper layer is noticeably less than that from an absolutely black body.

Later, Vinnikov (1965b), using data on the integrated function of transmission of the atmospheric gases, obtained for determination of emission the
formula

$$I_s = \sigma T_H^4 + (\sigma T^4 - \sigma T_H^4)\frac{P(m_0) + P(m_H)}{2}(1 - c_H n_H - c_C n_C - c_B n_B), \quad (2.93)$$

in which m_0 and m_H are the mass of water vapor in the whole atmosphere
and in the air layer above the tropopause; P is the function of transmission;
c_H, c_C, and c_B are coefficients equal to the heights of the upper surfaces of
clouds of the lower, middle, and upper layers, respectively, relative to the
height of the tropopause; the cloudiness data are represented by the values
when the earth is observed from space. This formula has been used for determination of outgoing emission in calculations of the radiation balance of the
earth–atmosphere system, carried out during preparation of a map for
"Атлас теплового баланса земного шара (Atlas of the Heat Balance
of the Earth)" (1963).

Considerable difficulty in climatological calculations of the outgoing
emission both from radiation nomograms and by formulas (2.91–2.93)
might appear in connection with the necessity of using materials from aerological observations. In many regions of the globe, the amount of such data
is insufficient, and this inevitably lowers the accuracy of the corresponding
calculations.

Having available the calculations of absorbed radiation and outgoing
emission, one can determine the radiation balance of the earth-atmosphere
system by the formula

$$R_s = Q_s(1 - \alpha_s) - I_s \tag{2.94}$$

(where Q_s is the solar radiation at the outer boundary of the atmosphere),
and can then calculate the radiation balance of the atmosphere by the
formula

$$R_a = R_s - R, \tag{2.95}$$

where R is the radiation balance at the earth's surface, which in most cases
can be determined more accurately than the balance of the earth–atmosphere
system.

The question of the gain of sensible heat in the atmosphere by condensation
of water vapor can be comparatively easily solved for the atmosphere as a
whole. The difference between the amounts of water that are condensed in
the atmosphere and evaporated from the surfaces of droplets (or ice crystals)
in clouds and fog is, on the average, equal to total precipitation. Therefore,
for the whole atmosphere, the heat input owing to condensation for a more
or less long period of time is equal to the product of the amount of precipitation by the latent heat of vaporization.

It is much more difficult to calculate the heat input from condensation in restricted regions and short periods of time. In this case, the heat input by condensation in the atmosphere (or the reverse in sign, heat expenditure for evaporation of cloud particles) is proportional to the difference between precipitation and the increase (or decrease) of the amount of water vapor in a vertical column of air as a result of evaporation (or condensation growth) of the cloud particles.

The change in the amount of water vapor caused by atmospheric processes of condensation and evaporation is rather difficult to determine by direct methods. Utilization of the atmospheric water balance for its calculation does not provide good results either, because in this situation it often represents a small difference between large values that are determined with considerable error.

Thus, accurate calculation of the income of the heat of condensation in the atmosphere for short periods of time and restricted regions is difficult. One might consider, however, that long-term means of this value in particular regions are in most cases close to the product of the latent heat of evaporation by the amount of precipitation.

Exceptions to this rule are possible under conditions of a heterogeneous underlying surface, when the influence of mountains or coastlines may lead to a disparity between the amount of precipitation in a given region and the difference between condensation and evaporation in the atmosphere.

At present, it is hard to estimate the possible magnitude of such differences and the corresponding magnitudes of errors in calculations of the heat of condensation.

To determine the gain or loss of heat associated with a change in the heat content of the atmosphere B_a, it is possible to use the procedure proposed by Rakipova (1957), for which it is necessary to have data on the vertical distribution of air temperature and pressure within the troposphere. Utilization of data relating to higher levels usually has little influence on the results of the computations.

In calculating the component B_a, one must remember that because of the comparatively small heat capacity of the atmosphere it is, as a rule, noticeably less than the principal components of the atmospheric heat balance. Therefore, in many cases one can either neglect this component or take it into account in the most approximate way.

The determination of the income or outgo of heat associated with horizontal movement in the atmosphere is a rather difficult task. In climatological calculations of the heat balance, the heat-balance equation (2.96) is usually used for this purpose:

$$F_a = R_s - L(E - r) - B_s - F_0. \qquad (2.96)$$

Calculation of the value F_a as the residual member of the balance usually provides satisfactory results if there are sufficiently accurate data of all the other balance components.

Such a condition is not always easily fulfilled. It is also best, at the same time, to use the heat-balance equation as a control on the accuracy of computing all its components by independent methods. Therefore, there is great interest in attempts to determine the component F_a by direct methods, using the data of routine meteorological observations.

The value of the income or outgo of heat resulting from horizontal movement in the atmosphere is associated with the activity of the two different processes—advection by averaged motion and macroturbulent transfer.

In her study of 1957, Rakipova worked out a method for calculating the values of mean advection. In this study, the general equation of the heat transfer written in spherical coordinates was linearized and the included functions presented in the form of sums of zonal values and deviations from them.

Using this linearized equation, Rakipova obtained a formula that associated the values of mean advection with the field of atmospheric pressure. Although calculations by this formula are rather cumbersome, it permitted the obtaining of interesting data that make clear the characteristics of mean advection.

Less success was obtained in elaborating methods for determining the income and outgo of heat due to macroturbulent exchange. The approximate values of the horizontal macroturbulent heat fluxes can be estimated if one considers them to be equal to the product of the mean horizontal temperature gradients in the atmosphere and the coefficients of horizontal exchange. In this case, however, it should be borne in mind that the coefficients of horizontal exchange are variables depending both on general meteorological conditions and the scale of the processes under investigation. The difficulty of accurate determination of the values of these coefficients leads to considerable error in calculations of the macroturbulent heat fluxes.

The income or outgo of heat owing to macroturbulence, contained in the equation of the atmospheric heat balance, is proportional to the derivative of the value of the macroturbulent flux in its direction. It is evident that because the available data on the values of this flux are rather inaccurate, it is difficult to calculate this derivative with sufficient accuracy. Thus, the problem of working out a climatological method for calculating the macroturbulent gain or loss of heat is not yet solved.

Evaluations made by Rakipova (1957) show that, although under mean conditions the effect of macroturbulence on the gain (or loss) of heat in the atmosphere is noticeably less than that of mean advection, it is still substantial. As a result, a more or less accurate determination of the value of F_a by a direct method is at present difficult to carry out.

5. Accuracy of Determination of the Components
of the Heat Balance

Although the problem of the accuracy of calculations of the components of the heat balance is of great importance for the climatology of the heat balance, it has, until recently, been inadequately clarified in the scientific literature. Because of this fact, in discussing material on heat balance one often encounters controversial viewpoints on the probable error in the data under consideration. In some cases, there is a tendency to imply an underestimation of this error, and in others it has been greatly overestimated without sufficient basis.

All this speaks for the necessity of a more or less detailed analysis of the accuracy of climatological calculations of the components of the heat balance. It is of great interest to contrast the accuracy of data on the heat balance with that of climatological materials for the basic meteorological elements.

We shall indicate that to evaluate the errors of existing methods for determination of the components of the radiation and heat balances, it is possible to use four methods:

1. Comparison with one another of the results of different independent methods for calculating the components of the heat balance.
2. Comparison of calculations of balance components with measurements of them made by special instruments.
3. Evaluation of the error in calculating all the components of the balance by closing the equation of balance, when all components have been determined independently.
4. Evaluation of probable errors in calculations, by making an analysis of the formulas used.

Of these methods, the third is especially important, being based on the obvious certainty of fulfilling the law of the conservation of energy. This method for checking calculations of the balance components was used in a paper of the author (Budyko, 1946c) and in a number of subsequent investigations.

Applying the second of the above methods as a check, one must bear in mind that contemporary methods for instrumental measurements of components of the balance are inevitably associated with definite errors. Thus, in particular, the probable error in measuring total short-wave radiation with available instruments for more or less long periods may amount to several per cent.

The problem of errors in measuring the radiation balance with balance meters of different designs was studied by Kirillova and Kucherov (1953), Lebedeva and Sivkov (1962), and other authors. It can be inferred from their conclusions that the probable error in measurements of the radiation balance for comparatively long periods of time is characteristically of the order of 5–10%. The accuracy of measurements of other heat-balance components (particularly the latent-heat flux and the sensible-heat flux) with the aid of special instruments may vary over a wide range, depending on the type of instruments, observational conditions, and values of the measured fluxes.

Let us turn now to an appraisal of the accuracy of calculations of the principal components of the radiation and heat balances.

The chief component of the radiation balance—the total short-wave radiation—is measured at many actinometric stations, which greatly simplifies the checking of climatological calculations of this value. Comparisons of measured and calculated values of total short-wave radiation have been made in many investigations. We give here the results of such a comparison made for the purpose of checking the world maps of radiation on the continents, constructed in the Main Geophysical Observatory. Comparison of the results of calculations with data from the summary of measured means made by by T. G. Berliand (1961) showed that the disparity between measured and calculated values for monthly means is, on an average, less than 10%, and the coefficient of correlation between them is 0.98 (refer to Fig. 17). It is clear that a certain number of the disparities are connected with the short duration of observations at some actinometric stations. Taking this circumstance into account, it is possible to consider that even a rather schematic procedure of calculating total short-wave radiation permits the determination of monthly and annual means with an error of the same order as the error in instrumental measurements.

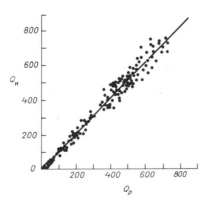

Fig. 17 Comparison of measured (Q_N) and calculated (Q_p) values of incident solar radiation (cal cm^{-2} per 24 hr).

The problem of assessing the accuracy of calculations of the radiation balance at the earth's surface is more complicated than that of estimates of short-wave radiation. Available observations and calculations show that the radiation balance varies substantially at different types of underlying surface in one and the same region. The great "microclimatic" variability of the radiation balance can be explained by the significant influence that albedo and temperature of the underlying surface have on it. To illustrate this influence, we give here the data from calculations of radiation balance, made by the procedure stated above, for three regions: Cape Shmidt (the Arctic), Sverdlovsk (forest zone), and Ashkhabad (desert zone).

For the first region, calculations of radiation balance were made for conditions of tundra, light-colored stony soil, and the sea surface, which, even in summer, is covered to a considerable extent with floating ice. For the region of Sverdlovsk, calculations were carried out for conditions of the meteorological plot, a clover field, and bare fallow. For the region of Ashkhabad, the radiation balance was calculated for the desert and an irrigated field.

The results of calculations are presented in Table 13.

TABLE 13

RADIATION BALANCE OF DIFFERENT SURFACES

(kcal cm^{-2} $month^{-1}$)

Region	Surface	May	June	July	August
Cape Shmidt	Tundra	—	5.0	6.4	3.7
	Stony soil	—	4.7	4.5	2.5
	Sea	—	2.3	1.9	0.9
Sverdlovsk	Meteorological site	5.5	7.0	6.7	4.2
	Clover field	5.0	5.9	5.6	3.5
	Bare fallow	7.2	8.5	8.2	5.5
Ashkhabad	Desert	5.4	6.7	6.4	6.1
	Irrigated field	8.2	10.4	10.5	10.0

As can be seen from the above materials, the values of the radiation balance at different types of underlying surface in the same region may differ from each other by several times. This fact must be taken into account both when constructing maps of the radiation balance and when comparing the results of measurements with calculated values.

Until recently, there were no data from long observations of the radiation balance. Now, at many actinometric stations of the USSR and in a number of places in other countries, systematic measurements of the radiation balance are being made. Comparison of components of the radiation balance from observational data with calculated values found earlier by the use of independent methods offers great interest.

For such a comparison, we have used observational data from 27 stations, some of which are situated in the territory of the USSR and the others in the United States, Western Europe, Asia, and Australia.

The results of comparison of measured and calculated annual sums of the balance at all the stations are presented in Fig. 18. Monthly sums of the balance are presented in Fig. 19. As is seen from Figs. 18 and 19, the measured and calculated values of the radiation balance match well on the average. The mean value of the discrepancy between them for the annual balance

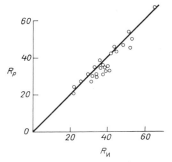

Fig. 18   Comparison of measured ($R_\text{и}$) and calculated (R_p) annual sums of the radiation balance (kcal cm^{-2} yr^{-1}).

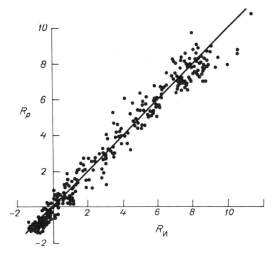

Fig. 19   Comparison of measured ($R_\text{и}$) and calculated (R_p) monthly sums of the radiation balance (kcal cm^{-2} month^{-1}).

equals 2.9 kcal cm^{-2} yr^{-1}, and for the monthly balances, 0.54 kcal cm^{-2} month^{-1}. In the first case, the discrepancy is less than 5% of the largest annual value, in the second case, of the order of 5% of the largest monthly value of the radiation balance.

The coefficients of correlation between the measured and calculated values equal 0.92 for the annual, and 0.98 for the monthly, sums of the radiation balance.

Taking into account the fact that the discrepancy between the results of calculations and the measurements, aside from calculation errors, must be to a considerable extent explained by errors in measurements, microclimatic variability in the radiation balance, and limited periods of observation, the agreement of the two independent methods for determination of the radiation balance should be admitted to be extremely satisfactory.

Of great interest is the question of checking the results of calculations relating to the indices of the radiation regime on the oceans. The first comparison of calculated values of the radiation balance on the oceans with observational data was performed by Albrecht (1952), who used for this purpose data of measurements of the radiation balance that he had taken during his trip in the Indian Ocean. A good agreement of the measured and calculated values of the radiation balance was established by Albrecht, but it did not permit, however, the drawing of any general conclusions as to the reliability of calculated indices to the oceanic radiation regime, because only a limited amount of observational data were at Albrecht's disposal.

Recently, the quantity of observations of the radiation regime on the oceans has grown sharply, which has enabled us to conduct a broad comparison of the calculation data obtained earlier with the new observational material. Such a comparison was made in the studies of Strokina (1967b, 1968) in respect to the short-wave radiation means and the radiation balance for different oceanic regions from the "Атлас теплового баланса земного шара (Atlas of the Heat Balance of the Earth)" (1963) and the data of ship observations in the Atlantic, Indian, and Pacific Oceans.

The results of the comparison of calculated and measured indices of the radiation regime for the oceans obtained by Strokina are presented in Figs. 20 and 21. It is seen from these figures that the measured and calculated values of total short-wave radiation and radiation balance agree satisfactorily. The coefficients of correlation between them are 0.91 for short-wave radiation and 0.95 for the radiation balance.

It appears that in this case, there is a small systematic discrepancy between measured and calculated values of short-wave radiation—the measured being somewhat larger than the calculated values. This discrepancy is, presumably, explicable by the fact that the procedure for calculating short-wave radiation which was developed for land conditions provides slightly

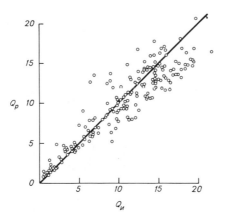

Fig. 20   Comparison of measured (Q_{H}) and calculated (Q_{P}) monthly values of incident solar radiation on the oceans (kcal cm^{-2} month^{-1}).

underestimated values for oceans, where the air transparency is, on the average, higher than it is over land.

Of much importance for checking the accuracy of calculations of radiation balance at land and water surfaces is the method of independent determination of all the heat-balance components. From this it is possible to estimate the mean error in determining all the heat-balance components. It is possible to calculate the relative value of this error by computing the ratio of the algebraic sum of all the heat-balance components to the sum of their absolute values.

On the basis of the results of the first work in which all heat-balance components were determined by independent methods for one of the stations in North America and for the southern part of the European territory of the

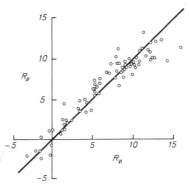

Fig. 21   Comparison of measured (R_{H}) and calculated (R_{P}) monthly values of the radiation balance of the ocean (kcal cm^{-2} month^{-1}).

USSR (Budyko, 1946a, 1947), the mean error in determining the sum of the components of the balance was calculated. In neither case did it exceed 5%.

Compared to land conditions, verification of the accuracy of calculated values of components of the heat balance of individual ocean regions by the method stated seems more complicated, because one of the components for the oceans (gain or loss of heat as a consequence of the activity of currents) is hard to determine by a direct method.

However, for the series of annual maps of the ocean heat balance constructed by the scientific workers of the Main Geophysical Observatory, it is possible to estimate the upper limit of the mean error in calculation by closing the equation of balance.

This value can be found on the basis of the following considerations. If the mean total error in the determination of the radiation balance, the conversion of heat in evaporation, and the sensible-heat flux on the oceans had been larger than the mean value of gain or loss of heat due to currents F_0, then the latter would have been impossible to determine as a residual component of the heat balance. In other words, the map of this value calculated from the balance equation would not have been in accord with the actual distribution of warm and cold currents.

Since, however, the map of income and outgo of heat owing to ocean currents that was designed by the scientific workers of the Main Geophysical Observatory corresponds well to the distribution of most currents, it is clear that the mean total error in calculating the three principal components of the balance is less than the mean value of F_0.

Thus, the relative mean error in calculating the heat-balance components for the oceans is less than the ratio of the mean value of F_0 to the sum of the mean value of the radiation balance, heat converted in evaporation, and sensible-heat exchange. Since, on the basis of the above data, this ratio turns out equal to 12%, the mean error in calculations of the sums of the absolute values of the balance components presumably does not exceed 12%.

Calculations of heat conversion in evaporation for both land and water bodies can be checked by closing the equation of water balance.

The procedure of determining evaporation and the latent-heat flux on the basis of the relationship equation has been tested in a number of studies. The most complete checking of calculations of evaporation accomplished by the relationship equation was carried out with the available material on the water balance of the different continents (Budyko and Zubenok, 1961). For this purpose, evaporation was calculated by the water-balance equation (as the difference between precipitation and run-off) and determined from the relationship equation.

In this comparison, data were used for different continents and about 1200 different regions. Areas situated north of 60° N were excluded from examination because, owing to considerable errors in the measurements of solid precipitation, more or less accurate determination of the annual total evaporation by means of the water balance turns out to be impossible.

Comparison of evaporation values found by independent methods showed the mean discrepancy between them to be close to 10%, which is approximately equal to the value of the probable error in determining evaporation by the water-balance method. At the same time, in some cases this difference is presumably of a systematic character and depends on the features of the annual cycle of evaporation and precipitation (refer to Chapter VI of this book).

The problem of accuracy in calculations of land evaporation made by the method based on the relation between evaporation and soil moisture was discussed in papers of Zubenok (1966a, 1968) and Kuz'min (1966). These papers present the evaporation values in single months, found with the calculation model described earlier, in comparison with the results of observations conducted at heat-balance stations, where evaporation was determined on the basis of the radiation balance and the vertical gradients of temperature and humidity.

This comparison showed that in regions of sufficient moisture, the measured and calculated values of evaporation correspond well to each other (correlation coefficients above 0.9). In regions of insufficient moisture, the correlation coefficients decrease slightly, which is presumably to be explained by the large influence on evaporation of micro- and mesoclimatic variability of moisture conditions in these regions.

In the study by Kuz'min it was pointed out that the probable errors in calculating evaporation according to this calculation scheme grow larger with a decrease in the duration of the period for which evaporation is determined. For the annual period, these errors are comparatively small (on an average, less than 10%); for monthly periods they reach 20%.

The problem of errors in calculations of the turbulent fluxes of heat and water vapor from water bodies can be investigated by analyzing the accuracy of the various assumptions on which the calculation formulas are based. We will not repeat here the results of such an analysis, because they are given in Section 2 of this chapter and in Section 3 of Chapter III of this book.

On the basis of the data stated above and other available material, we draw the following conclusions concerning the accuracy of contemporary methods for calculating the components of the radiation and heat balances at the earth's surface.

The error in the monthly and annual means of radiation on continents obtained with the use of climatological calculation methods is approximately 5–10%.

When the relative error in calculations of the radiation balance is being estimated, one must remember that both the annual and monthly means of the radiation balance approach zero under certain conditions. Therefore, it is advisable to compare the error in calculation of annual values of the radiation balance with the amplitude of their variations, and for monthly values with the maximum value of the radiation balance in the annual cycle. The relative error in calculations of the radiation balance for land, calculated in such a way, is on the average less than 10%. The annual values of heat converted in evaporation from land (latent-heat flux) are determined with an average error of the order of 5–10%. Taking into account these magnitudes of error, it is possible to evaluate the mean error in calculation of the turbulent sensible-heat flux on land, which proves to be slightly larger than that in calculation of the radiation balance.

The errors in calculations of the components of the heat balance for the oceans are presumably somewhat larger than those for the land, but the order of magnitude of these errors is probably about the same.

It should be indicated that for different regions of the globe, the values of the probable errors in calculations of the heat-balance components should differ markedly, especially because of the different reliability of the basic meteorological data used in the calculations. The largest errors are noted in the high latitudes and also in the less explored regions of the oceans (especially in the Southern Hemisphere). It is possible to conclude that the probable relative error of several components of the heat balance at the earth's surface obtained by modern calculation methods does not often exceed that of the climatological norms of several basic meteorological elements (such as cloudiness or precipitation). At the same time, in terms of detail, data available on the heat balance are still inferior to material available for many meteorological elements.

The problem of possible errors in determination of the components of the heat balance of the atmosphere is, at present, but little developed.

In Fig. 22 are presented the latitudinal means of the annual values of the radiation balance of the earth–atmosphere system, found by use of the map designed by Vinnikov for the Атлас теплового баланса земного щара (Atlas of the Heat Balance of the Earth)" (1963) (line 1). This figure also represents the distribution of the same value as calculated by Vinnikov from measurements taken by satellite (Vonder Haar and Suomi, 1969—line 2; Bandeen et al., 1965—line 3). It is evident that the direct measurements of the radiation balance agree satisfactorily with the results of the earlier indirect calculations. Comparison of the corresponding maps shows that the data obtained by observations from satellites confirms many peculiarities of the spatial distribution of the radiation balance of the earth–atmosphere system established earlier by calculation methods.

At the same time, however, the agreement of calculations and measure-

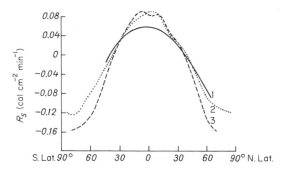

Fig. 22 Dependence of the radiation balance of the earth–atmosphere system on latitude.

ments relating to characteristics of the radiation regime of the earth–atmosphere system is inferior to the agreement for conditions at the earth's surface. This is associated with the lesser accuracy in determination of these indices, whether by available calculation methods or by instruments carried by satellites.

REFERENCES

Аверкиев М. С. (1956). Возможные месячные и годовые суммы прямой солнечной радиации на горизонтальную поверхность при различной прозрачности атмосферы для широт 40—70°. Вестн. МГУ, сер. геогр., № 2.

Averkiev, M. S. (1956). Greatest possible monthly and yearly totals of direct-beam solar radiation on a horizontal surface for different transparencies of the atmosphere at latitudes from 40° to 70°. *Vestn. Mosk.Univ. Geog. Ser.*, **11**, No. 2.

Аверкиев М. С. (1958). Суммарная радиация и ее компоненты при безоблачном небе и зависимость от прозрачности атмосферы для широт 40—70°. Вестн. МГУ, сер. биол.-почв., геол., геогр., № 4.

Averkiev, M. S. (1958). Total incoming solar radiation and its components with cloudless sky and in relation to transparency of the atmosphere at latitudes from 40° to 70°. *Vestn. Mosk. Univ. Ser. Biol. Pochvoved. Geol. Geogr.* **13**, No. 4.

Айзенштат Б. А. (1951). О непосредственном определении компонент теплового баланса поверхности земли. Инф. сб. № 1. Динамическая и сельскохозяйственная метеорология. Гидрометеоиздат, Л.

Aizenshtat, B. A. (1951). On the direct determination of components of the heat balance at the earth's surface. *USSR Gl. Upr. Gidrometeor. Sluzhby, Inform. Sb.*, Leningrad, No. 1, pp. 65–74. MGA 4.1-118.

Актинометрический справочник. Зарубежные страны. 1964. Под ред Т. Г. Берлянд. Гидрометеоиздат, Л.

"Aktinometricheskii Spravochnik. Zarubezhnye Strany. (Actinometric Handbook for Foreign Countries)" (T. G. Berliand, ed.). Gidrometeoizdat, Leningrad, 1964.

Актинометрический Ежегодник. Гидрометеоопздат, Л.

"Actinometric Yearbook." Gidrometeoizdat, Leningrad.

Алпатьев А. М. (1950). Рациональное использование осадков—основа преодоления засухи. Сб. «Агроклиматические условия степи Украинской ССР и пути их улучшения». Изд. АН СССР, Киев.

Alpat'ev, A. M. (1950). The rational utilization of precipitation—a basis for overcoming droughts. *In* "Agroklimaticheskie Usloviia Stepi Ukrainskoi SSR i Puty Ikh Uluchsheniia (Agroclimatic Conditions of the Steppes of the Ukrainian SSR and Means for Their Improvement)." Izdat. Akad. Nauk Ukr. SSR, Kiev.

Алпатьев А. М. (1954). Влагооборот культурных растений. Гидрометеоиздат, Л.

Alpat'ev, A. M. (1954). "Vlagooborot Kul'turnykh Rastenii (Moisture Exchange in Crop Plants)." Gidrometeoizdat, Leningrad. MGA 7.3-242 10 I-83.

Атлас теплового баланса. (1955). Под ред. М. И. Будыко. Изд. ГГО, Л.

"Atlas Teplovogo Balansa (Atlas of the Heat Balance)" (M. I. Budyko, ed.). Izdat. Gl. Geofiz. Observ., Leningrad. 1955. MGA 8.5-19 11A-25.

Атлас теплового баланса земного шара. (1963). Под ред. М. И. Будыко. Междуведомственный геофизический комитет, М.

"Atlas Teplovogo Balansa Zemnogo Shara (Atlas of the Heat Balance of the Earth)" (M. I. Budyko, ed.). Akad. Nauk SSSR, Prezidium. Mezhduvedomstvennyi Geof. Komitet, 1963; Guide to the "Atlas of the Heat Balance of the Earth," U.S. Weather Bur., WB/T No. 106. U.S. Weather Bur., Washington, D.C., 1964.

Багров Н. А. (1954). Планетарное альбедо Земли. Труды ЦИП, вып. 35.

Bagrov, N. A. (1954). Planetary albedo of the Earth. *Tr. Tsent. Inst. Prognozov* No. 35.

Берлянд М. Е., Берлянд Т. Г. (1952). Определение эффективного излучения Земли с учетом влияния облачности. Изв. АН СССР, сер. геофиз., № 1.

Berliand, M. E., and Berliand, T. G. (1952). Determining the net long-wave radiation of the Earth with consideration of the effect of cloudiness. *Izv. Akad. Nauk SSSR Ser. Geofiz.* No. 1.

Берлянд Т. Г. (1948). Радиационный и тепловой баланс Европейской территории СССР. Труды ГГО, вып. 10.

Berliand, T. G. (1948). Radiation and heat balance of the European USSR. *Tr. Gl. Geofiz. Observ.* **10**.

Берлянд Т. Г. (1956). Тепловой баланс атмосферы северного полушария. Сб. «А. И. Воейков и современные проблемы климатологии». Гидрометеоиздат, Л.

Berliand, T. G. (1956). The heat balance of the atmosphere of the Northern Hemisphere. *In.* "A. I. Voeikov i Sovremennye Problemy Klimatologii," (M. I. Budyko, ed.) Gidrometeorizdat, Leningrad; Translated in "A. I. Voeikov and Problems in Climatology: Selected Articles," pp. 57–83. *Isr. Program Sci. Trans.*, Jerusalem, 1963.

Берлянд Т. Г. 1960. Методика климатологических расчетов суммарной радиации. Метеорология и гидрология, № 6.

Berliand, T. G. (1960). Methods of climatological computation of total incoming solar radiation. *Meteorol. Gidrol.* No. 6, 9–12. MGA 12:1486.

Берлянд Т. Г. (1961). Распределение солнечной радиации на континентах. Гидрометеоиздат, Л.

Berliand, T. G. (1961). "Raspredelenie Solnechnoi Radiatsii na Kontinentakh (Distribution of Solar Radiation on the Continents)." Gidrometeoizdat, Leningrad. MGA 17.4-1.

Бирюкова Л. А. (1956а). О методике климатологического расчета суточного хода суммарной и поглощенной радиации. Труды ГГО, вып. 66.

Biriukova, L. A. (1956a). On methods of climatological computation of the daily march of incoming and absorbed solar radiation. *Tr. Gl. Geofiz. Observ.* **66**, 33–36. MGA 10:1618.

Бирюкова Л. А. (1956б). Некоторые особенности суточного хода суммарной радиации и радиационного баланса в разных климатическах областях СССР. Труды ГГО, вып. 66.

Biriukova, L. A. (1956b). Some characteristics of the daily march of incoming solar radiation and the radiation budget in different climatic regions of the USSR. *Tr. Gl. Geofiz. Observ.* **66**, 10–16. MGA 10:1618.

Бортковский Р. С., Бютнер Э. К. (1969). Расчет коэффициента теплообмена над морем. Изв. АН СССР. Физика атмосферы и океана, № 5.

Bortkovskii, R. S., and Biutner, E. K. (1969). Calculation of the coefficient of heat exchange at sea. *Izv. Akad. Nauk SSSR Fiz. Atmos. Okeana* **5**, No. 5, 494–503. MGA 21.3-490; *Izv. Atmos. Oceanic Phys.* **5**, No. 5, 277–282 (1969).

Бортковский Р. С., Бютнер Э. К. (1970). Проверка модели турбулентного теплообмена над морем по экспериментальным данным. Изв. АН СССР. Физика атмосферы и океана, № 1.

Bortkovskii, R. S., and Biutner, E. K. (1970). Test of a model of the turbulent heat exchange over sea with experimental data. *Izv. Akad. Nauk SSSR Fiz. Atmos. Okeana* **6**, No. 1, 37–44. MGA 22.4-368; *Izv. Atmos. Oceanic Phys.* **6**, No. 1, 18–22 (1970).

Браславский А. П., Викулина З. А. (1954). Нормы испарения с поверхности водохранилищ. Гидрометеоиздат, Л.

Braslavskii, A. P., and Vikulina, Z. A. (1954). "Normy Ispareniia s Poverkhnosti Vodokhranilishch (Norms of Evaporation from the Surface of Reservoirs)." Gidrometeoizdat, Leningrad. MGA 7.3-15.

Бройдо А. Г. (1957). Некоторые результаты исследования интегрального коэффициента турбулентного перемешивания. Метеорология и гидрология, № 9.

Broido, A. G. (1957). Some results of an investigation of the integral coefficient of turbulent mixing. *Meteorol. Gidrol.* No. 9, 27–30. MGA 10.3-216.

Бройдо А. Г. (1958). Связь коэффициента внешней диффузии с параметром устойчивости приземного слоя атмосферы. Труды ЛГМИ, вып. 8.

Broido, A. G. (1958). The relation of the coefficient of external diffusion with a parameter of stability of the layer of the atmosphere near the ground. *Tr. Leningrad. Gidrometeorol. Inst.* **8**.

Будыко М. И. (1945). О некоторых характеристиках турбулентности в приземном слое воздуха. Труды НИУ ГУГМС, сер. 1, вып. 7.

Budyko, M. I. (1945). Some characteristics of turbulence in the layer of air near the ground. *Tr. Gl. Upr. Gidrometeorol. Sluzhby Nauch. Issled. Uchrezhdeniia* [1], **7**.

Будыко М. И. (1946а). Измерение естественного испарения. Труды НИУ ГУГМС, сер. 1, вып. 34.

Budyko, M. I. (1946a). Measurements of natural evaporation. *Tr. Gl. Upr. Gidrometeorol. Sluzhby Nauch. Issled. Uchrezhdeniia* [1], **34**, 83–92. MGA 7.5-196 10H-5.

Будыко М. И. (1946б). Турбулентный обмен в нижних слоях атмосферы. Метеорология и гидрология, № 2.

Budyko, M. I. (1946b). Turbulent exchange in the lower layers of the atmosphere. *Meteorol. Gidrol.* No. 2.

Будыко М. И. (1946в). Методы определения естественного испарения. Метеорология и гидрология, № 3.

Budyko, M. I. (1946c). Methods of determining natural evaporation. *Meteorol. Gidrol.* No. 3.

Будыко М. И. (1946г). Распределение метеорологических элементов в приземном слое воздуха. Изв. АН СССР, сер. геогр. и геофиз., т. 10, № 4.

Budyko, M. I. (1946d). The distribution of meteorological elements in the layer of air near the ground. *Izv. Akad. Nauk SSSR Ser. Geogr. Geofiz.* **10**, No. 4.

Будыко М. И. (1947). О водном и тепловом балансах поверхности суши. Метеорология и гидрология, № 5.

Budyko, M. I. (1947). On the water and heat balances of land surfaces. *Meteorol. Gidrol.* No. 5.

Будыко М. И. (1948). Испарение в естественных условиях. Гидрометеоиздат, Л.

Budyko, M. I. (1948). "Ispareniia v Estestvennykh Usloviiakh." Gidrometeorizdat, Leningrad; "Evaporation Under Natural Conditions." OTS 63-11061. Isr. Program Sci. Transl., Jerusalem, 1963. MGA 16.2-17.

Будыко М. И. (1950). К теории гидрометеорологической эффективности полезащитного лесоразведения. Сб. «Вопросы гидрометеорологической эффективности полезащитного лесоразведения». Гидрометеоиздат, Л.

Budyko, M. I. (1950). On the theory of hydrometeorological effectiveness of shelterbelts. *In* "Voprosy Gidrometeorologicheskoi Effektivnosti Polezashchitnogo Lesorazvedeniia (Problems of the Hydrometeorological Effectiveness of Shelter Belts)." (N. A. Bagrov, ed.) Gidrometeoizdat, Leningrad.

Будыко М. И. (1951). О влиянии мелиоративных мероприятий на испаряемость. Изв. АН СССР, сер. геогр., № 1.

Budyko, M. I. (1951). On the influence of reclamation practices on potential evapotranspiration. *Izv. Akad. Nauk SSSR Ser. Geogr.* No. 1, 16–35. MGA 3.6-130.

Будыко М. И. (1955). Об определении испарения с поверхности суши. Метеорология и гидрология, № 1.

Budyko, M. I. (1955). On the determination of evaporation from the land surface. *Meteorol. Gidrol.* No. 1, 52–58. MGA 10 I-115.

Будыко М. И. (1956). Тепловой баланс земной поверхности. Гидрометеоиздат, Л.

Budyko, M. I. (1956). "Teplovoi Balans Zemnoi Poverkhnosti." Gidrometeoizdat, Leningrad; "Heat Balance of the Earth's Surface," translated by N. A. Stepanova. U.S. Weather Bur., Washington, D.C., 1958. MGA 8.5-20 11B-25 13E-286.

Будыко М. И. (1967). Тепловой баланс атмосферы и равновесный градиент температуры. Сб. «Равновесный градиент температуры». Гидрометеоиздат, Л.

Budyko, M. I. (1967). Heat balance of the atmosphere and the equilibrium gradient of temperature. *In* "Ravnovesnyi Gradient Temperatury (Equilibrium Gradient of Temperature)" (M. I. Budyko and M. I. Iudin, eds.). Gidrometeoizdat, Leningrad.

Будыко М. И., Берлянд Т. Г., Зубенок Л. И. (1954а). Тепловой баланс поверхности Земли. Изв. АН СССР, сер. геогр., №. 3.

Budyko, M. I., Berliand, T. G., and Zubenok, L. I. (1954a). The heat balance of the surface of the Earth. *Izv. Akad. Nauk SSSR Ser. Geogr.* No. 3, 17–41. MGA 7H-61.

Будыко М. И., Берлянд Т. Г., Зубенок Л. И. (1954б). Методика климатологических расчетов составляющих теплового баланса. Труды ГГО, вып. 48.

Budyko, M. I., Berliand, T. G., and Zubenok, L. I. (1954b). The technique of climatological calculation of components of the heat balance. *Tr. Gl. Geofiz. Observ.* **48.**

Будыко М. И., Гандин Л. С. (1966). Об определении турбулентного теплообмена между океаном и атмосферой. Метеорология и гидрология, № 11.

Budyko, M. I., and Gandin, L. S. (1966). On determination of the turbulent heat exchange between ocean and atmosphere. *Meteorol. Gidrol.* No. 11, 15–25. MGA 18.7-436.

Будыко М. И., Ефимова Н. А. (1955). О точности карт составляющих теплового баланса. Труды ГГО, вып. 50.

Budyko, M. I., and Efimova, N. A. (1955). On the accuracy of maps of components of the heat balance. *Tr. Glav. Geofiz. Observ.* **50,** 111–119. MGA 8.5-19.

Будыко М. И. [и др.]. (1952). Изменение климата в связи с планом преобразования природы засушливых районов СССР. Гидрометеоиздат, Л.

Budyko, M. I., Drozdov, O. A., L'vovich, M. I., Sapozhnikova, S. A., and Iudin, M. I. (1952). "Izmenenie Klimata v Sviazi s Planom Preobrazovaniia Prirody Zasushlivykh

Raionov SSSR (Changing the Climate in Connection with the Plan for Transforming Nature in the Drought Regions of the USSR)" (Kh. P. Pogosian, ed.). Gidrometeoizdat, Leningrad. MGA 4.5-1.

Будыко М. И. [и др.]. (1961). Радиационный баланс северного полушария. Изв. АН СССР, сер. геогр., № 1.

Budyko, M. I., Efimova, N. A., Mukhenberg, V. V., and Strokina, L. A. (1961). The radiation budget of the Northern Hemisphere. *Izv. Akad. Nauk SSSR Ser. Geogr.* No. 1, 3–24.

Будыко М. И., Зубенок Л. И. (1961). Определение испарения с поверхности суши. Изв. АН СССР, сер. геогр., № 6.

Budyko, M. I., and Zubenok, L. I. (1961). The determination of evaporation from land surfaces. *Izv. Akad. Nauk SSSR Ser. Geogr.* No. 6, 3–17.

Будыко М. И., Зубенок Л. И., Строкина Л. А. (1956). Определение интегрального коэффициента турбулентной диффузии. Метеорология и гидрология, № 12.

Budyko, M. I., Zubenok, L. I., and Strokina, L. A. (1956). Determination of the integral coefficient of turbulent diffusion. *Meteorol. Gidrol.* No. 12, 34–35.

Будыко М. И., Тимофеев М. П. (1952). О методах определения испарения. Метеорология и гидрология, № 9.

Budyko, M. I., and Timofeev, M. P. (1952). On methods for determining evaporation. *Meteorol. Gidrol.* No. 9.

Будыко М. И., Юдин М. И. (1946). Условия термического равновесия в атмосфере. ДАН СССР, т. 53, № 7.

Budyko, M. I., and Iudin, M. I. (1964). The conditions of thermal equilibrium in the atmosphere. *Dok. Akad. Nauk SSSR* **53**, No. 7.

Будыко М. И., Юдин М. И. (1948). Тепловой обмен поверхности земли с атмосферой и равновесный градиент температуры. Метеорология и гидрология, № 1.

Budyko, M. I., and Iudin, M. I. (1948). Heat exchange of the surface of the earth with the atmosphere and the equilibrium gradient of temperature. *Meteorol. Gidrol.* No. 1.

Винников К. Я. (1965а). Альбедо системы земля—атмосфера и поле уходящей коротковолновой радиации. Труды ГГО, вып. 170.

Vinnikov, K. Ia. (1965a). Albedo of the system earth-atmosphere and the field of outgoing short-wave radiation. *Tr. Gl. Geofiz. Observ.* **170**, 207–211. MGA 17.7-273.

Винников К. Я. (1965б). Уходящее излучение системы земля—атмосфера. Труды ГГО, вып. 168.

Vinnikov, K. Ia. (1965b). Outgoing radiation of the system earth-atmosphere. *Tr. Gl. Geofiz. Observ.* **168**, 123–140. MGA 16.12–324.

Водные ресурсы и водный баланс территории СССР (1967). Междуведомственный комитет СССР по международному гидрологическому десятилетию, ГГИ. Гидрометеоиздат, Л.

Vodnye Resursy i Vodnyi Balans Territorii SSSR (Water resources and water balance of the USSR). *Mezhduvedomstvennyi Komitet SSSR po Mezhdunarodnomu Gidrolog. Desiatiletiiu, Gos. Gidrol. Inst. 1967.* Gidrometeoizdat, Leningrad, 1967. MGA 18.10-14.

Гаевский В. Л. (1961). Альбедо больших территорий. Труды ГГО, вып. 109.

Gaevskii, V. L. (1961). The albedo of extensive areas. *Tr. Gl. Geofiz. Observ.* **109**, 62–75.

Гальперин Б. М. (1949а). К методике приближенных расчетов сумм солнечной радиации. Метеорология и гидрология, № 4.

Gal'perin, B. M. (1949a). On methods of approximate calculation of total solar radiation. *Meteorol. Gidrol.* No. 4.

Гальперин Б. М. (1949б). Радиационный баланс Нижнего Поволжья за теплый период. Труды ГГО, вып. 18.

Gal'perin, B. M. (1949b). The radiation budget of the Lower Volga region in the warm season. *Tr. Gl. Geofiz. Observ.* **18**.

Гальперин Б. М. (1956). Методика приближенных расчетов прихода прямой солнечной радиации по данным станционных метеорологических наблюдений. Труды ЛГМИ, № 4.

Gal'perin, B. M. (1956). A method for approximate calculation of incoming direct solar radiation from data of routine meteorological observations. *Tr. Leningrad. Gidrometeorol. Inst.* No. 4.

Гойса Н. И. (1962). Некоторые закономерности суточного и годового хода радиационного баланса подстилающей поверхности и его составляющих. Труды УкрНИГМИ, вып. 31.

Goisa, N. I. (1962). Some features of the daily and annual marches of the radiation budget of the underlying surface and its components. *Tr. Ukr. Nauch. Issled. Gidrometeorol. Inst.* **31**, 60–81. MGA 14:3006; 16.1-215.

Грабовский Р. И. (1956). Атмосферные ядра конденсации. Гидрометеоиздат, Л.

Grabovskii, R. I. (1956). "Atmosfernye Iadra Kondensatsii (Atmospheric Condensation Nuclei)." Gidrometeoizdat, Leningrad. MGA 9.1-8.

Дьяченко Л. Н., Кондратьев К. Я. (1965). Распределение длинноволнового баланса атмосферы по земному шару. Труды ГГО, вып. 170.

D'iachenko, L. N., and Kondrat'ev, K. Ia. (1965). The global distribution of the long-wave radiation budget of the atmosphere. *Tr. Gl. Geofiz. Observ.* **170**, 192–201. MGA 17.7-263.

Евфимов Н. Г. (1939). Величина сумм эффективного излучения для некоторых пунктов СССР. Метеорология и гидрология, № 5.

Evfimov, N. G. (1939). Values of total net long-wave radiation at several points in the USSR. *Meteorol. Gidrol.* No. 5.

Ефимова Н. А. (1961). К методике расчета месячных величин эффективного излучения. Метеорология и гидрология, № 10.

Efimova, N. A. (1961). On methods of calculating monthly values of net long-wave radiation. *Meteorol. Gidrol.* No. 10, 28–33. MGA 13.9-523.

Зубенок Л. И. (1947). К вопросу об измерении температуры поверхности почвы. Труды ГГО, вып. 6.

Zubenok, L. I. (1947). On the problem of measuring the temperature of the soil surface. *Tr. Gl. Geofiz. Observ.* **6**.

Зубенок Л. И. (1966а). Обоснование метода расчета месячных сумм испарения. Материалы междуведомственного совещания по проблеме изучения и обоснования метода расчета испарения с поверхности суши и воды. Изд. ГГИ, Валдай.

Zubenok, L. I. (1966a). The basis of a method for calculating monthly sums of evaporation. *Mater. Mezhduvedomstvennogo Soveshchaniia po Probleme Izucheniia i Obosnovaniia Metoda Rascheta Ispareniia s Poverkhnosti Sushi i Vody (Proc. Interdept. Conf. Study of Bases of Methods of Calculating Evaporation from the Surfaces of Land and Water).* Izdat. Gos. Gidrol. Inst. Valdai.

Зубенок Л. И. (1966б). Роль испарения в тепловом балансе суши. Сб. «Современные проблемы климатологии». Гидрометеоиздат, Л.

Zubenok, L. I. (1966b). The role of evaporation in the heat balance of the land. *In* "Sovremennye Problemy Klimatologii (Contemporary Problems of Climatology)," (M. I. Budyko, ed.), pp. 57–66. Gidrometeoizdat, Leningrad. MGA 18.12-236.

Зубенок Л. И. (1968). Об определении суммарного испарения за отдельные годы. Труды ГГО, вып. 233.

Zubenok, L. I. (1968). Determination of evapotranspiration in individual years. *Tr. Gl. Geofiz. Observ.* **233**, 101–109. MGA 20.6-379.

Кастров В. Г. (1928). К вопросу об основной актинометрической формуле. Метеорол. вестн., № 7.

Kastrov, V. G. (1928). On the question of the basic actinometric formula. *Meteorol. Vestn.* No. 7.

Кириллова Т. В. (1952). О зависимости противоизлучения от степени облачности. Труды ГГО, вып. 37.

Kirillova, T. V. (1952). The dependence of downward long-wave radiation on the degree of cloudiness. *Tr. Gl. Geofiz. Observ.* **37.**

Кириллова Т. В. (1970). Радиационный режим озер и водохранилищ. Гидрометеоиздат, Л.

Kirillova, T. V. (1970). "Radiatsionnyi Rezhim Ozer i Vodokhranilishch. (The Radiation Regime of Lakes and Reservoirs)." Gidrometeoizdat, Leningrad.

Кириллова Т. В., Ковалева Е. Д. (1951). О введении поправок при определении эффективного излучения и противоизлучения по наземным данным. Труды ГГО, вып. 27.

Kirillova, T. V., and Kovaleva, E. D. (1951). The introduction of corrections in determining net and downward long-wave radiation from near-surface data. *Tr. Gl. Geofiz. Observ.* **27.**

Кириллова Т. В., Кучеров Н. В. (1953). Сравнение результатов измерения лучистых потоков по различным приборам. Труды ГГО, вып. 39.

Kirillova, T. V., and Kucherov, N. V. (1953). Comparison of the results of measuring radiative fluxes with different instruments. *Tr. Gl. Geofiz. Observ.* **39.**

Кондратьев К. Я. (1951). К вопросу о приближенном вычислении эффективного излучения с земной поверхности. Инф. сб. № 1. Динамическая и сельскохозяйственная метеорология. Гидрометеоиздат, Л.

Kondrat'ev, K. Ia. (1951). On the approximate calculation of net long-wave radiation at the earth's surface. *Inform. Sb. Leningrad Dinamicheskaia i Sel'skokhoziaistvennaia Meteorol.* **No. 1,** 88–90. MGA 3:600.

Кондратьев К. Я. (1954). Лучистая энергия солнца. Гидрометеоиздат, Л.

Kondrat'ev, K. Ia. (1954). "Luchistaia Energiia Solntsa (Radiative Energy of the Sun)." Gidrometeoizdat, Leningrad. MGA 8.5-8.

Кондратьев К. Я. (1956). Лучистый теплообмен в атмосфере. Гидрометеоиздат, Л.

Kondrat'ev, K. Ia. (1956). "Luchistyi Teploobmen v Atmosfere." Gidrometeoizdat, Leningrad. MGA 8.7-8; "Radiative Heat Exchange in the Atmosphere," (C. D. Walshaw, ed.), rev. enlarged ed., transl. by O. Tedder. Pergamon, Oxford, 1965. MGA 16.12-5.

Кондратьев К. Я. (1965). Актинометрия. Гидрометеоиздат, Л.

Kondrat'ev, K. Ia. (1965). "Aktinometriia." Gidrometeoizdat, Leningrad; Actinometry. *NASA Tech. Trans.* **TT F-9712** (1965). MGA 17.8-2.

Кондратьев К. Я., Филиппович О. П. (1952). Об уходящем излучении. Вестн. ЛГУ, сер. мат., физ., хим., № 6.

Kondrat'ev, K. Ia., and Filippovich, O. P. (1952). On outgoing radiation. *Vestn. Leningrad. Univ., Ser. Mat. Fiz. Khim.* No. 6.

Константинов А. Р. (1968). Испарение в природе. Изд. второе. Гидрометеоиздат, Л.

Konstantinov, A. R. (1968). "Isparenie v Prirode," 2nd ed. Gidrometeoizdat, Leningrad. MGA 20.11-12; "Evaporation in Nature," transl. of 1st ed. Isr. Program Sci. Transl., Jerusalem, 1966. MGA 18.10-13.

Кузин П. С. (1934). График испарения с поверхности речного бассейна и его применение к расчету среднего многолетнего стока. Зап. ГГИ, т. 12.

Kuzin, P. S. (1934). A graph of evaporation from the surface of a river basin and its application to the calculation of mean long-term runoff. *Zap. Gos. Gidrol. Inst.* **12.**

Кузин П. С. (1938). Об испарении с поверхности почвы. Труды ГГИ, вып. 7.

Kuzin, P. S. (1938). On evaporation from the surface of the soil. *Tr. Gos. Gidrol. Inst.* **7**.

Кузин П. С. (1940). Карта испарения с поверхности речных бассейнов Союза ССР. Метеорология и гидрология, № 11.

Kuzin, P. S. (1940). A map of evaporation from the surface of river basins of the Soviet Union. *Meteorol. Gidrol.* No. 11.

Кузин П. С. (1950). Испарение с суши на территории СССР. Труды ГГИ, вып. 26.

Kuzin, P. S. (1950). Evaporation from land in the USSR. *Tr. Gos. Gidrol. Inst.* **26**.

Кузьмин П. П. (1938). Теплоотдача моря в воздух путем конвекции. Метеорология и гидрология, №. 2.

Kuz'min, P. P. (1938). Heat transfer from sea to air by means of convection. *Meteorol. Gidrol.* No. 2.

Кузьмин П. П. (1947). Опыт исследования теплового и водного балансов снеготаяния. Труды ГГИ, вып. 1.

Kuz'min, P. P. (1947). Experimental investigation of the heat and water balances of snow melting. *Tr. Gos. Gidrol. Inst.* **1**.

Кузьмин П. П. (1948). Исследование и расчет снеготаяния. Труды ГГИ, вып. 7.

Kuz'min, P. P. (1948). Investigation and calculation of snow melting. *Tr. Gos. Gidrol. Inst.* **7**.

Кузьмин П. П. (1950). Метод определения максимальной интенсивности снеготаяния. Труды ГГИ, вып. 24.

Kuz'min, P. P. (1950). A method for determining the maximum intensity of snow melting. *Tr. Gos. Gidrol. Inst.* **24**.

Кузьмин П. П. (1966). Теоретическая схема оценки ошибок расчета испарения с поверхности суши. Материалы междуведомственного совещания по проблеме изучения и обоснования методов расчета испарения с поверхности суши и воды. Изд. ГГИ, Валдай.

Kuz'min, P. P. (1966). A theoretical model for evaluating errors in the calculation of evaporation from the soil surface. *Mater. Mezhduvedomstvennogo Soveshchaniia po Probleme Izucheniia i Obosnovaniia Metodov Rascheta Ispareniia s Poverkhnosti Sushi i Vody* (*Proc. Interdept. Conf. Study of Bases of Methods of Calculating Evaporation from the Surfaces of Land and Water*). Izdat. Gos. Gidrol. Inst. Valdai.

Лайхтман Д. Л. (1947). Трансформация воздушной массы под влиянием подстилающей поверхности. Метеорология и гидрология, № 1.

Laikhtman, D. L. (1947). Transformation of air masses under the influence of the underlying surface. *Meteorol. Gidrol.* No. 1.

Лебедева К. Д., Сивков С. И. (1962). О точности измерений радиационного баланса термоэлектрическими балансомерами. Труды ГГО, вып. 129.

Lebedeva, K. D., and Sivkov, S. I. (1962). On the accuracy of measurements of the radiation balance by thermoelectric balance-meters. *Tr. Gl. Geofiz. Observ.* **129**.

Львович М. И. (1945). Элементы водного режима рек земного шара. Труды НИУ ГУГМС, сер. IV, вып. 18.

L'vovich, M. I. (1945). Elements of the water regime of the rivers of the world. *Tr. Gl. Upr. Gidrometeorol. Sluzhby Nauch. Issled. Uchrezhdeniia* [4] **18**.

Малевский-Малевич С. П. (1970). Влияние «холодной пленки» на теплообмен океан—атмосфера. Труды ГГО, вып. 257.

Malevskii-Malevich, S. P. (1970). The influence of the "cold film" on the heat exchange ocean—atmosphere. *Tr. Gl. Geofiz. Observ.* **257**, 35–45. MGA 23.2-341.

Мезенцев В. С., Карнацевич И. В. (1969). Увлажненность Западно-Сибирской равнины. Гидрометеоиздат, Л.

Mezentsev, V. S., and Karnatsevich, I. V. (1969). "Uvlazhnennost' Zapadno-Sibirskoi Ravniny (Moisture Conditions of the West Siberian Plain)." Gidrometeoizdat, Leningrad.

Мухенберг В. В. (1962). Альбедо поверхности суши северного полушария. Ин-т геологии и географии АН ЛитССР. Научные сообщения, т. XIII.

Mukhenberg, V. V. (1962). Albedo of the land surface of the Northern Hemisphere. *Liet. TSR Mokslu Akad. Geol. Geogr. Inst. Moksliniai Pranesimai* **13**, 175–179.

Мухенберг В. В. (1963). Альбедо подстилающей поверхности территории Советского Союза. Труды ГГО, вып. 139.

Mukhenberg, V. V. (1963). Albedo of the underlying surface of the territory of the Soviet Union. *Tr. Gl. Geofiz. Observ.* **139**.

Обухов А. М. (1946). Турбулентность в температурно-неоднородной атмосфере. Труды Ин-та теоретической геофизики, т. 1.

Obukhov, A. M. (1946). Turbulence in the thermally inhomogeneous atmosphere. *Tr. Inst. Teor. Geofiz. Akad. Nauk SSSR* **1**, 95–115. MGA 1.1-98.

Ольдекоп Э. М. (1911). Об испарении с поверхности речных бассейнов. Труды Юрьевской обсерватории.

Ol'dekop, E. M. (1911). Ob Isparenii s Poverkhnosti Rechnykh Basseinov (On Evaporation from the Surface of River Basins). *Tr. Meteorolog. Observ. Iur'evskogo Univ. Tartu*, **4**.

Поляков Б. В. (1946). Гидрологический анализ и расчеты. Гидрометеоиздат, Л.

Poliakov, B. V. (1946). "Gidrologicheskii Analiz i Raschety (Hydrologic Analysis and Calculations)." Gidrometeoizdat, Leningrad.

Поляков Б. В. (1947). Измерение влажности почв и прогноз их просыхания. Труды ЦИП, вып. 4(31).

Poliakov, B. V. (1947). Measurement of soil moisture and forecasting of soil drying. *Tr. Tsent. Inst. Prognozov*, **4** (31).

Ракипова Л. Р. (1957). Тепловой режим атмосферы. Гидрометеоиздат, Л.

Rakipova, L. R. (1957). "Teplovoi Rezhim Atmosfery (Thermal Regime of the Atmosphere)." Gidrometeoizdat, Leningrad. MGA 10.9-9.

Руководство по производству наблюдений за испарением с сельскохозяйственных полей, ч. I. (1957). ГГИ. Гидрометеоиздат, Л.

"Rukovodstvo po Proizvodstvu Nabliudenii za Ispareniem s Sel'skokhoziaistvennykh Polei," Chapter I "(Manual for Observing Evaporation from Agricultural Lands)," Pt. I. Gos. Gidrol. Inst. Gidrometeoizdat, Leningrad, 1957.

Руководство по градиентным наблюдениям и определению составляющих теплового баланса. (1964). Гидрометеоиздат, Л.

"Rukovodstvo po Gradientnym Nabliudeniiam i Opredeleniiu Sostavliaiushchikh Teplovogo Balansa (Manual for Gradient Observations and Determination of Components of the Heat Balance)." Gidrometeoizdat, Leningrad, 1964.

Рыкачев М. А. (1898). Новый испаритель для наблюденнй над испарением травы. Зап. АН, т. VII, № 3.

Rykachev, M. A. (1898). A new evaporimeter for observations on the evaporation of grass. *Akad. Nauk. Zap.* **7**, No. 3.

Савинов С. И. (1925). Солнечная, земная и атмосферная радиация. Климат и погода, № 2—3.

Savinov, S. I. (1925). Solar, terrestrial, and atmospheric radiation. *Klimat i Pogoda* No. 2–3.

Савинов С. И. (1928). По поводу статьи Кастрова «К вопросу об основной актинометрической формуле». Метеорол. вестн., № 7.

Savinov, S. I. (1928). Apropos the article by Kastrov, "On the question of the basic actinometric formula." *Meteorol. Vestn.* No. 7.

Савинов С. И. (1933). Соотношения между облачностью, продолжительностью солнечного сияния и суммами прямой и рассеянной радиации. Метеорол. вестн., № 1.

Savinov, S. I. (1933). The relationships between cloudiness, duration of sunshine, and totals of direct and scattered radiation. *Meteorol. Vestn.* No. 1.

Сивков С. И. (1952). Географическое распределение эффективных величин альбедо водной поверхности. Изв. ВГО, т. 84, № 2.

Sivkov, S. I. (1952). The geographic distribution of effective values of the albedo of water surfaces. *Izv. Vses. Geogr. Obshchestva* **84**, (No. 2) 200–201. MGA 8G-103.

Солнеччая Радиация и Радиационный Баланс (Мировая Сеть). Всесмир. Метеорол. Орган. и Гиав. Геофиз. Обсерв, им. Воейкова, Гидрометеоиздат, Л. (Мес., 1964–.) Solar Radiation and Radiation Balance Data (The World Network). World Meteorol. Org. and Glav. Geofiz. Observ. im. Voeikova. Gidrometeoizdat, Leningrad (mon., 1964–.) [Russ. and Engl.]

Строкина Л. А. (1963). Теплообмен поверхности океана с нижележашими слоями воды. Метеорология и гидрология, № 1.

Strokina, L. A. (1963). Heat exchange of the ocean surface with the underlying water layers. *Meteorol. Gidrol.* No. 1, 25–30. MGA 14.9-419.

Строкина Л. А. (1967а). Определение изменения теплосодержания океанов. Труды ГГО, вып. 209.

Strokina, L. A. (1967a). Determination of variation in the heat content of the oceans. *Tr. Gl. Geofiz. Observ.* **209**, 58–69. MGA 19.10-726.

Строкина Л. А. (1967б). О сравнении рассчитанных и наблюденных величин радиационного баланса океанов. Труды ГГО, вып. 193.

Strokina, L. A. (1967b). Comparison of computed and observed values of the radiation budget of the oceans. *Tr. Gl. Geofiz. Observ.* **193**, 44–46. MGA 19.9-368.

Строкина Л. А. (1968). Изучение радиационного режима океанов. Метеорология и гидрология, № 10.

Strokina, L. A. (1968). Study of the radiation regime of the oceans. *Meteorol. Gidrol.* No. 10, 77–83. MGA 20.7-295.

Тимофеев М. П. (1963). Метеорологический режим водоемов. Гидрометеоиздат, Л.

Timofeev, M. P. (1963). "Meteorologicheskii Rezhim Vodoemov (The Meteorological Regime of Water Bodies)." Gidrometeoizdat, Leningrad. MGA 16.10-4.

Тооминг Х. Г. (1961). О дневном ходе альбедо поверхности, покрытой растительностью. Актинометрия и атмосферная оптика. Гидрометеоиздат, Л.

Tooming, Kh. G. (1961). The daily march of albedo of surfaces covered with vegetation. "Aktinometriia i Atmosfernaia Optika," pp. 236–237. Gidrometeoizdat, Leningrad; (*Tr. Mezhvedomstvennoe Soveshch. Aktinomet. Atmosf. Opt., 2nd, Leningrad, 1959*), MGA 14:258.

Троицкий В. А. (1948). Гидрологическое районирование СССР. Труды Комиссии по ест.-ист. районир. СССР, т. II, вып. 3.

Troitskii, V. A. (1948). Hydrologic regionalization of the USSR. *Tr. Kom. Est.-Ist. Raionirov. SSSR* Book 2, vyp. [3].

Украинцев В. Н. (1939). Приближенное вычисление сумм прямой и рассеянной радиации. Метеорология и гидрология, № 6.

Ukraintsev, V. N. (1939). An approximate calculation of total direct and scattered radiation. *Meteorol. Gidrol.* No. 6.

Федосеева А. И. (1953). Альбедо системы Земля—атмосфера и его распределение по земному шару. Труды ГГО, вып. 41.

Fedoseeva, A. I. (1953). Albedo of the earth-atmosphere system and its global distribution. *Tr. Gl. Geofiz. Observ.* **41**.

Цейтин Г. Х. (1953). К вопросу об определении некоторых тепловых свойств почвы. Труды ГГО, вып. 39.

Tseitin, G. Kh. (1953). On the question of determining some thermal properties of the soil. *Tr. Gl. Geofiz. Observ.* **39**.

Шехтер Ф. М. (1950). К вычислению лучистых потоков тепла в атмосфере. Труды ГГО, вып. 22.

Shekhter, F. M. (1950). On the calculation of radiative heat fluxes in the atmosphere. *Tr. Gl. Geofiz. Observ.* **22**.

Шулейкин В. В. (1935). Элементы теплового режима Карского моря. Труды Таймырской гидрографической экспедиции, ч. 2.

Shuleikin, V. V. (1935). Elements of the thermal regime of the Kara Sea. *Tr. Taimyrskii Gidrograf. Ekspeditsiia* Pt. 2.

Шулейкин В. В. (1941, 1953). Физика моря. Изд. АН СССР, Л.—М.

Shuleikin, V. V. (1941, 1953). "Fizika Moria (Physics of the Sea)." Izdat. Akad. Nauk SSSR, Leningrad and Moscow. MGA 13E-289.

Юдин М. И. (1948). Суточный ход температуры и конвективный теплообмен. Изв. АН СССР, сер. геогр. и геофиз., № 4.

Iudin, M. I. (1948). The diurnal march of temperature and convective heat exchange. *Izv. Akad. Nauk SSSR Ser. Geogr. Geofiz.* No. 4.

Юдин М. И. (1967). Турбулентный поток тепла в пограничном слое атмосферы. Сб. «Равновесный градиент температуры». Гидрометеоиздат, Л.

Iudin, M. I. (1967). Turbulent heat flux in the boundary layer of the atmosphere. *In* "Ravnovesnyi Gradient Temperatury (Equilibrium Gradient of Temperature)." (M. I. Budyko and M. I. Iudin, eds.) Gidrometeoizdat, Leningrad.

Ярославцев И. Н. (1952). Альбедо естественного покрова почвы в Ташкенте. Изв. АН СССР, сер. геофиз., № 1.

Iaroslavtsev, I. N. (1952). Albedo of the natural soil cover at Tashkent. *Izv. Akad. Nauk SSSR Ser. Geofiz* No. 1, 85–88. MGA 8G-96.

Albrecht, F. (1940). Untersuchungen über den Wärmehaushalt der Erdoberfläche in verschiedenen Klimagebieten. *Wiss. Abh. Reichsamt Wetterdienst*, **8**, No. 2.

Albrecht, F. (1951). Die Methoden zur Bestimmung der Verdunstung der natürlichen Erdoberfläche. *Arch. Meteorol. Geophys. Bioklimatol. Ser. B* **2**, Pt. 1–2.

Albrecht, F. (1952). Strahlung- und Wärmehaushaltsuntersuchungen während einer Seereise durch den Indischen Ozean im Juni 1949. *Berr. Deut. Wetterdienstes* **7**, No. 42.

Angot, A. (1883). Recherches théoriques sur la distribution de la chaleur à la surface du globe. *Ann Bur. Cent. Météorol. de France*, Paris. [Publ. 1885].

Asklöf, S. (1920). Über den Zusammenhang zwischen der nächtlichen Wärmeausstrahlung, der Bewölkung und der Wolkenart, *Georg. Ann.* **2**, no. 3, pp. 253–259.

Bandeen, W. R., Halev, M., and Strange, I. (1965). A radiation climatology in the visible and infrared from the TIROS meteorological satellites. *NASA Tech. Note* **NASA TN D-2534**.

Bernhardt, F., und Philipps, H. (1958). Die räumliche und zeitliche Verteilung der Einstrahlung, der Ausstrahlung und der Strahlungsbilanz im Meeresniveau., Pt. 1 *Abh. Meteorol. Hydrogr. Dienstes DDR* No. **45**.

Black, J. N. (1956). The distribution of solar radiation over the Earth's surface. *Arch. Meteorol. Geophys. Bioklimatol., Ser. B*, **7**, No. 2.

Bolz, H. (1949). Die Abhängigkeit der infraroten Gegenstrahlung von der Bewölkung. *Z. Meteorol.* **3**, Pt. 7.

Brunt, D. (1932). Notes on the radiation in the atmosphere, I. *Quart. J. Roy. Meteorol. Soc.*, **58**, no. 247, pp. 389–418.

Dieulafait, L. (1883). Evaporation de l'eau de mer dans la sud de France et en particulier dans le delta du Rhône. *C. R. Acad. Sci.* **96.**

Elsasser, W. H., and Culbertson, M. F. (1960). "Atmospheric Radiation Tables." Meteorol. Monogr. Am. Meteorol. Soc., Boston.

Fritz, S. (1949). The albedo of the planet Earth and of clouds. *J. Meteorol.* **6**, No. 4.

Fritz, S. (1958). Seasonal heat storage in the ocean and heating of the atmosphere. *Arch. Meteor. Geophys. Bioklimatol. Ser. A*, **10**, Pt. 4.

Garstang, M. (1965). Sensible and latent heat exchange in low latitude synoptic scale systems. *Proc. Sea-Air Interaction Conf., Tallahassee, Fla., 1965*, U.S. Weather Bureau, Tech. Note 9-SAIL-1, Washington, D.C.

Giblett, M. A. (1921). Some problems connected with evaporation from large expanses of water. *Proc. Roy. Soc. Ser. A* **99**, No. 701.

Holzman, B. (1943). The influence of stability on evaporation. *Ann. N.Y. Acad. Sci.* **44.**

Jeffreys, H. (1918). Some problems of evaporation. *Phil. Mag.* [6], **35**, No. 207.

Kimball, H. (1928). Amount of solar radiation that reaches the surface of the earth on the land and on the sea, and methods by which it is measured. *Mon. Weather Rev.* **56**, No. 10.

Kondrat'ev, K. Ya., and Niilisk, H. J. (1960). The new radiation chart. *Geofis. Pura Appl.* **49**, 197–207.

Kraus, E. B., and Morrison, R. E. (1966). Local interactions between the sea and the air at monthly and annual time scales. *Quart. J. Roy. Meteorol. Soc.* **92**, No. 391.

Linke, F. (1934). "Meteorologisches Taschenbuch." Akad. Verlagsges., Leipzig.

London, J. (1957). A study of the atmospheric heat balance. Final Rep. Contract No. AF 19(122)—165, New York Univ., New York.

Malkus, J. (1962). Climatology of energy exchange and the global heat and water budgets. *In* "The Sea," (M. N. Hill, ed.) Wiley (Interscience), New York.

Manabe, S., Bryan, K. (1969). Climate and the ocean circulation. *Mon. Weather Rev.*, **97**, No. 11.

Milankovich, M. (1930). "Mathematische Klimalehre und astronomische Theorie der Klimaschwankungen." Gebrüder Borntraeger, Berlin (*Hdbuch. Klimatol.*, Bd. 1, Teil A) (Русский перевод: М. Миланкович. Математическая климатология и астрономическая теория колебаний климата. ОНТИ, М., 1938.)

Montgomery, R. B. (1940). Observations of vertical humidity distribution above the ocean surface and their relation to evaporation. *Pap. Phys. Ocean. Meteorol.* **7**, No. 4.

Montgomery, R. B. (1947). Problems concerning convective layers. *Ann. N.Y. Acad. Sci.* **48.**

Mosby, H. (1936). Verdunstung und Strahlung auf dem Meere. *Ann. Hydrog. Marit. Meteorol.* **64**, Pt. 7.

Prandtl, L. (1932). Meteorologische Anwendungen der Strömungslehre. *Beitr. Phys. Freien Atmos.* **19**, No. 3. *Bjerknes Festschrift.*

Priestley, C. H. B. (1959). "Turbulent Transfer in the Lower Atmosphere." Univ. Chicago Press, Chicago, Illinois.

Radiation instruments and measurements. 1958. "Annals of the International Geophysical Year." Vol. V, pt. VI. Pergamon, Oxford.

Raschke, E., Möller, F., and Bandeen, W. (1968). The radiation balance of the earth—atmosphere system over both polar regions obtained from radiation measurements of the Nimbus II meteorological satellite. *Sver. Meteorol. Hydrol. Inst. Meddelanden Ser. B*, No. 28.

Robinson, G. D. (1966). Another look at some problems of the air-sea interface. *Quart. J. Roy. Meteorol. Soc.* **92**, No. 394.

Rossby, C.-G. (1932). A generalization of the theory of the mixing length with applications to atmospheric and oceanic turbulence. *Mass. Inst. Techol. Meteorol. Pap.* **1**, No. 4.

Rossby, C.-G. (1936). On the momentum transfer at the sea surface. *Pap. Phys. Ocean. Meteorol.* **4**, No. 3.

Rossby, C.-G., and Montgomery, R. B. (1935). The layer of the frictional influence in wind and ocean currents. *Pap. Phys. Ocean. Meteorol.* **3**, No. 3.

Schmidt, W. (1915). Strahlung und Verdunstung an freien Wasserflächen; ein Beitrag zum Wärmehaushalt des Weltmeers und zum Wasserhaushalt der Erde. *Ann. Hydrog. marit. Meteorol.* **43**, Pt. 3 and 4.

Schmidt, W. (1917). Der Massenaustausch bei der ungeordneten Strömung in freier Luft und seine Folgen. *Akad. Wiss. Wien Math. Naturwiss. Naturwiss. Kl. Abt.* 2A **126**.

Schmidt, W. (1925). "Der Massenaustausch in freier Luft und verwandte Erscheinungen." H. Grand, Hamburg.

Schmidt, W. (1935). Turbulence near the ground. *J. Roy. Aeronaut. Soc.* **39**.

Sutton, O. G. (1934). Wind structure and evaporation in a turbulent atmosphere. *Proc. Roy. Soc. Ser. A*, **146**.

Sutton, O. G. (1953). "Micrometeorology." McGraw-Hill, New York. (Русский перевод: Сеттон. Микрометеорология. Гидрометеоиздат, Л., 1958.)

Sverdrup, H. U. (1936a). Das maritime Verdunstungsproblem. *Ann. Hydrog. Marit. Meteorol.* **44**, Pt. 2.

Sverdrup, H. U. (1936b). The eddy conductivity of the air over a smooth snow field. *Geofys. Publ.* **11**, No. 7.

Sverdrup, H. U. (1937). On the evaporation from the oceans. *J. Mar. Res.* **1**, No. 1.

Taylor, G. I. (1915). Eddy motion in the atmosphere. *Phil. Trans. Roy. Soc. Ser. A.* **215**.

Thornthwaite, C. W., and Holzman, B. (1939). The determination of evaporation from land and water surfaces. *Mon. Rev. Weather* **67**, No. 1.

Thornthwaite, C. W., and Holzman, B. (1942). Measurement of evaporation from land and water surfaces. Tech. Bull. No. 817. U.S. Dept. of Agricult. Washington, D.C.

Turc, L. (1955). Le bilan d'eau des sols. Paris [Univ.], Thèse dactylogr. (Русский перевод: Тюрк. Баланс почвенной влаги. Гидрометеоиздат, Л. 1958.)

Vonder Haar, T. H., and Suomi, V. E. (1969). Satellite observation of the Earth's radiation budget. *Science* **163**, 667–669.

Wu, J. (1969). Wind stress and surface roughness at air-sea interface. *J. Geophys. Res.* **74**, No. 2.

Wundt, W. (1937). Beziehungen zwischen Mittelwerten von Niederschlag, Abfluss, Verdunstung und Lufttemperatur für die Landfläche der Erde. *Deut. Wasserwirtschaft* Pt. 5–6.

Ångström, A. (1916). Über die Gegenstrahlung der Atmosphäre. *Meteorol. Z.* **33**, No. 12, pp. 529–538.

Ångström, A. (1920). Application of heat radiation measurements to the problems of evaporation from lakes and the heat convection at their surface. *Geogr. Ann.* **2**.

Ångström, A. (1922). Note on the relation between time of sunshine and cloudiness in Stockholm 1908–1920. *Arch. Mat. Astron. Fys.* **17**, No. 15.

Ångström, A. (1957). On the computation of global radiation from records on sunshine. *Ark. Geof.* **2**, Pt. 5.

III

Heat Balance of the Globe

1. Geographical Distribution of the Components of the Heat Balance

Determination of norms of the heat-balance components

As a result of numerous studies aimed at the determination of the components of the heat balance in different geographical regions, we now possess considerable material permitting us to investigate in detail the geographical distribution of all the principal balance components. One can use for this purpose both data of actual observations of the several balance components and also calculation results obtained by using the methods described in the previous chapter.

The most extensive observational materials relate to the radiation balance at the earth's surface, and especially to the total solar radiation.

As indicated earlier, total short-wave radiation has been measured for many years at a number of stations. Data from mass observations of the radiation balance started, in general, to accumulate in the 1950s, during the period of preparation and activity of the International Geophysical Year.

A considerable portion of the available observational data on elements of the radiation regime relates to comparatively short periods of time. Nevertheless, these data are widely used for determining norms [or long-term means] of monthly and annual values of total short-wave radiation and the radiation balance at the earth's surface. To clarify the accuracy of these norms, it is necessary to evaluate the variability of elements of the radiation regime.

The problem of variability of monthly and annual values of solar radiation has been discussed in several papers, the authors of which noted the comparative stability of the annual sums and the somewhat larger variability of monthly values, especially in winter. In some studies, conclusions were drawn concerning the duration of an observational series that would ensure definitive accuracy in calculating norms of radiation-regime indices.

The first study of this kind was carried out by Gorlenko (1933), who, as a result of analyzing observational data on short-wave radiation, came to the conclusion that 2–3 yr of observations are enough to ensure an error smaller than 10% in calculating norms of monthly sums.

Goisa (1959), after examining data from the 20-yr period of observations at Karadag, established the fact that the monthly means of total short-wave radiation obtained from a 10-yr series of observations were determined with an error comparable to the probable error in measurement.

The problem of accuracy in calculating mean monthly and annual sums of short-wave radiation was considered in a most detailed way by Tarnizhevskii (1959). On the basis of 10–15 yr of observations conducted at Karadag, Pavlovsk, Tashkent, and Odessa, and using Student's criterion, Tarnizhevskii established the number of years ensuring the necessary accuracy of the monthly and annual means of direct, scattered, and total solar radiation at these points. According to his data, annual means of total radiation can be found with an accuracy up to 10% from a 3-yr series of observations at both Tashkent and Pavlovsk, notwithstanding the great difference in the climatic conditions of these places.

The same accuracy (10%) of the monthly means of total radiation for conditions of Tashkent is ensured by 3–4 yr of observations in summer and 7–10 yr in winter. For Pavlovsk, an observational period for obtaining of monthly sums with an accuracy of 10% in summer increases to 5–6 yr and in winter to 15–25 yr. However, it must be remembered that in winter, the errors in the mean monthly sums determined from a short series are small in absolute value. This permits using short observational periods for evaluation of the total radiation norms in many cases in winter as well as in summer.

T. G. Berliand (1961) calculated monthly and annual means of total short-wave radiation by separate 5-yr, 10-yr, and 20-yr periods, and also moving means for these periods, at a number of Soviet and foreign stations that represent the most diverse climatic conditions. By analyzing these data, Berliand concluded that a 10-yr period of observations ensures the accuracy necessary for most investigations. Under climatic conditions that vary little (low latitudes), a 7-yr series of observations might suffice for obtaining reliable monthly means of total short-wave radiation.

In the monograph, "Радиационный режим территории СССР (Radiation Regime of the USSR)" (Barashkova et al., 1961), monthly means of total short-wave radiation for 5-yr periods were compared with the means for

18–20 yr series of observations at several points. From this comparison, it became clear that in 70% of the cases the monthly means over single 5-yr periods did not deviate more than 5% from the means of the 18–20-yr period.

To evaluate the variability of total short-wave radiation, the author and Efimova (1964) used observations for 22 yr (1940–1961) at one of the best actinometric stations—Vysokaia Dubrava (in the region of Sverdlovsk). In Table 14 are given the monthly and annual means of radiation according to data from this station for the 22-yr period and for two 10-yr periods. Also presented are values of the root-mean-square (rms) deviation for each quantity in individual years.

The data of Table 14 show that the discrepancies between the radiation means for the 10- and the 22-yr periods are very small and lie, in general, within the limits of accuracy of measurement. From the values of rms deviations, we can draw the conclusion that variability of radiation monthly sums is small in comparison with its annual cycle. Taking into account the available maps of norms for total short-wave radiation, we may also infer that the variability of monthly sums is usually much less than the geographical variability over extensive areas.

Thus, total short-wave radiation is a meteorological element that is rather stable in time. For a reliable determination of its norms, 10-yr observational periods are quite sufficient, and for an orienting estimate of mean conditions of the annual cycle and of spatial variability, one might use much shorter periods.

The question of variability of monthly and annual sums of the radiation balance has been investigated less than the similar question for solar radiation, since mass observational data on the radiation balance appeared a comparatively short time ago.

Some conclusions about variability of the radiation balance are contained in a paper of Efimova (1956), analyzing the anomalies of monthly values of the radiation balance. She established the fact that the effect of cloudiness on the radiation balance in middle latitudes depends on the season. In winter, an increase of cloudiness is associated with a reduction in radiative losses of heat through the exchange of long-wave radiation, and monthly sums of the radiation balance increase. In summer, the radiation balance in most cases increases with a decrease in cloudiness; however, because the reduction of cloudiness leads not only to an increase in solar radiation but also to an increase in the net long-wave radiation [deficit], variations in the monthly values of the radiation balance do not turn out to be very great.

This study was done by the use of calculation methods for determination of anomalies in the radiation balance. At the present time, there is a possibility of evaluating the variability of monthly and annual sums of the

TABLE 14

MEAN MONTHLY AND ANNUAL VALUES OF TOTAL SHORTWAVE RADIATION AT VYSOKAIA DUBRAVA (NUMERATOR) AND ROOT-MEAN-SQUARE DEVIATIONS FOR SINGLE YEARS (DENOMINATOR) (in kcal cm^{-2} per month or year)

Years	Jan.	Feb.	Mar.	Apr.	May	June	July	Aug.	Sept.	Oct.	Nov.	Dec.	Year
1940–1961	$\frac{1.7}{0.17}$	$\frac{3.7}{0.40}$	$\frac{8.0}{0.81}$	$\frac{10.6}{1.20}$	$\frac{13.8}{1.51}$	$\frac{15.1}{1.08}$	$\frac{14.1}{1.33}$	$\frac{11.4}{1.04}$	$\frac{6.7}{1.02}$	$\frac{3.6}{0.54}$	$\frac{1.9}{0.28}$	$\frac{1.1}{0.12}$	$\frac{92}{3.95}$
1942–1951	$\frac{1.8}{0.19}$	$\frac{3.8}{0.35}$	$\frac{8.0}{0.97}$	$\frac{10.4}{1.15}$	$\frac{13.9}{1.81}$	$\frac{15.1}{1.10}$	$\frac{13.8}{1.19}$	$\frac{11.3}{1.16}$	$\frac{6.6}{0.76}$	$\frac{3.8}{0.48}$	$\frac{2.0}{0.30}$	$\frac{1.2}{0.10}$	$\frac{92}{3.82}$
1952–1961	$\frac{1.6}{0.11}$	$\frac{3.6}{0.42}$	$\frac{8.1}{0.58}$	$\frac{11.0}{1.18}$	$\frac{14.0}{1.11}$	$\frac{15.3}{1.12}$	$\frac{14.5}{1.24}$	$\frac{11.4}{0.92}$	$\frac{6.7}{1.35}$	$\frac{3.5}{0.58}$	$\frac{1.9}{0.22}$	$\frac{1.1}{0.10}$	$\frac{93}{3.51}$

radiation balance from observational data obtained at a number of stations. Budyko and Efimova (1964) used for this purpose the results of observations over a 10-yr period at three stations: Voeikov (in the region of Leningrad), Vysokaia Dubrava, and Kuibyshev. These stations are characterized by a high quality of observations, and represent different climatic areas of the USSR.

In Table 15 are given monthly and annual sums of the radiation balance at these stations for the 10-yr period and also the root-mean-square deviations of these values in single years from the 10-yr norms.

Analyzing the data from Table 15, one must bear in mind that the probable error of instrumental measurement of the radiation balance amounts to several tenths of a kilocalorie per square centimeter in the monthly sums, and to several per cent of the measured value in the annual sums. Taking this circumstance into account, one can infer that variability of the monthly sums of the radiation balance is small compared to their change in the annual cycle, and is comparable to the probable error of observation.

In this connection, a possibility appears of determining radiation-balance norms from short observational periods. Determining the monthly and annual means of the radiation balance from the above data for 5-yr periods and comparing them to the means for 10-yr periods, it is easy to establish that the differences are small and lie within the range of observational accuracy.

Assuming that the rms deviations of the observed values from the means decrease in inverse proportion to the square root of the number of years of observation, we can calculate the duration of the observational period necessary for the determination of annual values of the radiation balance with an error not greater than 5%. As a result of such a calculation from the data of Table 15, we find that this period is only 2–3 yr.

Thus, for the determination of norms of the radiation balance, observational periods of only a few years are sufficient. Approximate norms can be determined even from data of single years, the error of such a determination being small in most cases compared to the variation of the radiation balance during the annual march.

All these evaluations relate to cases in which long-term variations in characteristics of the radiation regime associated with changes of climate are absent. Available observational data show (refer also to Chapter V) that the secular movement of total short-wave radiation in the period of observations is negligible, and therefore taking account of it in determining norms of short-wave radiation is not necessary. Proceeding from this statement, one can consider that secular changes in the radiation balance are also of no importance for the determination of its norms. A different situation occurs with direct short-wave radiation, which in some cases has noticeable long-term

TABLE 15

MEAN MONTHLY AND ANNUAL SUMS OF RADIATION BALANCE (NUMERATOR) AND ROOT-MEAN-SQUARE DEVIATIONS FOR SINGLE YEARS (DENOMINATOR) (in kcal cm^{-2} per month or year)

Jan.	Feb.	Mar.	Apr.	May	June	July	Aug.	Sept.	Oct.	Nov.	Dec.	Year
					Voeikovo, 1952–1961							
$\frac{-0.5}{0.18}$	$\frac{-0.5}{0.29}$	$\frac{0.1}{0.40}$	$\frac{3.6}{0.82}$	$\frac{6.8}{0.82}$	$\frac{7.9}{0.88}$	$\frac{7.5}{0.69}$	$\frac{5.0}{0.86}$	$\frac{2.3}{0.40}$	$\frac{0.2}{0.14}$	$\frac{-0.6}{0.21}$	$\frac{-0.6}{0.30}$	$\frac{31.2}{2.62}$
				Vysokaia Dubrava, 1951–1961 (without 1960)								
$\frac{-1.1}{0.23}$	$\frac{-0.8}{0.37}$	$\frac{0.0}{0.25}$	$\frac{4.4}{0.88}$	$\frac{7.0}{0.58}$	$\frac{8.0}{0.54}$	$\frac{7.7}{0.74}$	$\frac{5.7}{0.47}$	$\frac{2.5}{0.49}$	$\frac{0.3}{0.24}$	$\frac{-0.9}{0.41}$	$\frac{-1.0}{0.37}$	$\frac{31.8}{2.14}$
					Kuibyshev, 1952–1961							
$\frac{-0.7}{0.30}$	$\frac{-0.4}{0.22}$	$\frac{1.0}{0.86}$	$\frac{5.7}{0.72}$	$\frac{8.2}{0.66}$	$\frac{9.1}{0.72}$	$\frac{8.5}{0.80}$	$\frac{6.4}{0.45}$	$\frac{3.2}{0.35}$	$\frac{1.0}{0.35}$	$\frac{0.4}{0.16}$	$\frac{-0.7}{0.47}$	$\frac{40.9}{2.84}$

variations. This element of the radiation regime, however, is not often used in investigations of heat balance, and so we do not dwell here on the question of determining norms of direct radiation.

The considerations stated above permit the evaluation of the least duration of a period that is necessary for the evaluation of norms for elements of the radiation regime with a required accuracy. In the paper of Budyko and Drozdov (1966), it was indicated that when considering the question of the appropriate duration of the averaging period, one must remember that the accuracy of norms for elements of the meteorological regime depends also on the homogeneity of the available series of observations. As a result of such an approach, one can determine the upper limit of the duration of periods that are suitable for use in calculating norms of the meteorological elements.

It is evident that existing types of meteorological observations are associated with systematic errors, depending on imperfections of the instruments and observational methods used, on the incomplete representativeness of meteorological stations, and on inadequacies in the training of observers.

The methods of climatological processing of observational data permit taking some of these errors into account and introducing proper corrections. Making allowance for the approximate character of such corrections, it is clear that they do not exclude systematic errors in observational data, which restrict the homogeneity of the series obtained.

The homogeneity of series of meteorological observations is also restricted by changes in the conditions of instrument installation, construction, and so on. With a sufficiently dense network of meteorological stations, the influence of conditions of instrument installation on their readings might be to some extent taken into account and eliminated by means of comparing readings at stations situated near each other. However, the possible accuracy of such corrections is limited by the closeness of the relation of readings at different stations. As a result, in the available series of meteorological observations, there remains a certain heterogeneity, which restricts the comparability of observational data in time and space.

Designating by σ_0 the rms variation caused by heterogeneity of the data of the meteorological observational series used, we note that though σ_0 does not coincide with the values of the systematic error of observations, it usually has the same order of magnitude.

Values of σ_0 for different meteorological elements have been determined in investigations in the methodology of climatological analysis.

It must be stressed here that, although many meteorological elements are observed with comparatively small systematic errors, such errors are always present and in all cases limit the homogeneity of series of meteorological observations used in climatological investigations.

It is evident that appropriate accuracy in determining climatological norms is restricted by errors caused by the heterogeneity of the observational series used. Neglecting the temporal coherence of the series used, it can be assumed that the error in determining the norm over a period of n years is equal to $\sigma/\sqrt{n}$, where σ is the variability of the element under examination. From this, we obtain $\sigma_0 \leqslant \sigma/\sqrt{n_0}$, where n_0 is the most appropriate duration of the averaging period. It follows that $n_0 \leqslant (\sigma/\sigma_0)^2$.

Let us use this formula for calculating the greatest length of averaging period for the determination of norms of total short-wave radiation and the radiation balance.

In Table 16 are presented values of the heterogeneity of corresponding observational series σ_0, of the heterogeneity of the radiation regime σ in the warm and cold seasons in middle latitudes, and the values of the duration of the most appropriate averaging periods n_0 found by use of this formula.

TABLE 16

DURATION OF AVERAGING PERIODS

	Season	σ_0 (kcal cm^{-2} month^{-1})	σ (kcal cm^{-2} month^{-1})	n_0 (yr)
Total short-wave radiation	Warm season	0.2	1.0	25
	Cold season	0.1	0.4	16
Radiation balance	Warm season	0.2	0.7	12
	Cold season	0.1–0.2	0.3	4

Such estimates provide maximum lengths of suitable averaging periods in climatological studies.

In many cases, the values of suitable averaging periods can be decreased by taking into account the specific purpose of an investigation in which calculated climatological norms are to be used. Thus, for example, for many practical purposes the required accuracy of data on monthly mean air temperature does not exceed 1°. Taking into account the variability of the monthly mean temperature, it is easy to discover that for most climatic regions such accuracy will be obtained with an averaging period of no more than several years.

At the same time, there are fields of application of meteorological data in which a heightened accuracy of determination of the norms of meteorological elements is required. These include problems of evaluating climatic variation, variations in hydrological regime, and others, where "norms" are used as kinds of indexes to changing hydrometeorological conditions.

We will not dwell on the problem of determining norms of other heat-balance components from observational data, because mass observational material is available mainly for elements of the radiation regime.

World maps of the components of the heat balance

Beginning in the 1940s, observational data on short-wave radiation and the radiation balance at the earth's surface have been used for determination of norms of these elements. In a number of works, maps of short-wave radiation and radiation balance in different areas have been constructed (Kalitin, 1945; Hand, 1953; Barashkova *et al.*, 1961; Pivovarova and Pleshkova, 1962; and others). Recently, maps of elements of the radiation regime of the earth–atmosphere system have been constructed on the basis of observations from satellites. Some of these maps characterize the radiation regime over a limited period of time (Rashke *et al.*, 1968; and others), and others provide norms for radiation-regime elements relating to a period of several years (Vonder Haar and Suomi, 1969).

It must be remembered that for a number of components of the heat balance of the earth's surface and atmosphere, there still are not any mass data from direct observations. Even for such well-studied elements of the radiation regime as total short-wave radiation and the radiation balance at the earth's surface, the available data of observations on the oceans and on parts of the land are insufficient for designing even schematic maps.

Under such conditions, calculation methods for determination of components of the radiation and heat balances have great importance. With the use of calculation methods, the norms of radiation and heat balance components are determined from available norms of the basic meteorological elements: cloudiness, air temperature and humidity, wind, and others, obtained as a result of observations conducted over long periods of time.

General employment of calculation methods for the determination of norms of heat-balance components in contemporary investigations has made it possible to construct a series of maps giving a detailed presentation of the geographical regularities in the heat balance at the earth's surface and in the atmosphere.

We note that calculation methods for designing climatic maps have long been used in climatological studies. In the very first works directed at studying the geographical distribution of the meteorological elements, methods for calculating values of the investigated elements were widely used along with direct generalization of observational data. Thus, for example, while the first world maps of the distribution of air temperature were constructed by Humboldt in 1817 (for the annual period) and by Dove in 1848 (for months) on the basis of observational data, approximately at the same time (in 1831)

Kaemtz designed temperature maps for months by means of calculations carried out according to Meyer's formula.

Later, in association with the rapid accumulation of observational data from meteorological stations, maps of the principal meteorological elements were mainly constructed on the basis of immediate generalization of observational data. In this case, however, the procedure for processing observational data used in map construction has been gradually improved, incorporating more and more complicated calculation methods. Utilization of such methods has actually led to the circumstance that modern maps of the distribution of the principal meteorological elements—air temperature, precipitation, and others—acquire to some extent the character of calculation. (This statement applies especially to maps of mountain regions.)

Thus, we cannot entirely set climatic maps of the principal meteorological elements against those of the components of the heat balance with regard to the method of construction. Both types actually are made by generalizing observational data from the basic network of hydrometeorological stations, and calculation methods are used in drawing all types of maps. The differences between maps of the basic meteorological elements and those of the heat balance reduce to the fact that the relative importance of calculation methods in constructing the heat-balance maps is greater than it is for constructing most of the common climatological maps.

The most complete presentation of regularities in the geographical distribution of the components of the heat balance at the earth's surface is to be had from the materials of the "Атлас теплового баланса земного шара (Atlas of the Heat Balance of the Earth)" (1963), prepared by the scientific workers of the Main Geophysical Observatory (GGO). This atlas contains world maps of mean annual and monthly total short-wave radiation, the radiation balance at the earth's surface, heat conversion in evaporation turbulent [sensible-] heat flux, and evaporation. In addition, the atlas includes maps of annual values of the vertical exchange of heat between the ocean surface and the underlying layers of water, radiation balance of the earth–atmosphere system, heat released by condensation of water vapor in the atmosphere, and heat transfer by horizontal movement in the atmosphere.

Using maps of this atlas, we will first take up the problem of the geographical distribution of values of total incoming solar radiation—the principal components of the radiation balance.

The geographical distribution of total incoming short-wave radiation is shown in Figs. 23 to 25. These maps have been designed on the basis of calculated data for radiation at 2100 points on land and 280 on the oceans, along with use of available observational data from actinometric stations. In the maps presented here (as well as in all other maps from the "Атлас

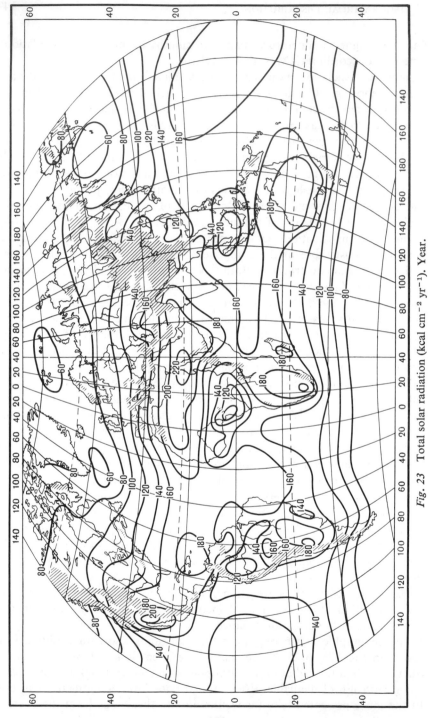

Fig. 23 Total solar radiation (kcal cm^{-2} yr^{-1}). Year.

150

тепловой баланса земного шара"), mountain regions without information are cross-hatched.

As is seen from Fig. 23, the annual values of total short-wave radiation
vary from values less than 60 kcal cm^{-2} yr^{-1} to those exceeding 220 kcal
cm^{-2} yr^{-1}. In high and middle latitudes, the distribution of short-wave
radiation has, in general, a zonal character, while in low latitudes, substantial deviation from a zonal distribution is observed. Low latitudes are characterized by a marked reduction of short-wave radiation values near the
equator, connected with increased cloudiness.

The largest values of total short-wave radiation are observed in the belts of
high pressure in the Northern and Southern Hemispheres, especially in the
desert regions of the continents. The maximum solar radiation is noted in
northeastern Africa, due to the very slight cloudiness above this area.

Diminished values of short-wave radiation are observed in regions of
monsoon climate (for example, the eastern coast of Asia) and other regions
of heavy cloudiness.

For a characterization of the distribution of short-wave radiation in
different months, Figs. 24 and 25 present maps of radiation in December and
June, the months with the smallest and greatest mean altitudes of the sun
for the corresponding hemisphere.

In the map of short-wave radiation in December, the zero isoline in the
Northern Hemisphere passes a bit north of the Arctic Circle in all longitudes.
At higher latitudes, the sun does not rise above the horizon in this month.

South of the zero isoline, short-wave radiation increases rapidly. Its distribution in the extratropical latitudes of the Northern Hemisphere has in
general a zonal character. In low latitudes, the zonal distribution breaks
down, and the areas of increased and decreased radiation are located in
accordance with the localized areas of lesser or greater cloudiness. Beginning
with low latitudes of the Northern Hemisphere and extending over the whole
Southern Hemisphere, zonal variations of total short-wave radiation in
December are not very great. The lack of significant reduction in radiation
with increased latitude in the Southern Hemisphere is explained by the
effect of day length, which compensates for the reduction of mean sun
altitude as latitude increases.

A similar picture is seen in the distribution of total solar radiation in
June (Fig. 25). In the Northern Hemisphere, radiation varies comparatively
little (though the areas of increased values in desert regions are well marked).
In middle and high latitudes of the Southern Hemisphere, radiation decreases
rapidly with the increase of latitude.

The distribution of total short-wave radiation in March and September
resembles the distribution presented in the annual map. At this time also, the
greatest values of radiation are observed in the regions of tropical deserts.

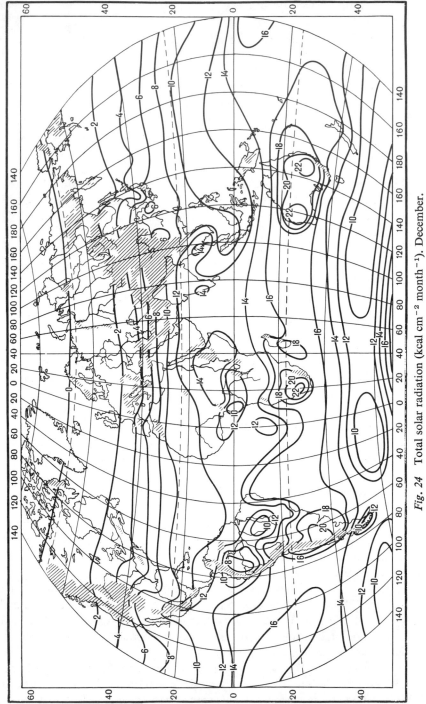

Fig. 24 Total solar radiation (kcal cm^{-2} month^{-1}). December.

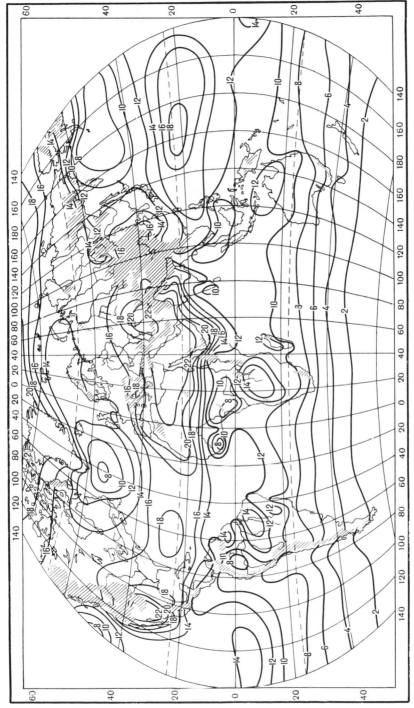

Fig. 25 Total solar radiation (kcal cm^{-2} month^{-1}). June.

153

In the rest of the months (January and February, April and May, July and August, October and November), the distributions of total short-wave radiation display a character intermediate between those discussed above.

Passing on to the problem of the spatial distribution of other components of the radiation balance, we note that the distribution of absorbed short-wave radiation is in most cases very similar to that of total incoming short-wave radiation. However, unlike the isolines of total incoming radiation, the isolines of absorbed radiation are usually discontinuous. In particular, at the boundary between land and water, the isolines of absorbed radiation as a rule are broken, in accordance with the discontinuity in the albedo of the underlying surface.

For most of the lands and oceans, the difference between the values of incoming and absorbed short-wave radiation is comparatively small (approximately 5–20%). This difference increases slightly for deserts and especially for areas covered with snow and ice. In consequence, where a boundary of snow or ice cover occurs at the surface of land or ocean, the values of absorbed radiation at this border change abruptly.

For study of the spatial distribution of net long-wave radiation (which defines the loss of heat by the exchange of long-wave radiation), it is possible to use the maps composed of material calculated for "Атлас теплового баланса земного шара." These calculations were carried out for 1460 points on land and 280 on the oceans, more or less evenly located over the surface of the globe (Efimova and Strokina, 1963).

These maps show that spatial changes in net long-wave radiation are, in general, smaller than those in total short-wave radiation. Such a phenomenon is to some extent explained by the fact that in most climatic zones, variations of temperature and absolute humidity are interconnected, absolute humidity increasing with a rise in temperature. Since a rise in temperature and an increase in absolute humidity influence net long-wave radiation in opposite directions, it therefore changes relatively little.

The greatest values of the annual sums of the net long-wave radiation are noted in the tropical deserts on land, where they reach 80–90 kcal cm^{-2} yr^{-1} (values of net long-wave radiation are positive when they correspond to deficit of heat). Here an enormous heating of the underlying desert surface in comparison with air temperature produces a great effect on the net long-wave radiation.

Near the equator, the net long-wave radiation is reduced in magnitude (30–40 kcal cm^{-2} yr^{-1}) and differs comparatively little between ocean and land. In land regions of extratropical latitudes, it is, on the average, somewhat larger than on oceans in the same latitudes, especially under arid conditions.

The spatial distribution of the radiation balance [radiation surplus] at the underlying surface is presented in Figs. 26–28.

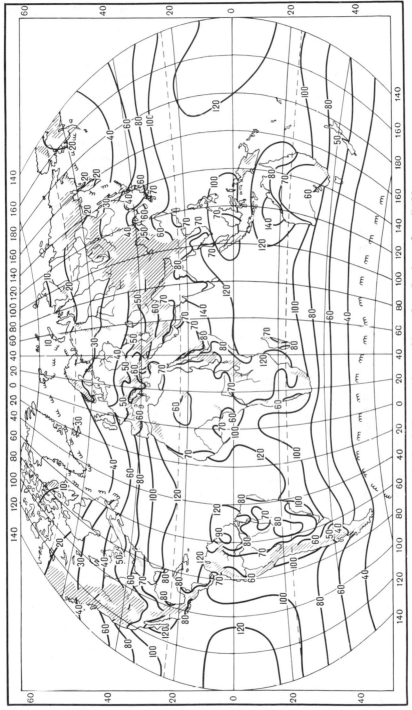

Fig. 26 Radiation balance at the earth's surface (kcal cm^{-2} yr^{-1}). Year.

In the map of annual sums of the radiation balance (Fig. 26), the abrupt variation at the change from land to sea and defined by a break in isolines is very noticeable. As a consequence of a lesser albedo of the ocean surface, the radiation balance here is as a rule greater than that at a land surface in the same latitude.

Of considerable importance is the fact that at all the surfaces of the oceans and lands, the annual sum of the surface radiation balance turns out positive. As established by modern investigations, a negative annual sum in the radiation balance is probably observed only in regions of permanent snow and ice cover.

The distribution of the radiation balance over the surface of the oceans exhibits, in general, a zonal character, as seen from the map in Fig. 26. Some deviations from zonality are noted, for example, in the regions of activity of warm and cold currents. These deviations may have different signs for the same type of current, because of the complex nature of the relations of the radiation balance with water and air temperatures, humidity, and cloudiness.

The comparatively small variation in values of the radiation balance at the surface of the oceans in low latitudes, and the rapid decrease of balance values in middle latitudes going from low to high latitudes, warrant attention.

The greatest value of radiation balance at the earth's surface is observed in the northern part of the Arabian Sea—more than 140 kcal cm^{-1} yr^{-1}.

The variation of annual values of the radiation balance on land also has, to some extent, a zonal character, but in a number of regions zonality is abruptly broken by the effect of differences in moisture conditions. It has already been indicated more than once in studies on the climatology of the heat balance that the radiation balance in arid land regions is reduced in comparison with regions of sufficient or surplus moisture in the same latitudes. The cause of this phenomenon lies in the significant increase, under conditions of an arid climate, in the loss of radiant energy as net long-wave radiation (due to the high surface temperature, little cloudiness, and relatively low humidity), and in the reflection of short-wave radiation.

Therefore, in Fig. 26, along with a general decrease in radiation balance with increasing latitude, there are well-marked domains of reduced radiation balance caused by the dryness of the climate. This regularity is observed, for example, in the Sahara, in the deserts of Central Asia, and in many other desert and arid regions. In monsoon regions, the annual values of the radiation balance at the land surface are also slightly reduced, as a consequence of the heavy cloudiness in the warm season.

The greatest annual values of the radiation balance on land are observed in the wet tropical regions, but even here they hardly reach 100 kcal cm^{-2}

yr^{-1}, which is noticeably less than the corresponding maximum for oceanic conditions.

Let us consider now the distribution of the radiation balance in December. As is seen from Fig. 27, the radiation balance in December is negative over a considerable portion of the surface of the Northern Hemisphere. It is interesting to note that the zero isoline of the radiation balance on both oceans and land is situated in approximately the same latitude—about 40° N. To the north of this latitude, the radiation balance on the oceans increases in absolute magnitude, reaching -2 kcal cm^{-2} month^{-1} and even larger negative values.

The negative radiation balance on land also increases in absolute value northwards, but the deficit here only reaches magnitudes around -1 kcal cm^{-2} month^{-1}. The reason for this difference lies in the fact that at the surface of the oceans in high latitudes, water temperature during the cold season is much higher than that of the land surface in the same latitudes. Therefore, the net long-wave radiation on the oceans turns out much greater than that on land, and the radiation balance is smaller.

Southward of the latitude of 40° N, the radiation balance on the oceans in December increases approximately zonally all the way to the Equator, where it reaches values of 8–10 kcal cm^{-2} month^{-1}. South of the Equator, the radiation balance on the oceans varies comparatively little, its greatest values (up to 12–14 kcal cm^{-2} month^{-1}) being observed for the most part in the regions of the Tropic of Capricorn. Southward, the radiation balance again diminishes slightly. On land between 40° N and the Equator, it also regularly increases towards the south, and south of the Equator it varies comparatively little, essentially from 6 to 10 kcal cm^{-2} month^{-1}.

General regularities of the distribution of the radiation balance in June in the Northern Hemisphere are analogous to those of its distribution in December in the Southern Hemisphere, and vice versa.

The zero isoline of the radiation balance on oceans and land in June goes approximately along 45° S. Northward of this parallel, the radiation balance (refer to Fig. 28) increases and on oceans reaches its greatest values in the regions of the Tropic of Cancer. (The maximum value, slightly exceeding 16 kcal cm^{-2} month^{-1}, is observed in the northern portion of the Arabian Sea.) North of the Tropic of Cancer, the radiation balance on the oceans first slightly declines but with the approach to the Arctic Circle starts increasing again, which can be explained by the increased length of summer days in high latitudes. The radiation balance on land in the Southern Hemisphere increases regularly in a northward direction up to the Equator; north of the Equator over large expanses of land, it varies relatively little.

In conclusion, it must be indicated that the data on radiation balance discussed above are macroclimatic characteristics, and define its mean values

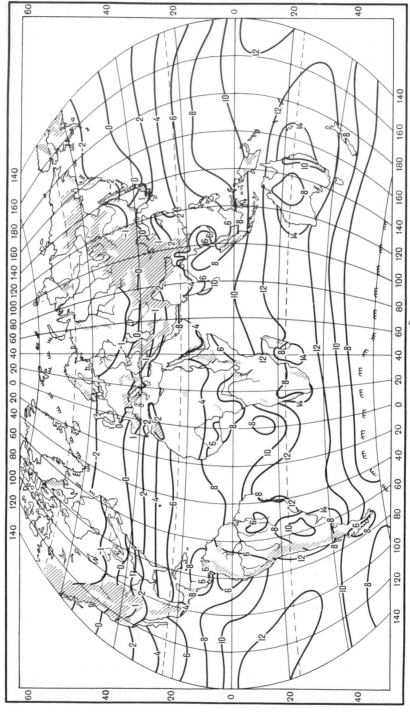

Fig. 27 Radiation balance at the earth's surface (kcal cm⁻² month⁻¹). December.

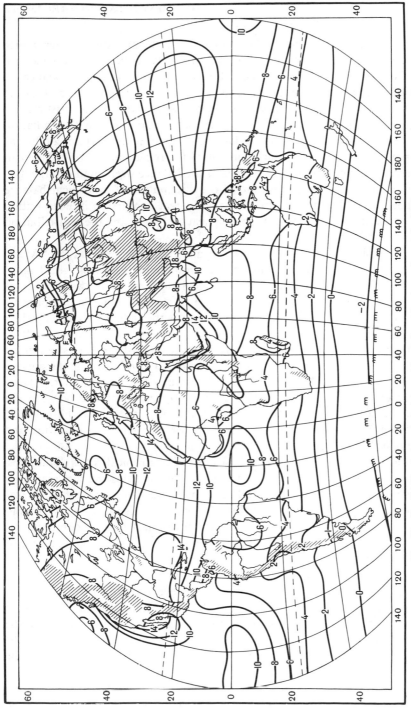

Fig. 28 Radiation balance at the earth's surface (kcal cm^{-2} month^{-1}). June.

for more or less large regions. As pointed out in the previous chapter, under land conditions, a great microclimatic variability in the radiation balance may be observed. Therefore, actual values of the radiation balance at individual sectors of the underlying surface in any geographical region of the continents may differ noticeably from mean background characteristics.

Although, for oceanic conditions, the spatial variability of the radiation balance is much less than it is for land, even here, under certain conditions (the presence of drifting ice, accumulation of seaweed, and so on), there can be observed sudden changes in values of the balance over small distances.

Let us turn now to the question of the distribution of other heat-balance components at the earth's surface, namely, heat conversion in evaporation [latent-heat flux], the turbulent sensible-heat exchange, and the redistribution of heat by currents.

In examining this question, we will again use the maps from the "Атлас теплового баланса земного шара." Corresponding series of world maps have been constructed on the basis of calculations made by the procedures stated in the previous chapter. Calculation of the heat-balance components was carried out for the same points for which the radiation-balance values were calculated.

The distribution of the annual values of the latent-heat flux is presented in Fig. 29. This map shows that the values of evaporation from the surface of land and water near a coastline differ greatly from each other. Such a phenomenon is presumably explained both by the difference between the values of potential evaporation on land and oceans, and by the effect of insufficient moisture in many land regions, which restricts evaporation and the flux of latent heat.

Figure 29 shows that the latent-heat flux in extratropical zones diminishes, on the average, with an increase of latitude, but that this average regularity is disturbed for both oceans and land by large azonal changes. In low latitudes, the distribution of the flux of latent heat also has a very complicated character. On the oceans, a decrease of this heat-balance component is observed near the Equator, in comparison with the regions of high atmospheric pressure.

The principal reason for azonal changes in the latent-heat flux on the oceans is the distribution of warm and cold ocean currents. All the major warm currents increase the flux noticeably, and the cold ones decrease it. These changes are clearly apparent in the regions of the warm currents of the Gulf Stream, Kuro Shio, and others, and also in regions of the cold currents, such as the Canary Current, the Benguela, the California, the Peru, the Labrador Current, and so on.

It is worth notice that because of the activity of currents raising or lowering the water temperature, the annual value of evaporation from the ocean surface in the same latitude may change by a factor of several times.

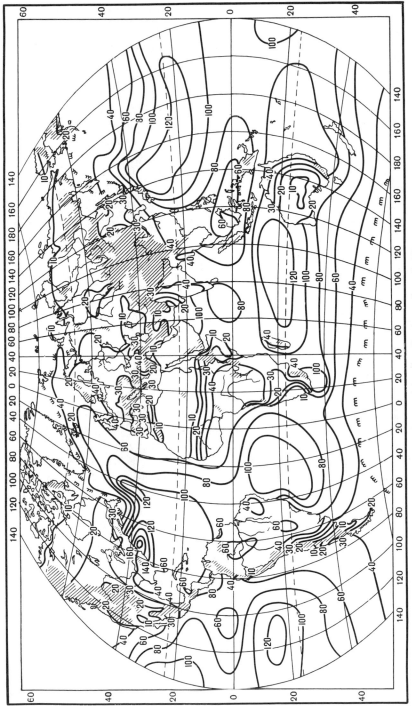

Fig. 29 Latent-heat flux (kcal cm^{-2} yr^{-1}). Year.

161

Besides ocean currents, azonal variations of evaporation and latent-heat flux are influenced by the conditions of atmospheric circulation that determine the regime of wind speed and humidity deficit above the ocean.

The distribution of the latent-heat flux from land surfaces differs more from the zonal pattern than the distribution on the oceans, owing to the enormous influence of climatic moisture conditions on evaporation.

With availability of sufficient amounts of soil moisture, evaporation and latent-heat flux are regulated mainly by the size of the radiation balance. Such conditions are observed in regions of the high latitudes and in humid regions of the middle and low latitudes.

In regions of insufficient humidification, evaporation is reduced because of the lack of soil moisture and, under desert and semidesert conditions, approaches the small value of annual precipitation in these regions. In Fig. 29 are seen areas of markedly reduced latent-heat flux in the principal arid regions of the globe. The greatest latent-heat flux is observed in several equatorial regions, where, with the abundance of moisture and great input of heat, it exceeds 60 kcal cm^{-2} yr^{-1}, which corresponds to the evaporation in a year of a water layer more than 1 m deep.

Much greater values can be reached by evaporation from the ocean surface, where the radiation balance is slightly greater than that for land and, of greater significance, the evaporating surface may receive a large additional amount of thermal energy due to redistribution of heat by marine currents. As a result, in some tropical and subtropical regions, annual evaporation from the ocean surface reaches values somewhat exceeding 2 m.

The maps of monthly values of the latent-heat flux (Figs. 30 and 31) point to the contrasting character of the annual march of evaporation on lands and oceans of the extratropical latitudes.

It is known that during the cold season, evaporation on land diminishes considerably, the evaporation maximum being observed at the beginning or in the middle of the warm season, depending on moisture conditions. To the contrary, ocean evaporation usually increases in the cold season in comparison with the warm season. The cause of this lies in the increase in the difference between water and air temperatures in the cold season, which causes the difference in the water-vapor concentration at the water surface and in the air to increase. Besides, in many oceanic regions, mean wind speeds in the cold season are higher than in the warm season, and this also increases evaporation during the cold season.

An important factor in the increase of heat outgo for evaporation in the cold season is the condition of heat inflow to the evaporating ocean surface, dependent on horizontal heat exchange in the hydrosphere.

Increased evaporation in the cold season is associated with the intensification of the activity of the warm currents, while cold currents reducing the flux of latent heat are especially active in the warm season.

The map of the latent-heat flux in December (Fig. 30) shows that the greatest values of evaporation in this season are observed on the oceans, in zones of activity of the warm currents of the Northern Hemisphere—the Gulf Stream and Kuro Shio.

In these regions, the flux reaches very large values, exceeding 15–20 kcal cm^{-2} $month^{-1}$. On most of the land surface in extratropical latitudes of the Northern Hemisphere, evaporation is very small, and the latent-heat outgo does not in general exceed 1 kcal cm^{-2} $month^{-1}$. In the Southern Hemisphere, the distribution of the flux of latent heat has a rather complicated character, its greatest values on the oceans and in humid regions of the continents being observed near the Tropic of Capricorn, where the radiation balance is especially great at this time.

The distribution of heat outgo for evaporation in June (Fig. 31) is characterized by reduced values in extratropical latitudes of the oceans of the Northern Hemisphere. These values are, on the average, less than those in corresponding latitudes on land. In low latitudes, evaporation from the oceans varies little; in the extratropical latitudes of the Southern Hemisphere, it declines appreciably with an increase in latitude.

Let us turn now to the problem of the geographical distribution of the turbulent flux of sensible heat.

The map, Fig. 32, shows the quantity of heat given out by the earth's surface into the air (positive values) or gained from the air (negative values) during a year. The fact that on the average over the year, the surface of all the continents (except Antarctica) and most of the ocean surface yield heat to the atmosphere attracts attention.

On the greater part of the ocean surface, the value of the turbulent sensible-heat flux is small compared to the principal components of the heat balance, and usually does not exceed 10–20% of their values. The flux reaches large absolute values in those regions where the water is, on the average, much warmer than the air, i.e., in the regions of the activity of powerful warm currents (the Gulf Stream), and in high latitudes where the sea still remains free of ice. Under such conditions, the turbulent heat flux can exceed 30–40 kcal cm^{-1} yr^{-1}.

Cold currents, lowering the water temperature, tend to decrease the heat flux from the ocean surface into the atmosphere, and increase that in the opposite direction.

In contrast to the oceans, where the turbulent sensible-heat flux, on the average, increases in absolute value in a profile from low latitudes into high, the flux on land varies in the opposite direction. At the same time, under land conditions, the value of the sensible-heat flux is strongly influenced by the moisture conditions of climate; in arid regions, the turbulent flux of sensible heat from the land surface into the atmosphere is much greater than in humid ones.

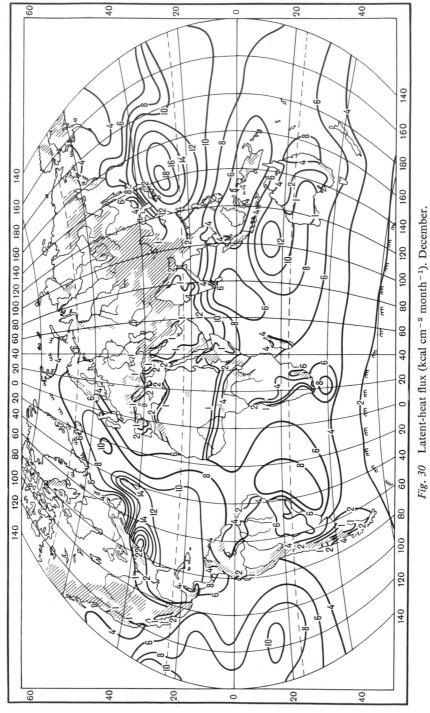

Fig. 30 Latent-heat flux (kcal cm⁻² month⁻¹). December.

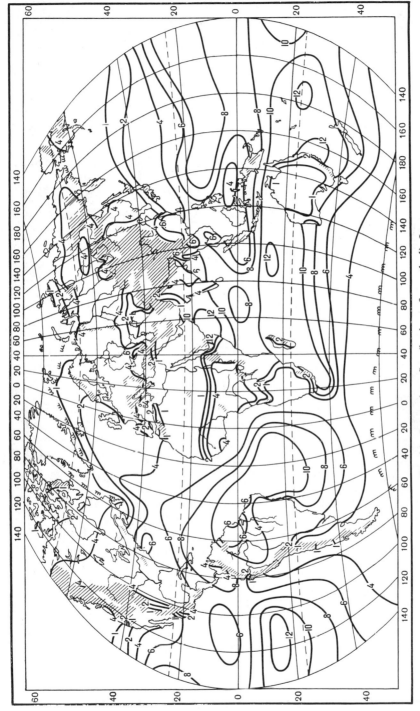

Fig. 31 Latent-heat flux (kcal cm⁻² month⁻¹). June.

165

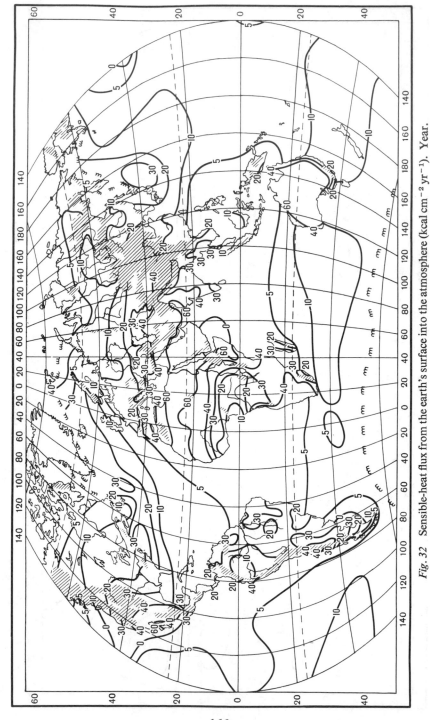

Fig. 32 Sensible-heat flux from the earth's surface into the atmosphere (kcal cm^{-2} yr^{-1}). Year.

166

In accordance with this, the greatest outgo of sensible heat by the turbulent flux on land is noted in the tropical deserts, where it can exceed 60 kcal cm^{-2} yr^{-1}. In humid tropical regions and especially in regions of middle and high latitudes, the heat flux is usually much less than this value.

In December (Fig. 33), the turbulent heat flux reaches large values in the northwestern portions of the Atlantic and Pacific Oceans, as a result of the activity of warm currents and also the development of heat exchange between the cold continental surface and the warmer ocean. In the regions of activity of the Gulf Stream and the Kuro Shio, the oceanic heat outgo in turbulent heat flux amounts to 4–8 kcal cm^{-2} month^{-1}.

In all other oceanic regions, the turbulent sensible-heat flux is small in absolute magnitude, and in some regions, including the zones of the Peru and Benguela cold currents, it turns out to be directed from the atmosphere to the ocean. On the Northern-Hemisphere continents north of 40–45° N, the sensible-heat exchange is also directed from the atmosphere to the earth's surface. A considerable outpouring of heat from the earth's surface to the atmosphere is observed in the tropical deserts, especially those of the Southern Hemisphere, where it can exceed 6–8 kcal cm^{-2} month^{-1}.

Another picture of the distribution of the turbulent sensible-heat flux on the oceans is observed in June (Fig. 34), when, in the northern portion of the Atlantic Ocean, near the coasts of North America, Europe, and Africa, there exist extensive zones where the turbulent heat flux is directed from the atmosphere to the ocean surface. A similar picture is also found over a considerable portion of the Pacific Ocean in the Northern Hemisphere.

It must be indicated, however, that at all these expanses, the turbulent flux is small in absolute value (less than 2 kcal cm^{-2} month^{-1}). This indicates that in the process of heat exchange between oceans and atmosphere, the oceans of the Northern Hemisphere lose much more heat during the cold season than they gain from the atmosphere during the warm season.

In the Southern Hemisphere in June, the oceans in middle and high latitudes lose comparatively little heat into the atmosphere. This is associated with the absence of large contrasts between the thermal state of continents and oceans.

Turbulent exchange of sensible heat on the continents in June is characterized by positive [upward] values of the heat flux in almost all latitudes (except the southern part of South America and a small area in southern Australia). In the deserts of the Northern Hemisphere, the heat loss from the earth's surface to the atmosphere amounts to 6–8 kcal cm^{-2} month^{-1}.

The maps of turbulent sensible-heat flux show that in some cases, the flux changes sign at the boundaries of continents and oceans. One of the causes of such a distribution lies in the formation of air masses that move from a heated to a colder underlying surface, or in the opposite direction.

Like the maps of the radiation balance, all the maps of latent and sensible

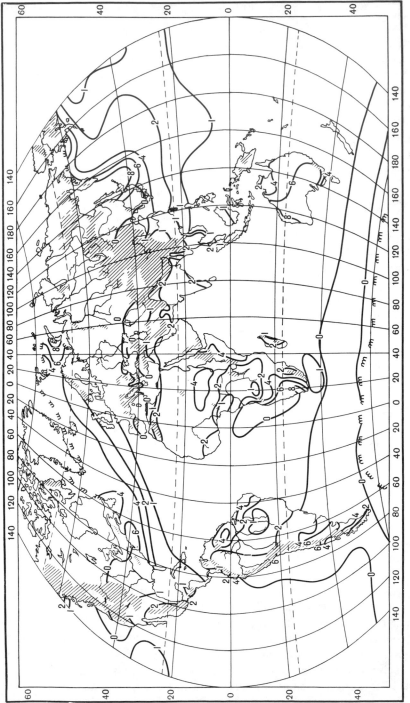

Fig. 33 Sensible-heat flux from the earth's surface into the atmosphere (kcal cm^{-2} month^{-1}). December.

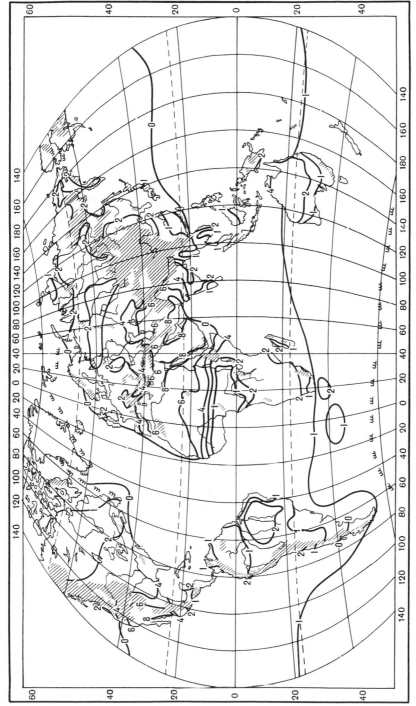

Fig. 34 Sensible-heat flux from the earth's surface into the atmosphere (kcal cm^{-2} month^{-1}). June.

169

heat flux examined here contain data on the mean values of the indicated heat-balance components over considerable portions of the earth's surface. As pointed out in the preceding chapter, evaporation in many regions is characterized by great spatial variability, especially noticeable in regions of unstable moisture status on the continents. Values of the turbulent sensible-heat flux vary similarly. Therefore, the values of the heat-balance components in the above maps have the character of background values, which may differ appreciably from those at individual points or in small regions.

Of great importance in the heat balance of the oceans is the income or outgo of heat resulting from horizontal heat exchange, due mainly to the activity of marine currents. Annual means of this quantity, determined as a residual component in the heat balance from materials of the above calculations of the heat-balance components, are presented in Fig. 35.

In examining this map, we must first of all point out that in the oceans, a great quantity of heat is redistributed between tropical and extratropical latitudes. In this redistribution, warm and cold currents play a large role. The map shows a correspondence between the areas of increased positive values of this quantity (which corresponds to the flow of heat from the ocean surface into the deeper layers) and regions of cold currents, and between the areas of the reduced and negative values of the quantity and regions of warm currents.

Such a correspondence is observed, for example, for warm currents (such as the Gulf Stream, Kuro Shio, Agulhas Current, and the southwestern Pacific) and for cold currents (such as the Canary Current, Benguela Current, California Current, and Peru Current).

At the same time, the distribution of isolines in Fig. 35 in some oceanic regions does not fully correspond to the location of the principal regions of warm and cold currents. This is partially explained by the fact that the value shown on the map represents, not a direct heat transfer by ocean currents, but just one of the consequences of this transfer—the mean heat flux from the oceanic surface to deeper layers. It should also be noted that some peculiarities of the isolines in Fig. 35 are presumably connected, to some extent, with insufficient reliability of the calculated values. Since these values were obtained as a residual component in the heat balance, it is evident that their calculations were influenced by the errors in the determination of all the other balance components, and that they receive the largest calculation error, in comparison with the other components. This circumstance probably influences the location of isolines, diminishing their reliability, most especially in several oceanic regions of the Southern Hemisphere, where the initial climatological data used for the calculations were no doubt insufficiently reliable.

Whereas for mean annual conditions the heat flux directed toward the

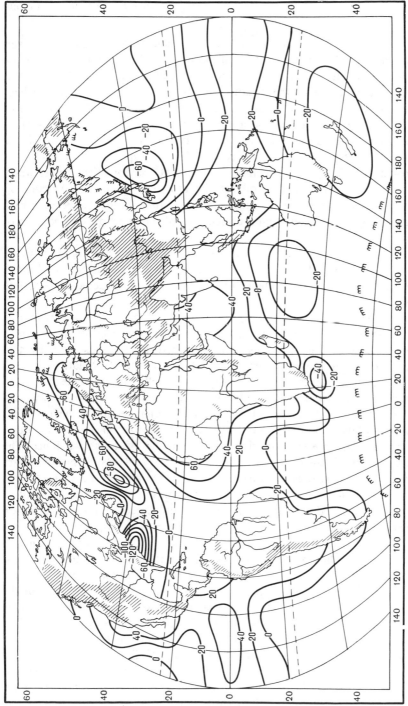

Fig. 35 Heat flux from the ocean surface to the underlying layers of water (kcal cm^{-2} yr^{-1}). Year.

171

ocean surface from the deeper layers is equivalent to a heat gain to a given
oceanic region influenced by the ocean circulation, for individual months the
flux directed to the ocean surface from the deeper layers is equal to the sum
of the heat gain due to the ocean circulation and the change in the heat
content of the water. Since changes in the heat content of the ocean water
during the annual cycle can be approximated from data on water-surface
temperature, it then becomes possible, with the aid of the heat-balance
equation, to determine the annual cycle of heat transport by currents.

Strokina (1963) calculated changes in the heat content of the upper water
layers of the North Atlantic during the annual march. This calculation
corroborated the fact that in middle latitudes the changes in oceanic heat
content are very significant and represent one of the principal components of
the oceanic heat balance.

Using data on the changes in heat content, Strokina determined for single
months the values of heat flux directed to the ocean surface, under the
influence of currents and macroturbulence, and constructed appropriate
maps.

One of these maps (for January) is presented in Fig. 36. It is seen from this
map that in winter, the ocean in the Gulf Stream system gives off an enormous
quantity of thermal energy. This is compensated, for the most part, by heat
coming from a zone situated between the Equator and 30° N latitude.

In subsequent papers by Strokina (1967a, 1969), monthly means of the
changes in heat content were determined for the entire world ocean, and
maps were constructed. These maps show that changes in the heat content
of the upper layers of ocean water in all latitudes may reach significant values,
comparable with those of the principal components of the heat balance. The
largest changes in heat content (more than 25 kcal cm^{-2} month^{-1}) are
observed in the northwest regions of the Pacific Ocean and the adjacent seas.

The maps from the "Атлас теплового баланса земного шара" permit us
also to get a general idea of the regularities in the geographical distribution
of the components of the heat balance of the earth–atmosphere system.

Figure 37 presents a map of the annual values of the radiation balance of
the earth–atmosphere system, constructed on the basis of calculated data at
260 points evenly distributed over the surface of the globe. In this map, the
zero isolines separate the tropical and subtropical latitudes where, on the
average, the income of radiant energy during a year is greater than its outgo,
from regions where the heat outgo due to long-wave emission is greater than
the absorbed solar radiation. These isolines lie near the 40th parallels in the
Northern and Southern Hemispheres. The general distribution of the yearly
values of the radiation balance has a zonal character, the observed deviations
from a zonal distribution being much less than the corresponding deviations
in the map of the radiation balance at the earth's surface.

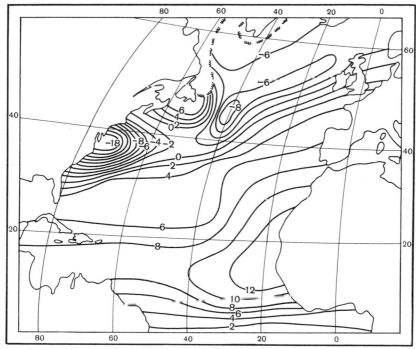

Fig. 36 Income or outgo of heat in the upper layer of water due to currents and macro-turbulence (kcal cm^{-2} month^{-1}) in the northern part of the Atlantic Ocean. January.

At the same time, this map shows a regular diminution of the radiation balance in desert regions of the continents. The deserts of North Africa and Arabia turn out to be a zone of negative radiation balance, while the radiation balance is positive in the corresponding latitudes of oceans and humid continental regions.

It is interesting to note that this paradoxical inference concerning the near-zero values of the radiation balance in some tropical deserts, which had been obtained as a result of calculations of the radiation regime of the earth–atmosphere system, was afterward corroborated by observational data from satellites.

Comparing the maps in Figs. 37 and 26, it is possible to get an idea of the regularities of the geographical distribution of the atmospheric radiation balance, which represents the difference between the radiation balance of the earth–atmosphere system and that at the earth's surface. It is seen from the data comprised in these maps that annual values of the atmospheric radiation balance in all regions of the globe are negative. Their latitudinal variation is appreciably less than that of the radiation balances of either the earth's surface or the earth–atmosphere system.

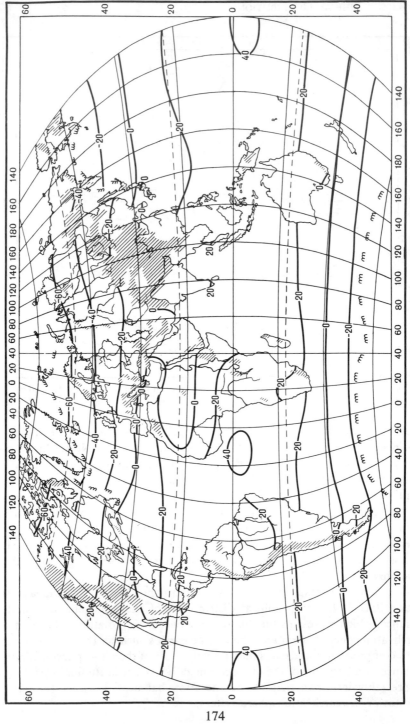

Fig. 37 Radiation balance of the earth–atmosphere system (kcal cm^{-2} yr^{-1}). Year.

In recent years, world maps of individual components of the atmospheric radiation balance, namely, the outgoing long-wave radiation (Vinnikov, 1965) and the net long-wave balance of the atmosphere (D'iachenko and Kondrat'ev, 1965), have been published. The maps by Vinnikov show that the monthly means of outgoing radiation vary, approximately, by a factor of 2, from 10 to 20 kcal cm^{-2} $month^{-1}$. Of interest is a conclusion, following from the data obtained by D'iachenko and Kondrat'ev, on the small variability in time and space of the net long-wave balance of the atmosphere, the monthly means of which are usually equal to 10–12 kcal cm^{-2} $month^{-1}$.

The net income or outgo of heat representing the difference between evaporation from the earth's surface and condensation of water vapor in the atmosphere has great importance in the heat balance of the earth–atmosphere system.

We discussed earlier the regularities of the geographical distribution of the heat outgo for evaporation. The features of the heat income from condensation are seen from the map, Fig. 38, which presents annual means of the heat gain in the atmosphere due to condensation of water vapor ("Атлас теплового баланса земного шара," 1963).

For construction of this map, the assumption was made that the heat income in each geographical region for the year is equal, on the average, to the product of the total precipitation by the latent heat of vaporization. The annual precipitation data necessary for calculation were taken from the world map of Kuznetsova and Sharova (1964).

The map in Fig. 38 shows that the heat income due to condensation, corresponding to the distribution of precipitation, reaches greatest values in the equatorial regions, decreases markedly in the zones of high pressure, increases in middle latitudes above the oceans, and then decreases again in approaching the poles.

From the equation of balance of the earth–atmosphere system and data on the other components, one can determine the value of heat income (or outgo) produced by horizontal movements in the atmosphere.

This calculation was carried out in making up the "Атлас теплового баланса земного шара" and resulted in construction of the map presented in Fig. 39. This map shows the annual sums of heat redistribution by air currents. In accordance with the adopted system of signs, positive values in this map represent regions of outgo and negative values those of heat input.

In this map, as well as in the map of the radiation balance of the earth–atmosphere system, the isolines break at the boundaries of oceans and continents. This is explained by the substantial difference of radiative and thermal characteristics between land and ocean surfaces.

As is seen from Fig. 39, heat transfer by air currents is a highly variable component of the heat balance, and this variability is quite complicated.

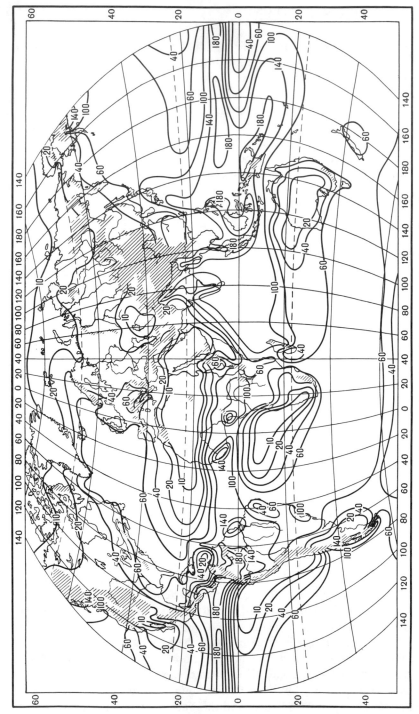

Fig. 38 Heat gain from condensation of water vapor (kcal cm^{-2} yr^{-1}). Year.

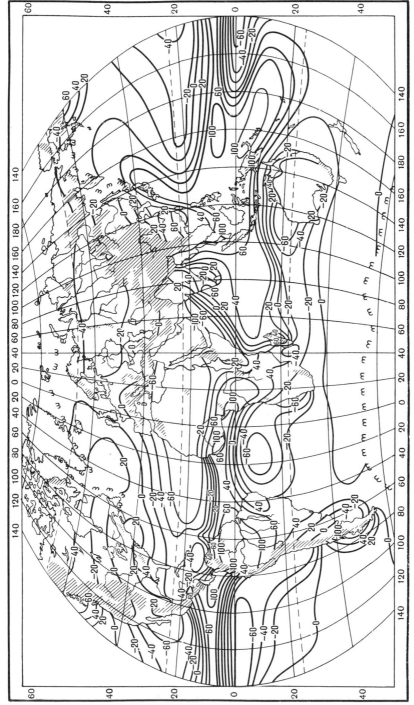

Fig. 39 Heat income due to horizontal motion in the atmosphere (kcal cm^{-2} yr^{-1}). Year.

177

The greatest surplus of thermal energy transferred by atmospheric advection into other areas is found in the equatorial zone. A certain amount of heat is also carried away from the [regional] atmosphere over tropical and subtropical regions of the continents, and from the atmosphere above midlatitude oceans. This surplus reaches and is expended mainly in the zones of high pressure above the oceans, over midlatitude continents, and in the high latitudes of both hemispheres.

The heat balance of polar regions

The study of the heat balance of the Arctic and Antarctic has, until just recently, involved considerable difficulty, owing to insufficient material of the required observations. Not long ago, and especially during the preparation and conducting of the International Geophysical Year, numerous data were obtained permitting study of the distribution of the heat-balance components in the polar regions.

Actinometric investigations in the Arctic were started by the end of the last century (Westman, 1903). During the first half of this century, observations of solar radiation were carried out during a number of polar expeditions, including those conducted during the drift of the "Maud," analyzed and published by Mosby (1932), observations by Kalitin (1921, 1924), who for the first time determined the value of radiation balance for one of the regions of the Arctic (Kalitin, 1929), the observations by Ångström (1933), by Wegener (1939), and others.

Systematic actinometric observations in the Arctic were begun during the period of the Second International Polar Year in 1932–1933, when seven actinometric stations in the Soviet section of the Arctic and several stations in other Arctic areas were organized.

The permanent actinometric network in the Arctic subsequently developed rather slowly, the number of functioning stations being sometimes reduced and sometimes increased. It was only in postwar years that this network embraced all the major regions of the north polar latitudes. At present, more than thirty permanent actinometric stations are functioning in the Arctic, most of them being situated in the Soviet sector. In addition, beginning in 1950, observations of the radiation regime have been carried out in the central Arctic on the Soviet drifting stations, "Северный Полюс."

At most of the permanent actinometric stations and at the drifting stations, all elements of the radiation balance, including long-wave radiation, are measured.

Among a number of works devoted to studying the radiation regime of the Arctic, the studies of Gavrilova (1959, 1963), Marshunova (1961), and Marshunova and Chernigovskii (1968) should be mentioned. We present here some maps of elements of the Arctic radiation regime constructed by Gavrilova on the basis of data calculated for 241 points, available observational data being utilized to make the parameters of the calculation formulas more accurate.

Figures 40–42 present maps of total short-wave radiation in the Arctic for the year, June, and December. Deviation of total radiation values from a zonal distribution in the maps for the year and June is explained by different conditions of cloudiness in different sectors of the Arctic. The distribution of radiation in December is almost exactly zonal because of the dominant effect of astronomic factors on radiation in this month.

We should call attention to a marked increase of radiation in June in the Central Arctic, compared to lower latitudes. This increase is explained by astronomical factors (the great length of daylight).

It should be indicated that under Arctic conditions, most of the incoming short-wave radiation comes in the form of scattered radiation, as a result of considerable cloudiness in the summer months and the high reflectivity of snow and ice.

The values of absorbed short-wave radiation in the Arctic depend substantially on the state of the underlying surface. While at a snow-free land surface and especially at the open ocean surface, absorbed radiation is only

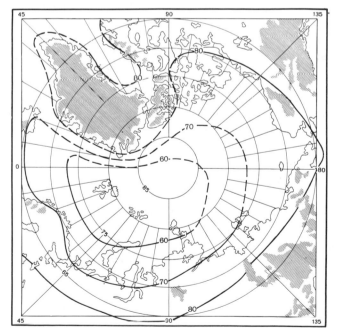

Fig. 40 Total solar radiation in the Arctic (kcal cm^{-2} yr^{-1}). Year.

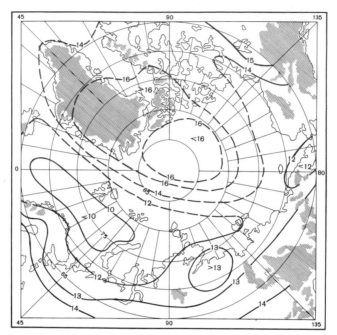

Fig. 41   Total solar radiation in the Arctic (kcal cm^{-2} month^{-1}). June.

slightly less than the incoming, at the surface of snow and ice cover, absorbed radiation is usually a small portion of incoming radiation.

A general idea of the annual cycle of albedo of the ocean surface in the Central Arctic and in a land region (Uedineniia Island) is given in Fig. 43.

It is seen from this figure that the albedo of ice cover remains high during the whole year, slightly diminishing only in the middle of summer, when the snow surface becomes wetter. On land in summer, during the period of snow melting and after its disappearance, the albedo decreases sharply, which leads to a considerable increase in absorbed radiation.

The values of the net long-wave radiation [deficit] in the Arctic, according to the studies of Gavrilova and Marshunova, on the average decrease slowly with an increase in latitude, in correspondence with a decrease in the temperature of the earth's surface. In winter, the value of net long-wave radiation is comparatively small over the extensive areas covered with ice and snow, and increases above the ocean surface in regions that are free of ice cover.

The annual totals of the net long-wave radiation [deficit] in the Arctic turn out to be considerably smaller than in middle latitudes. This is explained by the low temperatures of the earth's surface, by considerable cloudiness in summer, and also by temperature inversions in the cold season.

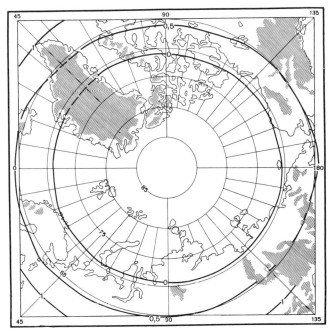

Fig. 42 Total solar radiation in the Arctic (kcal cm⁻² month⁻¹). December.

Maps of the radiation balance of the Arctic designed by Gavrilova are presented in Figs. 44–46. It is evident from the map for the year (Fig. 44) that, notwithstanding a large income of short-wave radiation, the annual sums of the radiation balance over broad expanses of the Central Arctic are close to zero. This is apparently due to the high values of albedo of the snow and ice cover.

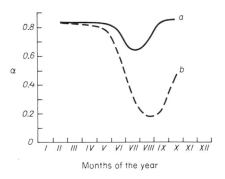

Fig. 43 Annual march of the albedo (α) of ocean and land surfaces (curves a and b, respectively) in the Arctic basin.

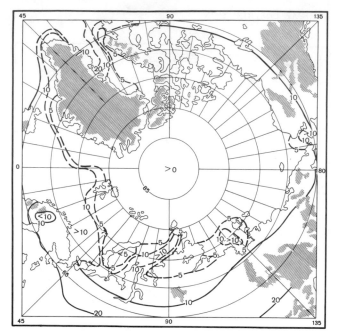

Fig. 44 Radiation balance of the Arctic (kcal cm^{-2} yr^{-1}). Year.

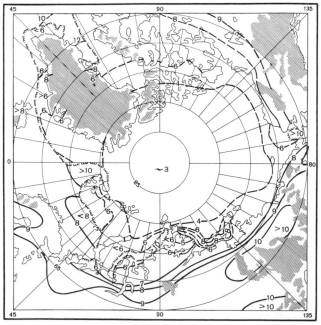

Fig. 45 Radiation balance of the Arctic (kcal cm^{-2} month^{-1}). June.

182

In the area of the peripheral Arctic seas, annual values of the radiation balance reach 5–10 kcal cm^{-2}; in regions with areas of open water in summer, the annual radiation balance increases to 15–20 kcal cm^{-2} and more.

The radiation balance in June (Fig. 45) is noticeably greater than zero over the whole Arctic. In this month, a pronounced contrast of balance values between the areas covered with ice and those free of it is observed. In December (Fig. 46), the radiation balance in the entire polar area is below zero, increasing in absolute magnitudes at ice-free ocean areas, where the net long-wave radiation is large.

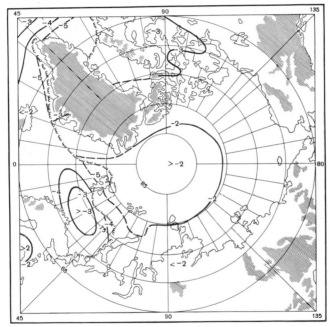

Fig. 46 Radiation balance of the Arctic (kcal cm^{-2} month^{-1}). December.

The geographic distributions of other components of the heat balance of the Arctic have been studied mostly in peripheral areas. Some heat-balance information for these areas can be obtained from the world maps given earlier.

The determination of heat converted in evaporation, the turbulent sensible-heat flux, and other heat-balance components for the Central Arctic is associated with considerable difficulty, owing to the relatively small values of the balance components under these conditions. Some information on this question will be provided in the second section of the following chapter.

The radiation regime and heat balance of the Antarctic, almost completely unexplored up to the recent past, have been examined in the studies of Loewe (1956), Liljequist (1957), Rusin (1961 and elsewhere), and other authors. As a result of these investigations, maps of the components of the Antarctic radiation and heat balances have been constructed. Figures 47–49 present maps of total short-wave radiation (year and January) and annual values of the radiation balance, compiled by Rusin *et al.* (1966), and published in the Soviet "Атлас Антарктики."

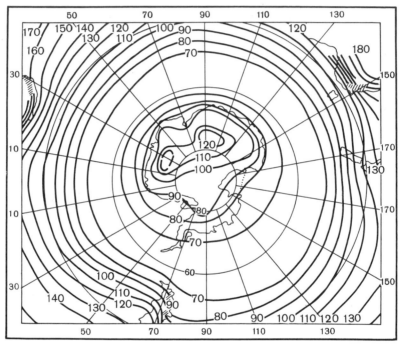

Fig. 47 Total solar radiation in the Antarctic (kcal cm^{-2} yr^{-1}). Year.

In the first of these maps (Fig. 47) is clearly seen an area of minimal values of total short-wave radiation in the zone of 60° S, and a pronounced increase of radiation on the Antarctic continent, associated with the extremely high transparency of the atmosphere in this region. This effect is still more distinctly seen in the map for January (Fig. 48), when the maximum values of total short-wave radiation in the center of Antarctica exceed 30 kcal cm^{-2} month^{-1}. In December, the corresponding value is a few per cent greater than in January, and constitutes the highest monthly values of total short-wave radiation observed on the globe.

According to data obtained by Rusin, the atmospheric transparency in the Antarctic is especially great in the central highland regions, where the transparency coefficient (the ratio of the flux of direct radiation incident upon a normal surface to the value of the solar constant) amounts to 0.9.

It is natural that under such conditions, the role of scattered radiation declines and, notwithstanding intensive reflection of the sun's rays from the snow surface with their subsequent scattering, the principal component of the total solar radiation is found to be direct-beam radiation.

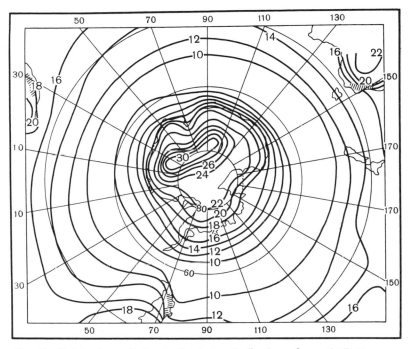

Fig. 48   Total solar radiation in the Antarctic (kcal cm^{-2} month^{-1}). January.

The annual values of the radiation balance (Fig. 49) are characterized by a rapid decrease in high latitudes due to the very high albedo of the snow and ice cover. The albedo of the Antarctic continent, according to Rusin's data, is equal on the average to 0.83–0.84, slightly decreasing in summer months in the coastal regions. Because of such high values of albedo, absorbed radiation in Antarctica is rather small and amounts in sum to about 15–20 kcal cm^{-2} yr^{-1}.

Net long-wave radiation in the Antarctic, in spite of the small values of counterradiation from a cold atmosphere with little cloudiness, is comparatively small because of the permanently low temperature of the radiating surface. However, over the period of a year, it proves to be greater than absorbed short-wave radiation, the result of which is that annual totals of the radiation balance in Antarctica are negative. The location of the zero isoline of the balance coincides closely with the coastline of the continent. It must be indicated that the negative values of the annual radiation balance are not only the consequence of the unique climatic conditions on this continent but are also, to some extent, a factor that substantially influences the stability of the regime of Antarctic glaciation.

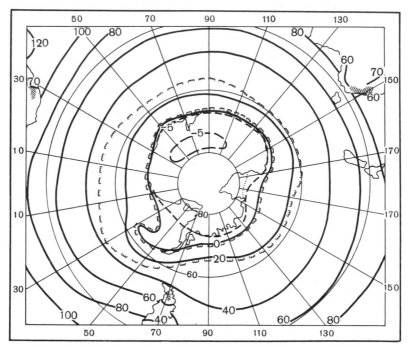

Fig. 49   Radiation balance of the Antarctic (kcal cm^{-2} yr^{-1}). Year.

During three to four summer months, the values of the radiation balance in Antarctica are positive. They reach their maximum in the coastal zone and slowly decrease toward the center of the continent. During most of the year, however, monthly values of the radiation balance are negative. The lowest values (up to -2 to -3 kcal cm^{-2} month^{-1}) are observed at the coast, while in the central regions in winter, the radiation balance is approximately equal to -1 kcal cm^{-2} month^{-1}.

The maps in Figs. 50 and 51, drawn by Strokina (1966), give some idea of the distribution of the turbulent sensible-heat flux and the latent-heat flux from the surface of the ocean encircling Antarctica. It is seen from these maps that both of the turbulent components of the heat balance decrease with an increase in latitude. It must be remembered, however, that near the coasts of the mainland the values of the latent-heat and sensible-heat fluxes increase appreciably, because this region receives quite cold and dry air out of the Antarctic continent. This heat outgo is especially great in regions where leads in the ice remain open throughout the year, where it may reach 100–200 kcal cm^{-2} yr^{-1} and still greater values. As a result, the general

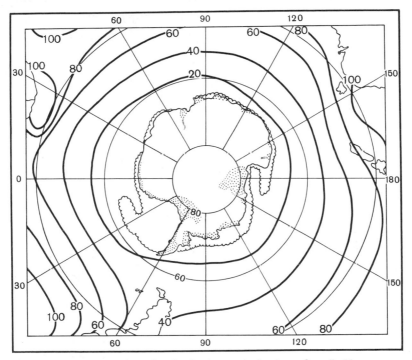

Fig. 50 Latent-heat flux in the Antarctic (kcal cm^{-2} yr^{-1}). Year.

decrease in the outgoing fluxes of latent and sensible heat with increase in latitude is replaced near the coast of Antarctica by a pronounced rise in these quantities. (This cannot be depicted in the maps presented here because of their small scale.)

The values of the turbulent fluxes of sensible and latent heat on the Antarctic continent are at present determined only approximately. According to the data obtained by Rusin, the turbulent sensible-heat flux in Antarctica over the course of the whole year is directed from the atmosphere toward the earth's surface. Annual values of this flux amount to -5 to -10 kcal cm^{-2}

yr^{-1}, except in the region of katabatic winds, where they may reach -15 to -20 kcal cm^{-2} yr^{-1}.

Heat conversion in evaporation in the central regions of Antarctica is small, and probably fully compensated by the heat income from condensation of water vapor on the snow surface. In the coastal zone, evaporation noticeably increases in regions of drainage wind activity, where heat loss for evaporation may amount to 10–15 kcal cm^{-2} yr^{-1}.

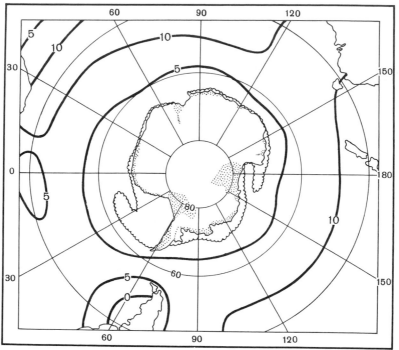

Fig. 51 Sensible-heat flux from the earth's surface into the atmosphere in the Antarctic (kcal cm^{-2} yr^{-1}). Year.

Considering the evaluations of components of the heat balance presented here, Rusin inferred the special importance of the turbulent sensible-heat flux as the fundamental source of energy in the heat balance of Antarctica. It follows from this conclusion that the thermal regime of Antarctica essentially depends on heat transfer by atmospheric advection from lower latitudes.

Comparing regularities in the heat balances of the central regions of the Arctic and Antarctic, we can conclude that in several respects they are similar.

In Antarctica, as in the central regions of the Arctic Ocean, all the components of the heat balance are, as a rule, rather small in comparison with their values in lower latitudes. The reason for this is the high albedo, which results in the fact that the energy basis of the heat balance—absorbed solar radiation—turns out to be very small. Thus, with appreciable annual and very large summer values of total solar radiation, the radiation balance in high latitudes is close to zero, which has a considerable effect on the conditions of air-mass transformation and is an important factor in the formation of the cold thermal regime of high latitudes.

The heat balance of mountain regions

The components of the radiation and heat balances on land depend substantially on the relief of the terrain. This influence is especially great in mountainous areas, where it is a consequence of both the general elevation of the surface and also of special exposures of slopes with respect to the direction of the sun's rays and to the position of adjacent hills covering part of the sky.

Study of the radiation regime in mountains began at the end of the 19th century. Among the first studies in this direction were those of K. Ångström (1901), who measured solar radiation on top of the Peak of Tenerife (3683 m), Allesandri's observations (1909) on Monte Rosa (4500 m), and Nezdiurov's observations (1909) conducted on Little Ararat (up to the height of 3800 m). Systematic measurements of short-wave radiation in mountains were first begun at Alpine health resorts, data of these observations having been generalized in papers of Dorno (1925), Götz (1926), and others.

Later, the Alpine regime of radiation was thoroughly studied in the papers of such Austrian scientists as Steinhauser (1939, 1951), Mörikofer (1935), Sauberer (1938, 1954, 1955), Sauberer and Dirmhirn (1951, 1958), Dirmhirn (1951), and other authors. Although the radiation regime of other foreign mountain regions is far too little investigated, data of more or less long observations, chiefly of short-wave radiation, are nevertheless available for some regions.

In the Soviet Union, the most detailed studies of the radiation regime of mountain regions have been carried out in the Caucasus (Voloshina, 1961; Gongodze and Sulakvelidze, 1953; Mosidze, 1956; Rukhadze, 1960; Tsutskiridze, 1960; Shikhlinskii, 1960; and others) and in Middle Asia (Aizenshtat, 1961; Veremeichikova, 1962; Danilova, 1954; Zuev, 1958; Drozdov and Nikolaenko, 1964; Karol', 1962; Kazanskii and Kolesnikova, 1961; Lopukhin, 1957, 1959; and others).

In some recent investigations, the heat-balance components at the earth's surface of mountain regions have been measured. Such observations were in most cases carried out on glaciers and associated with the study of their evolution.

Utilization of material of the above investigations permitted the working out of methods for calculating the components of the radiation and heat balances in mountains and applying them to a detailed study of the distribution of these components in mountain regions. Thus, for example, Shikhlinskii (1960, 1968) calculated and mapped total short-wave radiation, radiation balance, turbulent sensible-heat flux, and latent-heat flux for the territory of the Azerbaijan SSR.

In the study of Borzenkova (1965), applying specific methods for climatological calculation of heat-balance components, maps of radiation-balance components in the Caucasus were constructed. Vertical gradients of the values studied, which later were used for the construction of appropriate maps, were determined in this paper.

We present here maps of the annual values of total short-wave radiation (Fig. 52) and the radiation balance (Fig. 53) in the Caucasus that were constructed by Borzenkova.

As seen in the first map, short-wave radiation varies considerably in the territory of the Caucasus. These variations are due both to changes in terrain altitude and to differences in the regime of cloudiness.

Values of the radiation balance are less variable than those of solar radiation, up to altitudes of 2–2.5 km. Above this level, the radiation balance starts decreasing noticeably, and in the zone of permanent snow, it reaches values close to zero.

Using material of available investigations of the radiation regime and heat balance in mountain regions, it is possible to draw some conclusions about regularities of the income of solar energy and its transformation in mountain conditions.

In the mountains, total solar radiation usually increases with altitude, because of the increase of both direct and scattered radiation. It should be indicated, however, that scattered radiation increases with altitude only when clouds are present; in cloudless weather, the quantity of scattered radiation does not increase with altitude, but decreases. A pronounced increase in the amount of scattered radiation is observed in the zone with snow cover, as a result of the significant increase of radiation reflected from the earth's surface.

Net long-wave radiation also increases somewhat with altitude, at any rate up to an altitude of several kilometers. However, these changes are not very great, because the reduction of atmospheric counter-radiation in the mountains is, to a considerable extent, compensated by the reduction of radiation emitted from the earth's surface due to the lowering of its temperature.

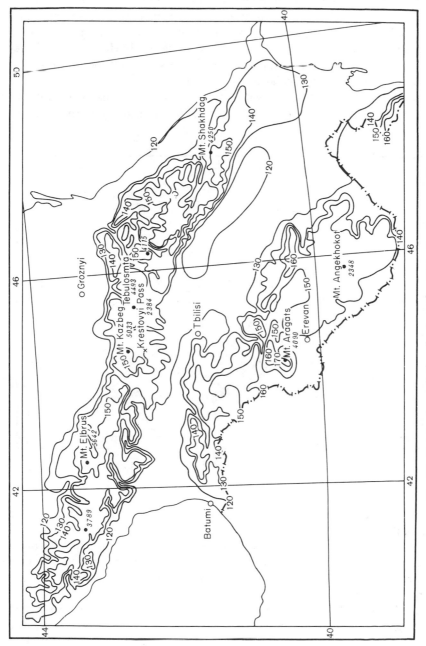

Fig. 52 Total solar radiation (kcal cm⁻² yr⁻¹) in the Caucasus. Year.

191

The radiation balance of mountain regions lying below the zone of snow or ice changes relatively little with altitude, since the increase in absorbed short-wave radiation is, to some extent, balanced by the increase in net long-wave radiation. With snow cover, the abrupt increase in albedo significantly reduces absorbed short-wave radiation, which leads to a considerable decrease in values of the radiation balance.

Variations of latent-heat flux with altitude depend on moisture conditions. In areas of surplus moisture, the conversion of heat by evaporation in

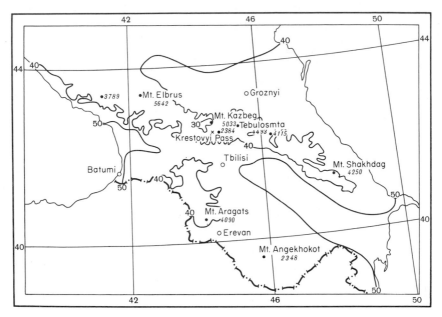

Fig. 53   Radiation balance (kcal cm^{-2} yr^{-1}) in the Caucasus. Year.

mountains decreases with altitude, because of the fall in temperature of the evaporating surface. In regions of insufficient moisture, the quantity of precipitation in mountains usually increases with height, which sometimes leads to an increase in latent-heat flux with height up to the level at which the effect of temperature reduction compensates the influence of the increase of precipitation.

The dependence of the turbulent sensible-heat flux on altitude is associated with the variations in the latent-heat flux, and in the snow-free zone, it is usually of a reverse character—an increase of latent-heat flux with altitude is accompanied by a decrease of the sensible-heat flux, and vice versa.

2. Variations of the Components of the Heat Balance in Time

The annual march of components of the heat balance

On the basis of the material comprised in "Атлас теплового баланса земного шара," it is possible to present the principal regularities of the changes in components of the heat balance during the annual march. Let us look first at the characteristics of the annual cycle of balance components at the surface of the land.

A typical annual march of the heat-balance components in the equatorial zone is presented in Fig. 54 (São Gabriel, South America). The graph in this figure shows that in the equatorial zone, the radiation balance [surplus] R

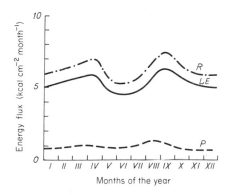

Fig. 54 Annual march of the components of the heat balance. São Gabriel, 0° 08′ S, 67° 05′ W. Equatorial continental climate.

changes comparatively little during the annual march. The two maxima—in spring and in fall—are associated with the increase of total short-wave radiation at the times of equinox, when in equatorial latitudes the mean altitude of the sun is greatest.

Because the soil is permanently moistened by abundant precipitation in the region of São Gabriel, the principal fraction of the energy of the radiation balance goes for evaporation. The annual march of the latent-heat flux LE is nearly parallel to the annual march of the radiation balance. The sensible-heat flux P is characterized by small values in every month. Its value increases at the end of a period of relatively low precipitation, when the heat outgo for evaporation becomes slightly reduced.

Other regularities of the annual march of the heat-balance components are shown in Fig. 55, illustrating climatic conditions of the equatorial monsoons on the east side of the continents (Saigon, Vietnam). A radiation balance maintaining high values throughout the year has a maximum at the end of winter and beginning of spring, when the region under consideration is occupied by dry tropical air with little cloudiness. The reduction of cloudiness increases total short-wave radiation considerably, which leads to an increase in the radiation balance.

Heat conversion in evaporation in Saigon is also great because of high annual precipitation, but it possesses a significant annual cycle. At the beginning of the dry period, when the soil has not yet dried out, the conversion to latent heat remains large. Then, in proportion to the drying of the soil, this conversion to latent heat falls off rapidly. At the end of the dry season, it has decreased to a fraction of what it was in the rainy season.

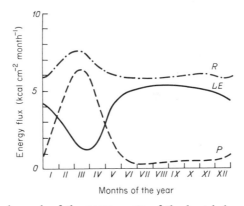

Fig. 55 Annual march of the components of the heat balance. Saigon, 10° 47′ N, 106° 42′ E. Equatorial monsoon climate.

It is interesting to note that the evaporation minimum is observed later than the maximum in the radiation balance. This is presumably to be explained by the dependence of evaporation on the state of soil moisture.

The annual march of the exchange of sensible heat is, in general, opposite to that of evaporation. The value of the turbulent sensible-heat flux is small in all months except in the dry period, when it becomes greater than the flux of latent heat.

Regions of the tropical zones are characterized by a great variety of regimes of components of the heat balance, depending on their location relative to the quasi-permanent pressure systems.

The annual march of components of the heat balance in regions of continental tropical climate is presented in Fig. 56 (Aswan, northeastern Africa).

Under typical conditions of tropical deserts, the annual march of the heat-balance components is defined by rather simple regularities. With insignificant cloudiness throughout the year, the variations in the radiation balance are conditioned principally by changes in sun altitude that occur during the annual march and lead to corresponding changes in total incoming short-wave radiation. The marked annual cycle in the radiation balance in this case shows the great influence of astronomical factors on the radiation balance even in comparatively low latitudes (about 24°). It should be noted that the greatest values of the radiation balance at Aswan are approximately equal to those at Saigon, although the corresponding values of total short-wave radiation differ considerably. This can be explained by the increased albedo in desert regions and mainly by the large values of net long-wave radiation at a strongly heated desert surface.

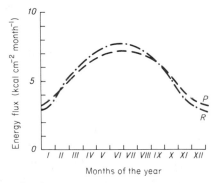

Fig. 56 Annual march of the components of the heat balance. Aswan, 24° 02′ N, 32° 53′ E. Tropical continental climate.

Since there is practically no precipitation in Aswan, the heat conversion in evaporation through the year is near zero. As a consequence, the sensible-heat outgo is very great and near the value of the radiation balance. (The small difference between these values is caused by the existence of a small heat exchange in the soil.)

Different conditions of the annual march of components of the heat balance are observed in the regions at the western periphery of the subtropical anti-cyclones. In these regions (refer to Fig. 57, where the annual march of heat-balance components at Payo-Obispo, Central America is presented), the amount of precipitation is significant, and the conversion of heat for evapora-tion is correspondingly large. During almost the whole year, the heat con-version for evaporation constitutes the greater part of the radiation balance, the outgo of sensible heat being small in comparison. Evaporation decreases slightly in spring, in the time of a short dry period, during which the soil loses part of its moisture. Simultaneously, the value of the sensible-heat outgo increases markedly.

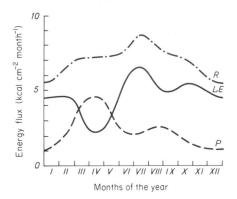

Fig. 57   Annual march of the components of the heat balance. Payo-Obispo, 18° 30′ N, 88° 20′ W. Tropical climate of the western periphery of the oceanic anticyclones.

In regions on the eastern periphery of the oceanic anticyclones, desert conditions are observed which are not very different from those of continental tropical deserts. An example of the annual march of components of the heat balance in this climatic type is presented in Fig. 58 (Mossamedes, southwestern Africa).

As seen from this figure, the radiation balance in Mossamedes, like that in Aswan, varies in correspondence to changes in the mean altitude of the sun (its maximum being in the Southern Hemisphere summer). Conversion of heat in evaporation is negligible in Mossamedes, and the flux of sensible heat is close to the radiation balance.

In the subtropical zones, climatic conditions also are very diverse, in dependence on regularities in the circulation processes. Corresponding to this, the balance components change also.

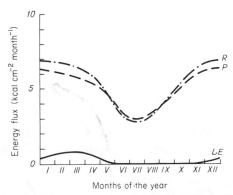

Fig. 58   Annual march of the components of the heat balance. Mossamedes, 15° 12′ S, 12° 09′ E. Tropical climate of the eastern periphery of the oceanic anticyclones.

A typical picture of the annual march of heat-balance components in a subtropical continental climate is presented in Fig. 59 (Aidin, central Asia). In this case, the annual march of the radiation balance, conditioned by astronomical factors, is very marked, and the radiation balance approaches zero in the winter months. Heat conversion in evaporation is small, because of the small amount of precipitation. Therefore, in the warm season, the sensible-heat flux reaches high values.

Another type of the annual march of heat-balance components is seen for the conditions of the western coasts of continents in subtropical climates.

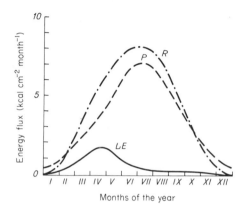

Fig. 59 Annual march of the components of the heat balance. Aidin, 39° 23′ N, 54° 50′ E. Subtropical continental climate.

Under conditions of an arid summer and humid winter, typical of the Mediterranean climate, a unique annual march of latent-heat and sensible-heat flux is observed. In these regions, heat outgo for evaporation rapidly increases in spring along with the increase in the radiation balance, and then sharply falls with the drying of the upper layers of the soil. A small secondary maximum of evaporation is observed at the end of autumn, when the soil is becoming moist again. It is soon replaced, however, by a winter minimum, caused by the deficit in the radiation balance. In these conditions, the turbulent flux of sensible heat has a high maximum in summer and at the beginning of autumn.

In the subtropical monsoon climate on islands near the eastern coasts of the continents, as is seen from Fig. 60 (Miyazaki, Japan), the maximum in the radiation balance is shifted toward the end of summer. This is caused by heavy cloudiness in the summer monsoon. The large amount of precipitation provides for high amounts of latent-heat flux, which are close to the values

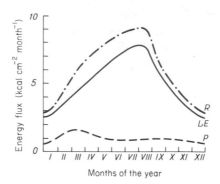

Fig. 60   Annual march of the components of the heat balance. Miyazaki, 31° 56′ N, 131° 26′ E. Subtropical monsoon climate.

of the radiation balance. The sensible-heat outgo throughout the year is comparatively small.

In middle latitudes, the regularities of the annual march of the components of the heat balance are also different under different conditions of atmospheric circulation. In the interior regions of the continents, the radiation balance possesses a distinct summer maximum, which, in the Northern Hemisphere, comes in June (refer to Fig. 61, where data for Barnaul are given). In spring and autumn, the radiation balance changes rapidly, and in the cold season it is characterized by negative values, which in absolute terms are much smaller than the summer maximum. The period with negative values of radiation balance corresponds more or less to the period of snow cover on the ground, although there is not complete coincidence between them.

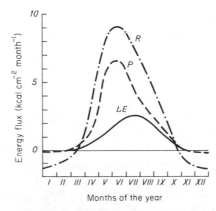

Fig. 61   Annual march of the components of the heat balance. Barnaul, 53° 20′ N, 83° 42′ E. Continental climate of the middle latitudes.

The annual march of heat used in evaporation under these climatic conditions resembles that of the radiation balance. In this case, the difference between the values of latent-heat flux and radiation balance in the warm season is larger, the greater the moisture deficit of a given place is. Variations in the outgo of sensible heat during the annual cycle are characterized by a summer maximum, which increases with an increase in dryness of the climate. In winter, the sensible-heat flux is directed from the atmosphere to the earth's surface, but its absolute values are smaller than in summer.

The difference between the times when components of the heat balance reach their maxima deserves attention. The maximum outgo of heat for evaporation can be observed earlier or later than the maximum in the radiation balance. The date of this maximum depends on the annual march of precipitation and the associated change in soil moisture. If the maximum in the latent-heat flux precedes the radiation-balance maximum, then the maximum in the sensible-heat flux is commonly observed after that in the radiation balance, and vice versa.

In the zone of monsoon climates of the eastern coasts of the middle-latitude continents, the annual march of heat-balance components depends on the monsoon circulation (refer to Fig. 62, Grossevichi). In this case, heavy cloudiness in summer reduces the maximum value of the radiation balance. The curve of the latent-heat flux has a unique shape, with a maximum in August. In winter, the heat balance of this region has features like those of the heat balance in the same latitudes in a continental climate.

In higher latitudes and conditions of a subarctic continental climate, the heat-balance components have an annual march similar to that in conditions of the continental climate of middle latitudes (refer to Fig. 63, Turukhansk).

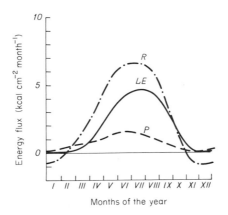

Fig. 62 Annual march of the components of the heat balance. Grossevichi, 47° 58′ N, 139° 32′ E. Monsoon climate of the middle latitudes.

In this zone, the highest values of the radiation balance slightly exceed those in lower latitudes, although the length of the period with positive values of the radiation balance is found to be shorter. As a consequence, the curve of the annual cycle of the radiation balance acquires a more pointed shape. Under these conditions, the curve of the annual cycle of the flux of latent heat has a similar shape.

It is interesting to note that in the Subarctic, the sensible-heat flux directed upward in the warm season is still larger in absolute magnitude than that directed from the atmosphere to the underlying surface in the cold season.

The above material shows that the greatest monthly totals of the radiation balance on continents vary comparatively little from equatorial latitudes to the Subarctic. The principal cause of this lies in the fact that in higher latitudes,

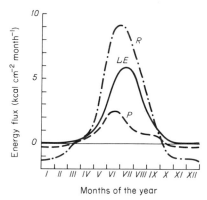

Fig. 63   Annual march of the components of the heat balance. Turukhansk, 65° 47′ N, 87° 57′ E. Subarctic continental climate.

the smaller maximum height of the sun in summer is to some degree compensated by an increase in length of day. Thus, the variation in annual totals of the radiation balance with latitude, which is outstanding in middle and high latitudes, is not due to a decrease in maximum values of the balance but to a reduction in the duration of the period with positive values.

The annual marches of two other basic components of the heat balance on land—the latent-heat flux and the sensible-heat flux—are closely connected with moisture conditions.

With surplus moisture in the soil throughout the year, the latent-heat flux is close to the value of the radiation balance, the sensible-heat flux being small and (with a positive radiation balance) usually indicating an outgo of heat from the underlying surface into the atmosphere.

With the existence of dry periods leading to a noticeable drying of the soil, the decline in the latent-heat flux relative to the radiation balance is greater, the more the soil dries. Simultaneously, the sensible-heat flux increases. In this situation, the beginning of the decline in the latent-heat flux and of the growth in the sensible-heat flux comes slightly behind the time a rainless period sets in, because at the beginning of this period the soil usually still retains a considerable amount of moisture.

Under land conditions, the monthly sums of the soil-heat flux from the surface to the lower layers are, as a rule, considerably smaller in absolute terms than the maximum monthly totals of the principal components of the heat balance. At the same time, in those periods when the principal balance components are small in absolute value (for example, in winter months), the values of the heat flux in the soil are quite comparable in size with these components.

The curve of the annual march of the soil-heat flux resembles a sine curve, characterized in the warm season by heat used for warming the soil and in the cold season by the gain of heat at the surface from the cooling of the soil. The amplitude of the annual march of the soil-heat flux, as already pointed out in Chapter II, is closely connected with the annual amplitude of air temperature variation. In consequence, in many tropical regions where air temperature varies little during the annual cycle, the monthly sums of heat flux into [and out of] the soil are small throughout the year.

Monthly values of the soil-heat flux reach their greatest magnitude under conditions of continental climates of the middle and high latitudes. However, in these cases, the maximum monthly values of this flux remain appreciably less than those of the radiation balance. This distinguishes the conditions of the exchange of heat between the surface and the lower layers on land from the corresponding situation on the oceans.

The components of the heat balance at the surface of Antarctica possess a completely unique annual march. Figure 64 presents appropriate data at Mirnyi station, situated at the periphery of the Antarctic continent. It is seen from this figure that under conditions of continental glaciation, the heat-balance components are small in absolute value throughout the entire year. The annual cycle of the latent-heat flux is similar to that of the radiation balance, but the total amount of heat used for evaporation over the whole year is greater than the total amount in the radiation balance. During the whole year, the flux of sensible heat is directed from the atmosphere to the earth's surface, reaching its maximum absolute value in winter.

The annual marches of heat-balance components at different climatic zones of the oceans will be considered in the same order as for the land.

We shall illustrate the annual march of the heat-balance components in the equatorial zone of the oceans by data for the central region of the Atlantic Ocean (latitude 0°, longitude 30° W). It is seen from the data presented in Fig. 65 that in this region, the radiation balance changes comparatively little

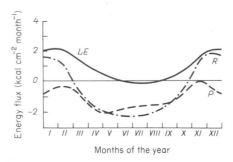

Fig. 64 Annual march of the components of the heat balance. Mirnyi, 66° 33′ S, 93° 01′ E. The Antarctic.

throughout the year. Heat converted in evaporation represents a considerable portion of the radiation balance, and the sensible-heat flux, which is small throughout the year in absolute value, is directed from the ocean's surface to the atmosphere.

In this region, the heat flux directed from the water surface into the deeper layers reaches its greatest values in spring and autumn, when the heat income from the radiation balance appreciably exceeds the heat outgo in the latent-heat sensible-heat fluxes. A surplus of heat received by the water masses at these times must presumably be transported from the region under consideration to higher latitudes as a result of the activity of currents and macro-turbulence.

The annual march of the heat-balance components under conditions of the oceanic climate of the equatorial monsoon zone is presented in Fig. 66 (a region of the Arabian Sea, latitude 15° N, longitude 70° E).

In this case, the annual course of the radiation balance is substantially influenced by an increase of cloudiness in summer, when there is a period of advection of equatorial air masses. The increase of cloudiness reduces total

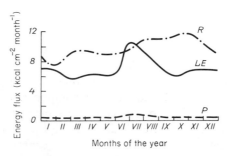

Fig. 65 Annual march of the components of the heat balance. Atlantic Ocean, 0° latitude, 30° W. Equatorial climate.

short-wave radiation and the radiation balance, in the annual cycle of which appears a secondary summer minimum. The turbulent flux of sensible heat is negligible throughout the year (which corresponds to the small differences between water and air temperatures); however, it increases slightly in winter, which is characteristic of monsoon climates.

In this region, the heat conversion in evaporation varies in an annual cycle that is inverse to the variation in the radiation balance. (We should note that such a regular feature is typical of the greater portion of the ocean surface.) In this case, the winter maximum can be explained by an inflow of dry trade-wind air, which noticeably increases the humidity deficit. The summer maximum is caused by a strong increase of wind speed during the active period of the equatorial monsoon.

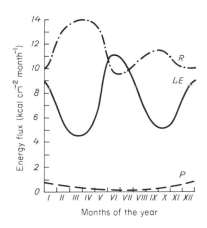

Fig. 66 Annual march of the components of the heat balance. Indian Ocean, 15° N, 70° E. Equatorial monsoon climate.

As a result of the considerable growth of the latent-heat flux in winter and in summer and the corresponding decrease in the radiation balance, there appears a heat flux directed from the lower water layers to the surface, though its absolute values remain relatively small. In contrast, great amounts of heat are transferred from the ocean's surface to the deeper layers in spring and autumn and then transported horizontally to other regions of the world ocean.

In the tropical belts of the oceans, the annual march of the heat-balance components is different in regions with different conditions of atmospheric circulation.

As is well known, warm ocean currents are found at the western periphery of the oceanic anticyclones.

We shall take as an example the region of the Mozambique Channel (latitude 20° S, longitude 40° E). The annual march of the heat-balance components in this area is given in Fig. 67.

Under these conditions, the radiation balance varies generally in accord with the annual march of short-wave radiation, and the latent-heat flux has the opposite pattern. The sensible-heat flux increases slightly in winter (Southern Hemisphere), when the activity of the warm current strengthens. At this season, heat fluxes in the latent and sensible forms noticeably exceed the radiation balance, which leads to the disbursal of a considerable amount of heat coming from deeper layers. Such a phenomenon is typical of the active area of warm currents transporting relatively heated water masses.

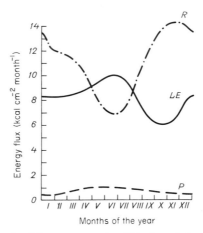

Months of the year

Fig. 67   Annual march of the components of the heat balance. Indian Ocean, 20° S, 40° E. Tropical climate of the western periphery of the oceanic anticyclones.

In contrast to conditions of the western periphery of the oceanic anticyclones are the cold currents at their eastern periphery. The annual course of the components of the heat balance changes correspondingly. We shall illustrate the annual course of the balance components in tropical regions of the western periphery of the oceanic anticyclones from data relating to the region of the Benguela Current in the southeastern Atlantic Ocean (latitude 20° S and longitude 10° E—refer to Fig. 68).

Heat conversion in evaporation is diminished here, compared to its value in the previous region, which is situated in the same latitude. The sensible-heat flux, small in absolute value, is directed in the Southern-Hemisphere summer from the atmosphere to the colder ocean surface.

Since the heat income from the radiation balance is greater than the heat used in evaporation through most of the year, then, for the region under

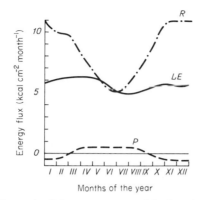

Fig. 68 Annual march of the components of the heat balance. Atlantic Ocean, 20° S, 10° E. Tropical climate of the eastern periphery of the oceanic anticyclones.

consideration, a large amount of thermal energy is transferred to the deeper water layers and is spent on heating the comparatively cold water masses transported by the current. This expenditure reaches especially great values in the Southern-Hemisphere summer.

Under conditions of the subtropical zone, the principal regularities in the annual march of heat-balance components at the ocean surface are, in general, similar to those for the corresponding regions of the tropical latitudes. A sharper annual cycle in the radiation balance, caused by considerable changes in the mean height of the sun during the year, warrants attention.

Typical curves for the annual march of heat-balance components at the ocean surface in middle latitudes are shown in Figs. 69 and 70. The first

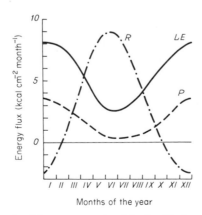

Fig. 69 Annual march of the components of the heat balance. Atlantic Ocean, 60° N, 10° W. Climate of middle-latitude regions in warm currents.

figure, relating to the northern Atlantic Ocean (latitude 60° N and longitude 10° W), defines the conditions of the heat balance in the area where a warm current, the Gulf Stream, is active.

At latitude 60°, the radiation balance at the ocean surface varies within very wide limits during the year, and its negative values in winter, unlike those for land conditions, cannot be considered small in absolute value.

Throughout the year, in this region, the turbulent flux of sensible heat is directed from the warmer ocean surface to the atmosphere, its values being much greater in winter than in summer. Heat outgo in evaporation is also very large in winter. The ocean surface must therefore get a great amount of heat from deeper layers during the winter months, in order to make up for the outgo in evaporation and sensible heat and the radiative heat loss.

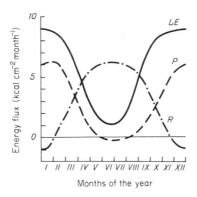

Fig. 70   Annual march of the components of the heat balance. Pacific Ocean, 45° N, 160° E. Monsoon climate of the middle latitudes.

The heat gained in this situation partly comes from the cooling of the upper layers of water and partly from the enormous energy resources of the Gulf Stream.

The annual march of the components of the heat balance changes when warm-current activity is combined with the effect of the monsoon climate of middle latitudes. Figure 70, representing data of the northwest part of the Pacific Ocean (southwest of the Kurile Islands—45° N and 160° E), shows that in these circumstances the sensible-heat flux becomes negative in the warm season, and in the cold is directed from the ocean toward the atmosphere. It is evident that the change of the sensible-heat flux reflects the influence of the monsoon circulation on the heat exchange.

In the region under consideration, as well as in the previous case, the ocean surface gets a significant quantity of heat from deeper layers in winter months, to a considerable degree the consequence of using the energy of the warm current, Kuro Shio. In opposition to this, the gain of heat from the radiation balance in summer greatly exceeds the expenditure for evaporation, which leads to a heating of the upper water layers and promotes the transfer of surplus heat to other oceanic regions by means of horizontal heat conductivity.

In conclusion, we make some deductions about general regularities in the annual cycle of components of the heat balance on the oceans.

The annual march of the radiation balance on oceans is, in general, similar to that on land areas that are under conditions of a humid climate.

Turbulent exchange of sensible heat on the oceans depends essentially on the activity of warm and cold ocean currents, which alter the temperature of the water surface. In regions of cold currents, the sensible-heat flux directed from the atmosphere to the underlying surface usually has small absolute values; in regions of warm-current activity, the heat flux directed from the water surface to the atmosphere may reach very large values.

It must be pointed out that in both cases (contrary to land conditions), the annual march of the sensible-heat flux is poorly connected with that of the radiation balance, but depends to a considerable extent on variations of the ocean current regime in its annual march.

A similar regularity is observed also in the annual march of the heat conversion for evaporation from oceans. As indicated above, in conditions of humid areas, the annual cycle of heat conversion for evaporation is close to that of the radiation balance. In contrast to this, the variations of heat conversion for evaporation during the annual cycle on oceans are usually in reverse to those of the radiation balance. At the same time, the annual sums of heat converted in evaporation on the oceans, when averaged over rather large areas, are in most cases very close to the sums of the radiation balance.

In regard to annual marches of components of the heat balance for land and oceans, conditions of the heat exchange between the surface and lower layers differ most of all. On land, this heat-balance component is usually small in individual months and near zero for the year; on oceans, it may amount to very large values both for the year and in particular individual months. Such a characteristic, caused by the great horizontal and vertical heat conductivity in water bodies, is the main cause of the difference between oceanic and continental climates.

The daily march of the components of the heat balance

Most of the material on the diurnal variation in the members of the balance has been obtained during short periods of expedition observations, which hampers their utilization in studying mean climatological regularities.

Among the experimental investigations of the diurnal march of heat-balance components, attention should be paid to the work carried out at the station of the physics of the boundary layer, in Koltushi (Leningrad region). Utilizing observational data obtained at Koltushi and analyzed by Ogneva (1955), Fig. 71 shows for July the mean diurnal cycle of the radiation balance R, the latent-heat flux LE, the sensible-heat exchange P, and the heat inflow A into and out of the soil.

It is seen from this figure that the diurnal variation of the heat-balance components in the warm season is analogous to the annual variation of balance components for similar climatic conditions of middle latitudes.

In the daytime, relatively large positive values of the radiation balance are converted to latent heat, sensible heat, and heat exchange in the soil. In this situation, the latent-heat flux is noticeably larger than the sensible-heat flux (typical of humid climate conditions), and the heat inflow into the soil is considerably less than either the latent-heat flux or the sensible-heat flux.

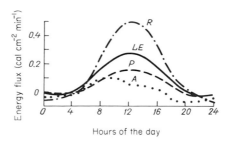

Fig. 71   Daily march of the components of the heat balance in the Leningrad region. July.

At night, the negative radiation balance is comparatively small in absolute value, the heat outgo for evaporation is close to zero, and the outgo of radiative heat is compensated by the gain of heat from the turbulent sensible-heat flux and heat outflow from the soil.

In the spring and autumn months, as Ogneva's data show, the amplitude of the diurnal march of the heat-balance components diminishes with the decrease in the maximum altitude of the sun. In winter, the amplitude of the mean diurnal variation of all the heat-balance components is rather small.

We shall give here some data on the diurnal variation of the heat-balance components in arid climatic conditions, for comparison with the conditions of humid mid-latitude climates considered above. For this purpose, we employ observational data obtained during the GGO expedition to Pakhta Aral (Central Asia), in July 1952 (Aizenshtat *et al.*, 1953). Although the period of observations of the expedition was rather limited, we can nevertheless feel certain that, because of the stability of desert and semidesert climate in summer, the observational material obtained during this expedition is typical of mean long-term conditions.

The diurnal march of components of the heat balance at Pakhta Aral is presented in Fig. 72. In this case also, the similarity between the regularities of the annual and diurnal cycles of the heat-balance components is quite apparent. As in the annual march, the diurnal march in summer is characterized by positive values of the radiation balance that are disposed of for sensible-heat flux and heat inflow into the soil; the turbulent sensible-heat flux noticeably exceeds in magnitude the heat flow into the soil. At night, a comparatively small radiative outgo of heat is compensated by the gain of heat from the soil and the air. Heat conversion by evaporation is close to zero because of the lack of moisture in the soil.

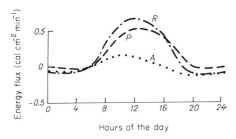

Fig. 72 Daily march of the components of the heat balance in the semidesert of Central Asia. July.

The difference between annual and diurnal cycles of the balance components is caused in this case by differences in the relative duration of the period with negative values of the radiation balance. In the diurnal cycle, this period is close to 12 hr, while in the annual cycle of the deserts of Central Asia, negative values of the radiation balance are observed during only a small part of the year—a few winter months.

Since, in lower latitudes, negative monthly values of the radiation balance are not observed at all, it is clear that for tropical and subtropical latitudes, the above similarity between annual and diurnal cycles is broken.

Besides data on the diurnal variation of heat-balance components obtained as a result of using special methods for balance observations, calculations have been made in a number of studies on the basis of network observations of the basic meteorological elements. Utilization of calculation methods to determine changes in the balance components during the diurnal cycle has expanded the possibilities of studying the climatological regularities of the heat-balance components.

Biriukova (1956), on the basis of calculations of diurnal variation in heat-balance components for climatic zones of the USSR, came to a number of conclusions concerning characteristic features of the diurnal marches under different climatic conditions.

Using calculation methods set forth in Chapter II of this book, Biriukova constructed graphs of the diurnal variation of the components of the heat balance in various climatic zones. We will not give these graphs here, but merely state the principal conclusions from this paper.

It follows from Biriukova's data that in the forest zone of middle latitudes in summer, the radiation balance is positive during the greater part of the 24-hour period (14–15 hr). In wintertime the radiation balance in this zone may remain negative throughout the 24 hours.

Under forest zone conditions, the greatest rates of latent-heat flux are usually observed in the afternoon, while the maximum sensible-heat outgo is often observed at earlier hours.

In more southern regions associated with the steppe zone, the radiation-balance maximum during the diurnal cycle in summer is slightly greater than that in the forest zone, but the duration of the period with a positive radiation balance is somewhat less.

In the steppe zone, the passage of the radiation balance through zero occurs at higher sun altitudes than in the forest zone. This is to be explained by the increased values of net long-wave radiation in the more southerly latitudes in the summer period.

In the winter period in a number of regions of the steppe zone, the radiation balance in daytime may maintain positive values during 4–6 hr of the 24.

For the still more southerly regions of the desert zone, very high maxima of total short-wave radiation are typical in summertime. In this situation, however, the corresponding maxima of the radiation balance are relatively reduced (because of the very great values of net long-wave radiation) and usually do not exceed those in the steppe zone.

Under conditions of the deserts of Central Asia, the radiation balance in the midday hours is, as a rule, positive during the whole year. The transition of radiation-balance values in the desert zone past zero occurs at solar altitudes that are higher than in the steppe and forest zones.

Material on the diurnal variation of components of the heat balance on oceans has been obtained by Strokina, who processed observational data from several weather ships for this purpose.

The results of Strokina's calculations are presented in Figs. 73 and 74, which characterize the diurnal march of the heat-balance components in the northern part of the Atlantic Ocean (latitude 44° N, longitude 41° W) for mean conditions in February and August.

In both cases, the latent- and sensible-heat fluxes between the ocean

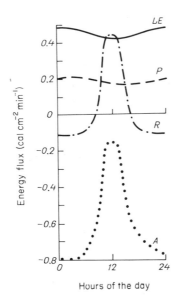

Fig. 73 Daily march of the components of the heat balance at the ocean surface (44° N, 41° W). February.

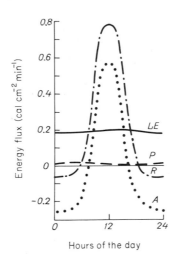

Fig. 74 Daily march of the components of the heat balance at the ocean surface (44° N, 41° W). August.

surface and the atmosphere change very little during the diurnal cycle. The changes in the radiation balance lead to considerable changes in the heat exchange between the ocean surface and lower layers.

It is seen from these figures that the diurnal regularities of all components of the heat balance on oceans (except the radiation balance) differ noticeably from the corresponding regularities on land.

Aperiodic variations in the components of the heat balance

Aperiodic variability in heat-balance components during long periods of time is a factor in climatic change and, for shorter periods, a factor of variations in weather.

The long-term variations in the balance components are usually small in comparison with the means of the balance components, which hampers their investigation.

Thus, for example, let us consider the case of a 5° rise in the temperature of the upper 100-m layer of the ocean, which corresponds to a very great shift in climatic conditions. If such a temperature variation occurred during a century, it would correspond to an increase in heat content of the water by 0.5 kcal cm^{-2} yr^{-1}, a small value in comparison with the principal components of the heat balance of the ocean. In reality, such variations in ocean temperature usually occur over much greater periods of time; as a result the corresponding yearly changes in components of the heat balance are extremely small.

Notwithstanding this fact, some fluctuations in energy regime associated with changes in climate can be investigated on the basis of observational data. In Chapter V of this book, material defining the secular trend of solar radiation incident on the earth's surface is presented. Some results of calculations of changes in components of the heat balance that have taken place during large climatic variations are also presented.

In contrast to the long-term variability of heat-balance components, the study of changes in heat-balance components by individual days, weeks, and months meets with considerably smaller difficulties, because the values of the corresponding changes are often comparable in size with the means of the balance components.

The first study of monthly anomalies of components of the heat balance was carried out by Efimova in the paper (1956) mentioned at the beginning of this chapter, in which values of radiation-balance anomalies in single months were calculated and mapped for the European territory of the USSR. Efimova pointed out that the relationships of anomalies in the radiation balance with anomalies in cloudiness are different in summer and winter.

Along with this, Efimova established a rather close relationship between anomalies of the radiation balance and those of air temperature. (An increase in radiation balance is usually followed by a rise in temperature.)

Zubenok (1968) calculated the values of evaporation in single months at several points in the USSR. On the basis of these data, it was found possible to evaluate the variability in monthly evaporation (and also in latent-heat flux). The coefficients of variation of these values found by Zubenok varied from 0.1 to 0.4, their value in regions of insufficient moisture being greater than in regions of surplus moisture.

Of great interest is the problem of the variability of the components of the oceanic heat balance, for the fluctuations in heat content of the upper layers of the ocean exert a great influence on large-scale atmospheric processes.

In recent years, calculations of the anomalies of the oceanic heat balance have been carried out. They have been based on utilization of the same methods as those that have been used for determining and mapping the norms of heat-balance components.

Among the pieces of research having this orientation, we must mention those of Roden (1959) and Arkhipova (1960). The first of these presented evaluations of anomalies in the heat-balance components for the region of the California current, which were obtained from data on the variability of individual meteorological elements influencing the balance components. Such evaluations are rather approximate, since the magnitudes of anomalies of the heat-balance component are determined by the variability, not of individual meteorological elements, but of their combinations, which must be considered when studying the anomalies.

More accurate calculations of anomalies of the heat balance on the oceans were carried out in Arkhipova's papers, in which monthly values of the heat-balance components over a 10-yr period were determined from observational data from weather ships in the northern part of the Atlantic Ocean. In her papers, information on mean and maximum values of the anomalies of components of the heat balance was obtained, and several regularities that characterize the stability of the anomalies in time and space were indicated.

To get more detailed data about the anomalies in the components of the heat balance on oceans, a similar investigation was carried out by Budyko, Kagan, and Strokina (1966). In this work, a calculation of the heat-balance components was made from observational data obtained from nine weather ships situated in the northern part of the Atlantic Ocean between 35 and 66° N and between 2° E and 51° W over the period 1951–1960. This calculation used material of meteorological observations from the summary of Pflugbeil and Steinborn (1963), which included the data of eight observational times in each 24 hours.

From these data, values of the radiation balance, sensible-heat flux, and latent-heat flux in each month were calculated, by use of procedures employed in drawing maps in "Атлас теплового баланса земного шара

(Atlas of the Heat Balance of the Earth)" (1963). In addition, monthly values of the changes in heat content of the upper 100-m layer of water were determined by means of the method stated in the previous chapter of this book. From the values found for components of the heat balance, means in each month of the 10-yr period were determined and found to be quite close to similar values calculated from data of the long-term observational period. This permitted the determination of anomalies of the heat-balance components as the difference between values for individual calendar months and the means over the 10-yr period of observations.

Table 17 presents absolute values of the anomalies in the heat-balance components, meaned over the period of observations and averaged for all nine weather ships. It is seen from this table that anomalies of radiation balance are comparatively small—less than 10% of the radiation-balance values in summer months. In winter, the absolute values of these anomalies becomes smaller and their relative sizes increase, in relation with the considerable annual range of the radiation balance in middle latitudes.

Slightly greater are the anomalies of the latent-heat flux, which during the year amount to about 20% of the means. Still greater is the variability of the sensible-heat flux, the anomalies of which exceed 30% in the winter months and reach still greater relative values in summer. This is associated with the smallness of the absolute magnitudes of the sensible-heat flux during the warm season.

The variations in heat content of the upper layers of water from month to month are very large. The anomalies are in absolute magnitude about 50% of the mean value of the variation in heat content.

In individual regions of the Atlantic Ocean, the mean anomalies in the components of the heat balance might be appreciably greater than the values given in Table 17. In particular, the variability of heat-balance components in the region where observations were made by ship D, situated in the stream of the North Atlantic current (44° N, 41° W) is very great.

A great variation in the amount of heat gained or lost in the upper layers of the ocean leads to great variations in values of the oceanic heat content in the same month of different years.

It is seen from analysis of this material that the anomalies in values of the heat content of the upper oceanic layer are characterized by a noticeable stability in time. It has been established that in many situations, the sign of the anomaly in a certain ocean region remains unchanged for several months, a positive correlation between anomalies being observed, on the average, for a period of about three months. This is, for example, apparent from the data of Table 18, which presents values of the autocorrelation coefficient (r_τ) between values of oceanic heat content in different months, in relation to the interval of time (τ). Since the calculation procedure used does not

TABLE 17

ANOMALIES OF MONTHLY VALUES OF COMPONENTS OF THE HEAT BALANCE[a] (kcal cm^{-2} month^{-1})

Heat balance components	Jan.	Feb.	Mar.	Apr.	May	June	July	Aug.	Sept.	Oct.	Nov.	Dec.
Radiation balance	$\frac{0.3}{-1.0}$	$\frac{0.4}{0.4}$	$\frac{0.4}{2.8}$	$\frac{0.7}{5.9}$	$\frac{0.9}{7.6}$	$\frac{0.6}{8.3}$	$\frac{0.8}{8.1}$	$\frac{0.6}{6.7}$	$\frac{0.4}{4.1}$	$\frac{0.3}{1.6}$	$\frac{0.3}{-0.3}$	$\frac{0.3}{-1.1}$
Latent-heat flux	$\frac{2.2}{11.4}$	$\frac{2.0}{11.0}$	$\frac{1.7}{9.3}$	$\frac{1.5}{7.2}$	$\frac{1.5}{5.2}$	$\frac{0.9}{4.0}$	$\frac{0.9}{3.8}$	$\frac{1.3}{5.6}$	$\frac{1.5}{7.9}$	$\frac{2.1}{9.6}$	$\frac{1.9}{10.9}$	$\frac{2.3}{11.8}$
Sensible-heat flux	$\frac{1.7}{5.0}$	$\frac{1.6}{4.4}$	$\frac{1.3}{3.3}$	$\frac{0.9}{1.9}$	$\frac{0.7}{0.9}$	$\frac{0.4}{0.6}$	$\frac{0.4}{0.2}$	$\frac{0.4}{0.6}$	$\frac{0.6}{1.2}$	$\frac{1.0}{2.2}$	$\frac{1.0}{3.2}$	$\frac{1.4}{4.6}$
Change in heat content	$\frac{2.1}{-4.6}$	$\frac{1.7}{-2.2}$	$\frac{2.2}{0.4}$	$\frac{1.8}{3.1}$	$\frac{2.1}{6.1}$	$\frac{2.6}{9.1}$	$\frac{3.1}{9.3}$	$\frac{3.4}{4.9}$	$\frac{2.4}{-2.1}$	$\frac{2.5}{-7.9}$	$\frac{2.4}{-9.2}$	$\frac{2.0}{-7.5}$

[a] Numerator—anomaly; denominator—norm.

215

TABLE 18

Autocorrelation Coefficients of the Heat Content of the Ocean r_τ
and the Changes in Heat Content $r_{1\tau}$ in Relation
to the Interval of Time τ

Coefficient	τ (months)				
	0	1	2	3	4
r_τ	1.00	0.71	0.28	0.08	0.00
$r_{1\tau}$	1.00	0.21	−0.38	−0.20	−0.10

permit us to calculate the heat content itself, but rather its variations from month to month, the autocorrelation between the values of heat content has been calculated from data on the autocorrelation of variations in the heat content $r_{1\tau}$ (lower line in Table 18).

The maps of anomalies of the different components of the heat balance of the ocean as well as the calculations that have been done show that the anomalies of the changes in heat content, the flux of latent heat, and the exchange of sensible heat usually spread over extensive areas. The positive correlation between values of the anomalies of these heat-balance terms obtains on the average over a radius of 1700 km. Figure 75 shows values (averaged for a year) of the coefficients of correlation between the anomalies of latent-heat flux that were obtained from different weather ships, in relation to the distance between them (ρ). Similar dependences are also observed for the other heat-balance components.

The interrelations between anomalies of the components of the heat balance have a definite interest. Calculations have shown that there exists a relation-

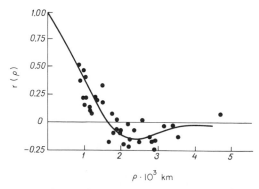

Fig. 75   Values averaged over the year of the coefficients $r(\rho)$ of correlation between the anomalies of the latent-heat flux from the data of different weather ships, in relation to the distance ρ between them.

ship between the anomalies of the latent-heat flux and those of the upward sensible-heat flux. On the average, this relationship is characterized by a correlation coefficient of $+0.8$. There are also relationships between the anomalies of the variations in ocean heat content and those of the latent-heat flux, which are inverse. In absolute values, the correlation coefficients are small (about -0.2, on the average). This is caused by the fact that the variations in heat content are determined not only by conditions of the thermal interaction between ocean and atmosphere but also by the heat transport by horizontal movements in a deep layer of water.

It must be borne in mind that the values of the correlation coefficients indicated above have been obtained from data that might contain certain errors. These errors are associated both with the procedure of measuring the hydrometeorological elements and with that of calculating the components of the heat balance. Therefore, the relations existing in nature should be characterized by higher correlation coefficients than those obtained here.

The data given on the variability of anomalies in components of the heat balance in the North Atlantic show that in a number of cases, these anomalies possess considerable stability in space and time. This confirms the possibility of using information on the oceanic heat balance when studying nonstationary atmospheric processes of large scale.

The variability of components of the heat balance for periods shorter than a month has so far been little studied.

Among studies in this direction we must mention the one of T. G. Berliand (1968), who collected a large amount of material on the interdiurnal variability of solar radiation and the radiation balance at many stations. On the basis of these data, maps were constructed of mean values of interdiurnal variability of solar radiation (for different months) in the Northern Hemisphere. Berliand pointed out that interdiurnal variability of the radiation balance is closely connected with the variability of solar radiation and, on the average, has about half its value.

3. Heat and Water Balances of the Earth

Heat balance

The material on geographical distribution of components of the heat balance set forth at the beginning of this chapter permits us to determine the components of the heat balance both of the earth as a whole and of its different latitudinal zones.

Such calculations were made earlier by Dines (1917), Alt (1929), Baur and Philipps (1934), Lettau (1954), and Houghton (1954).

In these studies, the terms of the heat balance were calculated either for the whole earth or for mean conditions of latitudinal zones. In papers of members of the Main Geophysical Observatory (Budyko *et al.*, 1954; Budyko *et al.*, 1962), the components of the heat balance at the earth's surface were determined from maps of heat-balance terms, which permitted specifying the mean values of these quantities.

We shall give here the results of calculation of the components of the earth's heat balance, based on utilization of the world maps in "Атлас теплового баланса земного шара" (1963).

On the basis of the material on the spatial distribution of the heat-balance components, latitudinal means were calculated, relating to the surface of continents, oceans, and the earth as a whole. The results of this calculation are presented in Table 19.

The data in this table show that only one component of the heat balance—the radiation budget [surplus]—possesses a similar latitudinal distribution on land and ocean. Both on the continents and on the oceans, the maximum values of the radiation budget are observed in the tropics, the latitudinal means within the limits of the tropical latitudes being almost constant.

The latitudinal changes in the difference between the values of the radiation surplus of land and ocean attract attention. This difference is at its maximum in the low latitudes, where it constitutes about one third of the value of the ocean radiation budget. With an increase of latitude, the radiation budgets of land and oceans draw nearer to one another, and in the latitudes from 50 to 70°, they become practically the same. One of the causes of this regularity lies in the increase in the mean albedo of water surfaces with the increase of latitude.

The latitudinal means of the latent-heat flux from land have their principal maximum at the equator, which shifts to decreased evaporation in the latitudes of the high-pressure belts. With a further increase of latitude in both hemispheres, there exists some increase in evaporation (more noticeable in the Northern Hemisphere), owing to a rise in precipitation in comparison with the arid zones of lower latitudes. With a still further increase of latitude, the latent-heat flux diminishes in association with the insufficient amount of heat.

On oceans, contrary to conditions on the continents, the maximum latitudinal means of the latent-heat flux are observed in the belts of high pressure. The fact that in latitudes of 50–70°, where the radiation budgets of land and ocean are approximately identical, the latent-heat flux from the ocean is much greater than it is from land is worthy of attention. This is obviously to be explained by the great amount of heat brought in by ocean currents and disbursed in evaporation.

The latitudinal means of the sensible-heat flux from the ocean increase

TABLE 19

LATITUDINAL MEANS OF COMPONENTS OF THE HEAT BALANCE AT THE SURFACE OF THE EARTH[a] (kcal cm^{-2} yr^{-1})

Latitude (degrees)	Ocean				Land			Earth			
	R	LE	P	F_0	R	LE	P	R	LE	P	F_0
70–60 N	23	33	16	−26	20	14	6	21	20	9	−8
60–50	29	39	16	−26	30	19	11	30	28	13	−11
50–40	51	53	14	−16	45	24	21	48	38	17	−7
40–30	83	86	13	−16	60	23	37	73	59	23	−9
30–20	113	105	9	−1	69	20	49	96	73	24	−1
20–10	119	99	6	14	71	29	42	106	81	15	10
10–0	115	80	4	31	72	48	24	105	72	9	24
0–10 S	115	84	4	27	72	50	22	105	76	8	21
10–20	113	104	5	4	73	41	32	104	90	11	3
20–30	101	100	7	−6	70	28	42	94	83	15	−4
30–40	82	80	9	−7	62	28	34	80	74	12	−6
40–50	57	55	9	−7	41	21	20	56	53	9	−6
50–60	28	31	8	−11	31	20	11	28	31	8	−11
Earth as a whole	82	74	8	0	49	25	24	72	60	12	0

[a] R is the radiation balance, LE is the latent-heat flux, P is the sensible-heat flux, and F_0 is the heat advection in the oceans.

regularly with increasing latitude. On land, these values are at their maximum in the high-pressure belts, somewhat reduced near the equator, and fall off sharply in high latitudes. The quite different kind of variation in these values on land and on the ocean defines the principal differences in the mechanism of air-mass transformation at the surface of continents and of oceans.

The distribution of the latitudinal means of heat input and outgo in the oceans due to the activity of currents shows that ocean currents carry away heat principally from the zone between 20° N and 20° S, the maximum of the thermal energy carried off by the currents being shifted slightly north of the Equator. This heat is transported into higher latitudes and disbursed in greatest quantities in the latitudinal zone from 50 to 70° in the Northern Hemisphere, where especially powerful warm currents are active.

The mean latitudinal distribution of the heat-balance components for the earth as a whole [land and sea] are characterized in different latitudinal zones by regularities typical of the continents or the oceans, depending on the relative areas of land and ocean in the different zones.

Means of the heat-balance components for individual continents and oceans are given in Table 20.

TABLE 20
HEAT BALANCE OF CONTINENTS AND OCEANS (kcal cm^{-2} yr^{-1})

Continents and oceans	R	LE	P	Continents and oceans	R	LE	P
Europe	39	24	15	Australia	70	22	48
Asia	47	22	25	Atlantic	82	72	8
Africa	68	26	42	Pacific	86	78	8
North America	40	23	17	Indian	85	77	7
South America	70	45	25				

It is seen from this table that in three continents (Europe, North America, South America) among the six, the greater part of the energy in the radiation balance is spent for evaporation. The three other continents (Asia, Africa, Australia) are characterized by the reverse relationship, which corresponds to prevailingly dry climatic conditions.

Mean heat-balance conditions of the three oceans differ very little. It is necessary to be aware of the fact that the sum of the fluxes of latent and sensible heat for each ocean is found to be close to the value of the radiation balance. This means that heat exchange between oceans resulting from the activity of ocean currents does not substantially affect the heat balance of each ocean as a whole. This result, natural from the physical point of view, presumably indicates the higher accuracy of these calculations of the oceanic heat balance in comparison with the earlier one (Budyko, 1956), in which the author did not succeed in closing the balance for each ocean separately. At the same time, we might suggest that the small excess of the radiation balance over the sum of the turbulent heat fluxes from the Atlantic Ocean corresponds to the real fact that a certain quantity of heat is transferred from the Atlantic to the Arctic Ocean. Since the difference lies within the limits of accuracy of the calculation, it is evident that this problem needs special investigation.

Table 20 includes no data on the heat balance of Antarctica and the Arctic Ocean because, in terms of accuracy, these data are slightly inferior to those for the other continents and oceans.

On the basis of the above data and available evaluations of heat-balance components for polar areas, the values of heat-balance components for all the continents, the world ocean, and the earth as a whole, have been calculated. The results of this calculation are presented in the last line of Table 19.

It follows from these data that on the oceans, about 90% of the energy of the radiation balance is spent for evaporation and only about 10% for direct turbulent heating of the atmosphere. On land, these two forms of disbursal of the radiative energy are characterized by almost identical values. For the whole earth, heat disbursed in evaporation makes up 83% of the radiation balance and in sensible-heat exchange, 17%.

These data may be compared with conclusions from several previous investigations in which the components of the heat balance of the earth as a whole were determined.

The results of such a comparison are seen in Table 21. All values presented in Table 21 are expressed in relative units in order to exclude any effect of differences in the evaluations of the solar constant on the results of the

TABLE 21

Heat Balance at the Surface of the Earth[a]

	Components of the balance				
Investigation	$Q(1 - \alpha)$	I	R	LE	P
Dines, 1917	42	14	28	21	7
Alt, 1929	43	27	16	16	0
Baur and Philipps, 1934	43	24	19	23	−4
Houghton, 1954	47	14	33	23	10
Lettau, 1954	51	27	24	20	4
Budyko, Berliand, and Zubenok, 1954	42	16	26	21	5
Budyko, Efimova, Zubenok, and Strokina, 1962	43	15	28	23	5

[a] Components of the heat balance are expressed in per cent of the quantity of solar radiation incident on the outer boundary of the atmosphere. I represents the net loss of heat by exchange of long-wave radiation.

calculations. It is apparent that the first calculation of heat balance of the earth's surface, made by Dines in 1917 by a very approximate method, led to results matching the last calculation well. Since the subsequent studies of Alt and also Baur and Philipps gave less accurate results, it might be considered that this coincidence is partially explicable by the outstanding physical intuition of Dines, and partially by chance.

The conclusions reached by Houghton and Lettau for most components of the balance are close to the results of our last calculation, though some heat fluxes (the net long-wave radiation of Lettau, and the sensible-heat exchange of Houghton) found in these studies differ markedly from the values we have obtained.

The results of our calculations also agree rather satisfactorily with the values of the heat balance of the Northern Hemisphere found in the study by London (1957).

We must dwell in more detail on the conclusions obtained in our calculations concerning the mean direction of the turbulent flux of sensible heat from the earth's surface to the atmosphere for the whole earth and in latitudinal zones situated between 70° N and 60° S for both land and oceans.

Not too long ago, there existed in meteorological literature, including textbooks, a viewpoint that the turbulent heat flux, on the average, is directed from the atmosphere to the earth's surface. This idea, first suggested by Schmidt (1921 and elsewhere), was supported by the results of heat-balance calculations made by Baur and Philipps (1935).

In their calculation of the heat balance of the underlying surface, Baur and Philipps determined the sensible-heat exchange, using a method offered by Schmidt, at two points, Batavia and Lindenberg, and then obtained the latitudinal distribution of this component by means of interpolation and extrapolation from these data.

In this case, Baur and Philipps did not use any actual data of heat converted in evaporation, and calculated its value as a residual component of the balance, not considering the redistribution of heat by ocean currents.

Such a method for calculation of heat balance components gives rise to some objections. First, proceeding from contemporary ideas, when determining the heat-balance components, one should consider factual material on evaporation, since heat conversion in evaporation is one of the most important components of the heat balance.

Secondly, the method offered by Schmidt for determination of turbulent heat flux, and based on the idea that this flux is proportional to the vertical gradient of potential temperature, cannot be considered correct. In calculations of Budyko and Iudin (1946, 1948), it was shown that the turbulent heat flux is proportional to the difference between the vertical temperature gradient and the equilibrium gradient, approximately equal to 0.6° per 100 m.

This difference departs considerably from the value of the potential-temperature gradient (data from later investigations on this subject are given in the collection "Равновесный градиент температуры (Equilibrium Gradient of Temperature)" (1967).

When solving the problem of the direction of the mean sensible-heat flux near the level of the earth's surface, one must take into consideration observational material on the temperature of the earth's surface. The development of observations of ocean-surface temperature has shown that over most of the equatorial oceans, the surface is warmer than the lower layer of air. Although in most cases the corresponding temperature difference is comparatively small and amounts to 1–2°, its sign shows, however, that on the greater part of the globe occupied by oceans, the sensible-heat flux is directed from the earth's surface into the atmosphere.

There are fewer corresponding data for the continents, and the quality of observations of land-surface temperature is often low. However, proceeding from the available observational data, we can deduce that except in cold-season conditions in middle and high latitudes, the daily mean temperature of the land surface is usually much higher than the temperature of the air, and in regions of insufficient moisture, the differences between surface and air temperatures may reach very large values.

Consequently, from the data of observations on the temperature of the earth's surface alone a conclusion can be drawn about the erroneous character of the Schmidt concept. A similar conclusion may be drawn also from the material of all the calculations of the heat balance at the earth's surface accomplished during the last decades. Thus we now possess three independent methods for determining the direction of the flux of sensible heat, related to computations of the heat balance, measurements of the difference in temperature between earth's surface and air, and measurements of the vertical gradient of temperature in the troposphere. All lead to the identical meaning, which indicates that the Schmidt paradox is fully explained.

Utilization of the material contained in the maps of "Атлас теплового баланса земного шара" permits obtaining data on the latitudinal means of the heat-balance components of the earth–atmosphere system and of the atmosphere. The results of suitable calculations are presented in Tables 22 and 23. It is seen from the data given in Table 22 that the relationships among the heat-balance components of the earth–atmosphere system differ noticeably in different latitudinal zones.

In the equatorial zone, a considerable supply of heat resulting from the phase transformations of water (that is, from the difference between the heat of condensation and the heat of energy converted for evaporation) $L(E - r)$ is added to the great supply of radiational energy R_s. These sources of heat provide for a large outgo of heat in atmospheric F_a and oceanic F_0 advection,

TABLE 22

LATITUDINAL MEANS OF THE COMPONENTS OF THE HEAT
BALANCE OF THE EARTH–ATMOSPHERE SYSTEM
(kcal cm^{-2} yr^{-1})

Latitude (degrees)	R_s	$L(E - r)$	F_a	F_0
70–60 N	-49	-8	-33	-8
60–50	-30	-15	-4	-11
50–40	-12	-9	4	-7
40–30	4	13	0	-9
30–20	14	31	-16	-1
20–10	23	11	2	10
10–0	29	-43	48	24
0–10 S	31	-14	24	21
10–20	28	16	9	3
20–30	20	32	-8	-4
30–40	9	19	-4	-6
40–50	-8	-8	6	-6
50–60	-29	-27	9	-11

TABLE 23

LATITUDINAL MEANS OF THE COMPONENTS OF THE HEAT
BALANCE OF THE ATMOSPHERE (kcal cm^{-2} yr^{-1})

Latitude (degrees)	R_a	Lr	P	F_a
70–60 N	-70	28	9	-33
60–50	-60	43	13	-4
50–40	-60	47	17	4
40–30	-69	46	23	0
30–20	-82	42	24	-16
20–10	-83	70	15	2
10–0	-76	115	9	48
0–10 S	-74	90	8	24
10–20	-76	74	11	9
20–30	-74	51	15	-8
30–40	-71	55	12	-4
40–50	-64	61	9	6
50–60	-57	58	8	9
Earth as a whole	-72	60	12	0

for which the comparatively narrow zone near the Equator is an extremely important energy source.

In higher latitudes, approximately up to 40°, with a positive radiation balance that diminishes with increasing latitude, a heat outgo for phase transformations of water is observed that amounts to considerable values. In a large part of this zone, the heat outgo for phase transformations is comparable with the value of the radiation surplus. As a result, the redistribution of heat by air and sea currents is small in comparison.

Higher than latitude 40° is situated the zone of negative radiation balance, which grows in absolute value with the increase in latitude. The radiation deficit in this zone is compensated by the income of heat transported by air and sea currents. In this situation, the relationship between the balance components that compensate the deficiency of radiative energy in different latitudinal belts turns out to be different. In the latitudinal zone 40–60°, the main heat source is the surplus of energy released in the process of water-vapor condensation over the heat used for evaporation at the earth's surface. In these latitudes, the income of heat redistributed by ocean currents is also of great importance.

Redistribution of heat in the atmospheric circulation becomes the main source of thermal energy in the higher latitudes and especially in the polar regions, where the gain of heat from condensation is small and the influence of ocean currents is either absent (the south polar zone) or weakened by the permanent ice cover (the north polar zone).

The data from Table 23 show that the latitudinal means of the radiation budget of the atmosphere vary less than the other heat-balance components. The negative values of the atmospheric radiation budget, which are large in absolute value and are observed in all latitudes, are compensated, for the most part, by the gain of heat from condensation.

The supply of heat from the earth's surface as a consequence of the sensible-heat exchange plays a lesser role, although its influence on the heat balance of the atmosphere is quite noticeable.

The values of the components of the heat balance of the whole earth are presented in diagrammatic form in Fig. 76.

From the total flux of solar radiation incident on the outer boundary of the troposphere and approximately equal to 1000 kcal cm^{-2} yr^{-1}, one fourth, on the average, which amounts to about 250 kcal cm^{-2} yr^{-1}, due to the spherical shape of the earth, comes to a unit area of the outer boundary of the troposphere.

Assuming the albedo of the earth to be equal to 0.33, we find that the short-wave radiation absorbed by the planet Earth amounts approximately to 167 kcal cm^{-2} yr^{-1}. This value is shown in Fig. 76 by the arrow $Q_s(1 - \alpha_s)$.

According to the above data, short-wave radiation equal to 126 kcal cm^{-2}

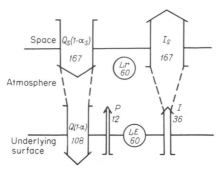

Fig. 76   Heat balance of the earth (components of the heat balance in kcal cm^{-2} yr^{-1}).

yr^{-1} arrives at the earth's surface. The mean albedo value of the earth's surface (determined by taking into account the differences in input of solar radiation in different regions) equals 0.14. Thus, at the earth's surface, a quantity of solar radiation amounting to 108 kcal cm^{-2} yr^{-1} (the arrow $Q(1 - \alpha)$ in Fig. 76) is absorbed and 18 kcal cm^{-2} yr^{-1} is reflected from the earth's surface.

The values given show that the atmosphere absorbs 59 kcal cm^{-2} yr^{-1}, considerably less than the earth's surface.

Since the radiation balance at the earth's surface equals 72 kcal cm^{-2} yr^{-1}, then it is evident that the net long-wave radiation at the level of the earth's surface is, on the average, 36 kcal cm^{-2} yr^{-1} (arrow I). The total value of long-wave radiation from the planet Earth, equal to the amount of absorbed short-wave radiation, is close to 167 kcal cm^{-2} yr^{-1} (arrow I_s).

The fact that the ratio of the net long-wave radiation from the earth's surface to the total emission from the earth (I/I_s) is considerably less than the corresponding ratio of the quantities of absorbed short-wave radiation $Q(1 - \alpha)/Q_s(1 - \alpha_s)$ is worthy of attention. This difference illustrates the enormous influence of the "greenhouse" effect on the thermal regime of the earth.

Because of the "greenhouse" effect, the earth's surface receives about 72 kcal cm^{-2} yr^{-1} radiative energy (the radiation surplus), which is partially spent for evaporation of water (60 kcal cm^{-2} yr^{-1} is shown in the form of the circle LE), and partially returned to the atmosphere by means of the sensible-heat flux (12 kcal cm^{-2} yr^{-1}, arrow P). As a result, the heat balance of the atmosphere is made up as follows:

1. The gain of heat from absorbed short-wave radiation, which amounts to 59 kcal cm^{-2} yr^{-1};
2. The gain of heat from condensation of water vapor (shown in Fig. 76 by the circle Lr), amounting to 60 kcal cm^{-2} yr^{-1};

3. The gain of heat from sensible-heat exchange at the earth's surface, amounting to 12 kcal cm^{-2} yr^{-1};
4. The outgo of heat as long-wave radiation into space, which equals the difference between the values I_s and I, i.e., 131 kcal cm^{-2} yr^{-1}.

The final value coincides with the sum of the first three components of the heat balance.

The water balance

Let us first discuss the problem of the water balance of the continents. Total precipitation on land has long been measured at numerous meteorological stations and posts. In consequence, the construction of precipitation maps for the continents on the basis of observational data is not associated with any major difficulty.

The annual precipitation means for the different continents, determined from the precipitation map constructed by Kuznetsova and Sharova (1964), are presented in Table 24. This table does not include data of precipitation in the Antarctic, which are, however, taken into account when calculating the precipitation mean for the total land surface.

TABLE 24
PRECIPITATION AND EVAPORATION ON THE CONTINENTS

Continent	Precipitation (cm yr^{-1})	Evaporation (cm yr^{-1})
Europe	64	39
Asia	60	31
North America	66	32
South America	163	70
Africa	69	43
Australia	47	42
All the land	73	42

We must indicate that the instruments used for measuring precipitation often underestimate the amount of precipitation received, especially when measuring the amount of snow that, due to wind effect, is not completely caught in the gauges.

Systematic errors in precipitation measurements are different for different instruments. When drawing the precipitation maps, attempts were made toward the correction of the most substantial errors of this kind, but the corrections adopted have usually been insufficient. In work of recent years, it has been established that in regions with a great amount of solid precipitation, the actual sums of precipitation might be several tens of per cent greater than the norms adopted earlier. The quantity of liquid precipitation is usually measured with smaller systematic errors, though sometimes they may amount to appreciable values. Therefore, the sums of precipitation presented in Table 24 are somewhat underestimated.

Because of the absence of mass observations of evaporation, the mean evaporation from the continent surface can be determined only by means of calculation methods. In Table 24, the evaporation values found with the use of the appropriate map from "Атлас теплового баланса земного шара" are presented.

As is seen from Table 24, the relationships between evaporation and pre- cipitation for single continents differ widely. While evaporation is close to the value of precipitation in Australia, evaporation is less than a half of total precipitation in South America and North America.

The difference between the annual sums of precipitation and evaporation on the continents is equal to the value of run-off. For many river basins, there exist observational data on run-off, though the accuracy of such obser- vations is not always high.

Using observational data and also applying some calculation methods, L'vovich has several times drawn world maps of annual sums of river run-off. The latest map of this kind was published in "Физико-географический атлас мира (Physico-Geographical Atlas of the World)" (L'vovich, 1964).

TABLE 25
RUN-OFF FROM THE CONTINENTS

Continents	f_1 (cm yr^{-1})	f_2 (cm yr^{-1})
Europe	29	25
Asia	29	29
North America	26	34
South America	44	93
Africa	16	26
Australia	5	5
All the land	25	31

In Table 25, the run-off values (f_1) for different continents found by use of this map are presented. In this table are also presented data of run-off from the continents obtained by Zubenok as a result of calculations done for the construction of the world map of evaporation for "Атлас теплового баланса земного шара" (f_2).

It might be noted that for some continents, the run-off values found by the different methods are quite close (Asia, Australia, Europe). For other continents, the difference is greater, reaching its maximum for South America, where the run-off values determined by various methods differ by more than a factor of 2.

It is not easy to estimate which values of run-off in these cases are more accurate. The high reliability of L'vovich's map for regions where accurate data of run-off measurements are available is undoubted. Where there are no such data or where their quality is low, the reliability of this map decreases.

It is probable that a considerable difference between the evaluations of run-off for South America, presented in Table 25, can be explained by this fact. It is known that the total run-off from this continent is, to a considerable extent, determined by the run-off of the Amazon, whose vast basin collects the greatest amount of water, in comparison with any other river of the globe. The earlier estimates of run-off in the Amazon basin yielded a value of about 50 cm yr^{-1}, which was taken into consideration in designing L'vovich's map. The new measurements yield a far greater value, about 100 cm yr^{-1} (Oltman, 1968). This value agrees well with the data that can be obtained with the use of the evaporation map from "Атлас теплового баланса земного шара."

We should note that consideration of the new data concerning the value of the Amazon's run-off would not only bring together the evaluations of run-off for South America in Table 25, but also reduce considerably the difference between the evaluations of run-off from all the land surface, presented in this table.

As is seen from Oltman's work, correction of the data on the run-off of the Amazon increases the run-off for the total land surface by approximately 10%, which equals about half of the difference between the two values of run-off from the continents presented in Table 25. Presumably, for the accurate evaluation of the total run-off from the continents, the obtaining of reliable data on run-off in other big rivers of the low latitudes, where the amount and quality of observations of run-off is often insufficient, would have great importance.

The water balance of the oceans is less studied than that of land, which to a considerable extent can be explained by the difficulty of determining the oceanic water balance on the basis of available observational material.

The water-balance equation of the world ocean for mean annual conditions can be presented in the form

$$r + f = E, \tag{3.1}$$

where r is precipitation, f is run-off from the continents into the oceans, and E is evaporation.

The same equation characterizes the water balance of single oceans or of individual oceanic regions, the component f representing, in such cases, the sum of river run-off and the horizontal redistribution of ocean water as a result of circulation in the hydrosphere.

The data on precipitation on the oceans, obtained in ship observations, describe only frequency of precipitation occurrence and do not contain information on precipitation quantities.

As a result of this, most maps of precipitation on the oceans have been designed on the basis of observational material obtained on islands and coastal stations. It is clear that from such material, it is difficult to determine reliably the value of precipitation for many oceanic regions remote from land. Besides, it has often been suggested that the data of observations on land near the coast give an appreciable systematic error when evaluating precipitation on the oceans, because near the coastline, there frequently develop updrafts increasing the amount of precipitation. Therefore, it has been suggested that the actual values of precipitation over oceans are less than the values obtained from observations at coastal and island stations.

World maps of the distribution of precipitation on the oceans have been constructed by Meinardus (1934), Schott (1926, 1935), Drozdov and Berlin (1953), Albrecht (1960), Kuznetsova and Sharova (1964), and other authors. Calculating the components of the ocean water balance with the use of maps available at that time, Wüst (1936) noticed that the income of water from precipitation and run-off considerably exceeds the evaporation from the oceans. From this, he concluded that for the above-mentioned reason, the actual values of precipitation on the oceans were 30% less than the values presented in the maps. Such a viewpoint was later taken into consideration in the papers of Jacobs (1951) and Möller (1951), who, in drawing maps of precipitation on the oceans, corrected the obtained results by the water balance, which substantially diminished the precipitation values.

Albrecht (1951) used the data of ship observations on the frequency of precipitation for determining precipitation on the oceans. With observational material obtained on land, he estimated the values of precipitation intensity at different latitudes, and then calculated the sums of precipitation on the oceans as the product of the intensity means for an appropriate area by the frequency of precipitation determined from observational data. Maps of precipitation for the Indian and Pacific Oceans were thus constructed for several months.

A similar method was used by Tucker (1961) for the construction of a precipitation map for the northern part of the Atlantic, and by Samoilenko (1966), who drew annual and monthly maps of precipitation for the Pacific.

It must be indicated that along with the utilization of observational data of precipitation, there exists the possibility of determining total precipitation on the oceans by calculation methods, with the use of empirical or theoretical relations that associate precipitation with other meteorological elements. For several reasons, the accuracy of such calculations cannot be high, which, however, does not exclude the possibility of applying them for comparison with the results of observations.

Mean values of evaporation from the ocean surface are determined by means of calculation methods. For this purpose, the following formula is generally used:

$$E = X(q_s - q), \tag{3.2}$$

where q_s is the saturation specific humidity at the temperature of the evaporating surface, q is the specific humidity at the level of ship observations, and X is a coefficient depending mainly on wind speed.

As was pointed out in Chapter II, in many works, beginning with the studies of Shuleikin (1935), it has been assumed that $X = \rho \chi u$, where ρ is the air density, χ is a constant coefficient, and u is the wind speed.

We can show that the value of evaporation from the ocean surface is closely connected with its radiation balance. The value of turbulent heat flux directed from the ocean surface into the atmosphere is determined by formula

$$P = c_p X(T_w - T), \tag{3.3}$$

where c_p is the heat capacity of the air at constant pressure, T_w is the temperature of the water surface, and T is the air temperature.

The heat-balance equation for the world ocean as a whole can be put in the form

$$R = LE + P, \tag{3.4}$$

where R is the radiation balance, and L is the latent heat of vaporization. From Eqs. (3.2–3.4), we find that for mean annual conditions, the heat-balance equation relating to the world ocean possesses the form

$$R = LX(q_s - q) + c_p X(T_w - T). \tag{3.5}$$

It was pointed out in the previous chapter that the sum of members of the right-hand side of this formula, determined for each physical moment of time and then averaged, differs little from the products of the mean value of the coefficient X by the mean differences in humidity and temperature.

Taking into account this fact, we obtain from Eqs. (3.2) and (3.5) the relation

$$E = \frac{R}{L}\left[1 + \frac{c_p(\overline{T_w - T})}{L(\overline{q_s - q})}\right]^{-1}. \tag{3.6}$$

Using observational data, it is possible to find that for the world ocean the value $c_p(\overline{T_w - T})[L(\overline{q_s - q})]^{-1}$ is much less than unity, and approximately equal to 0.1. Taking this into consideration, we find from Eq. (3.6) that total evaporation from the world ocean depends little on temperature and humidity of the air, is practically independent of wind speed, and is in general determined by the value of the radiation balance at the ocean surface. In this situation, the conversion of heat in evaporation makes up about 90% of the value of the radiation balance [surplus].

In further analysis, it must be borne in mind that for the world ocean, the value of river run-off is approximately an order smaller than the two other components of the water balance, namely precipitation and evaporation. Using data obtained by L'vovich (1964), we find the water gain from run-off into the world ocean to be equal to 10 cm yr^{-1}. According to other data, "Атлас тепловото баланса земного шара" (1963), this value is equal to 13 cm. The difference between the two values is insignificant compared with the accuracy of determining the principal components of the water balance.

Thus, the main object in studying the water balance of the ocean involves the estimation of precipitation and evaporation, which ought to match each other.

It is clear from the above that for this purpose, one can use several independent methods, including:

1. The determination of precipitation from observational data;
2. The determination of precipitation by means of calculation methods;
3. The determination of evaporation by Eq. (3.2), the coefficient of which is found without the use of radiation-balance data;
4. The determination of evaporation with the use of material on the radiation balance, the value of which has been found by means of calculation methods;
5. The determination of evaporation by means of material on the radiation balance, found from observational material.

Let us consider what kind of results we obtain in determining precipitation falling on the ocean surface on the basis of observational material.

The latest world map of the annual sums of precipitation on the oceans, constructed by Kuznetsova and Sharova, was published in the "Физико-географический атлас мира" ("Physico-Geographical Atlas of the World") (1964). This map was based principally on observational data of total precipitation on coastal and island stations. The value of precipitation on the surface of the world ocean per year, according to this map, is 114 cm.

It must be made clear how total precipitation on the oceans determined with the use of ship observations of precipitation frequency differs from the data of this map. The comparison of precipitation maps constructed in such a way with maps based on the data of observations on land point to considerable differences in individual oceanic regions.

Taking this into account, one might consider that the utilization of data from ship observations permits a more reliable determination of precipitation sums in regions distant from land, though the accuracy of the material obtained in this case is rather difficult to estimate. The methods for determining precipitation sums from ship observations are based not only on data of precipitation frequency but also of values of intensity, which, on the oceans, varies within a wide range. Since the intensity of precipitation on the oceans is determined from the data of observations on land, the intensity evaluations used in precipitation calculation may be characterized by appreciable random and systematic errors.

Random errors in determination of precipitation for various regions are, to a considerable extent, excluded when determining precipitation values for entire oceans or the whole world ocean. Such an inference is confirmed when comparing precipitation sums for the world ocean determined by various authors. Thus, for example, Albrecht (1960, 1961), using the data of ship observations, found annual values of precipitation on the Pacific and Indian Oceans. He then slightly altered these values to close the oceanic water balance. However, if we compare the values obtained by Albrecht immediately from observational data with similar values from the map of Kuznetsova and Sharova, we find that the precipitation sums for the Indian Ocean calculated by Albrecht are 3% lower and those for the Pacific Ocean are 8% higher than the data obtained from the map of Kuznetsova and Sharova.

The precipitation means for the northern part of the Atlantic Ocean found from Tucker's map (1961) are 30% less than the corresponding values according to Kuznetsova and Sharova. In contrast, the precipitation sum for the Pacific Ocean found by Samoilenko (1966) is 10% greater than the value obtained from the material of Kuznetsova and Sharova.

The results of these comparisons show that utilization of data of ship observations does not lead to appreciable changes in evaluations of the mean totals of precipitation falling on extensive expanses of the ocean. The greatest difference between the two types of precipitation maps relates to Tucker's investigation, which describes a comparatively small portion of the world ocean.

It might be considered that utilization of data from ship observations, which enables us to specify the spatial distributions of precipitation on oceans, does not solve the problem of exclusion of systematic errors in the precipitation values.

These errors may be related to two reasons. The first is the difference between the intensities of precipitation on land and oceans. It is possible that because of the great roughness of the land surface and the great intensity of thermal convection above the continents, the intensity of precipitation is, on the average, greater on land than on the oceans. In such a case, the available maps give overestimated values of precipitation on the oceans.

The second source of error might be the underestimation of values of precipitation measured with existing instruments. For the world ocean this error cannot be large, because the relative role of solid precipitation on the oceans is small. An approximate evaluation shows that the indicated error probably does not exceed 10%.

It is more difficult to determine the size of the error connected with the difference between the intensities of precipitation on land and ocean, which, generally speaking, might be more than 10%.

Application of existing calculation methods to the determination of precipitation on the oceans presumably does not permit us to estimate precipitation with a greater accuracy than can be obtained from observations. For this task, it is difficult, as yet, to use the methods of the general theory of climate, though in the latest investigations in this direction, data have been obtained on the amount of precipitation falling on the earth's surface. To calculate the sums of precipitation on the oceans, one could use the empirical relations between precipitation and other meteorological elements established in the papers of Gal'tsov and other authors.

Applying the empirical relation of total precipitation to the pressure field and humidity that was found by Gal'tsov (1962), Budyko and Strokina (1970) calculated precipitation amounts for the northern portion of the Atlantic Ocean on the basis of observational data obtained from weather ships. The map of precipitation drawn according to this data satisfactorily matches that of Kuznetsova and Sharova.

Such a comparison does not, however, solve the question of correctness of this or other maps of precipitation on the oceans, since the relation found by Gal'tsov is based on observations of precipitation on land. Using it for oceans may be associated with definite systematic errors.

Thus, for the determination of components of the water balance of the world ocean, estimation of the value of evaporation from the ocean has great importance.

For comparison of the results of using various methods for determining evaporation from the ocean surface, we shall use the world map of evaporation published in "Атлас теплового баланса земного шара (Atlas of the Heat Balance of the Earth)" (1963). On the basis of data from this map, evaporation from the world ocean surface per year equals 126 cm. Note that for the construction of this map the formula

$$E = \rho \chi u (q_s - q) \tag{3.7}$$

was used, and the value $\rho\chi$, assumed constant (equal to 2.5×10^{-6} g cm^{-3}), was found by closing the heat balance, that is, from the radiation balance of the ocean surface.

A number of maps of evaporation from the ocean surface have been constructed with the use of Eq. (3.7) or similar formulas, where $\rho\chi$ was considered to have a value changing within a limited range.

Let us consider what results the application of those formulas yields for the determination of evaporation, where the coefficient χ is given without the use of data on the radiation balance.

This group includes the formulas in which coefficients were found from closing the water-balance equation of inland water bodies, from measurements of the turbulent heat fluxes and humidity, by eddy fluctuations of the meteorological elements, and by other methods.

In the review by Robinson (1966), the results of seven papers of such an orientation, written by several authors, are given. Averaging the values of $\rho\chi$ obtained in these papers, we find its mean equal to $(1.8 \pm 0.3) \times 10^{-6}$ g cm^{-3}. It is evident that mean evaporation from the world ocean calculated at such a value of $\rho\chi$ will be 28% less than the value obtained from the map of "Атлас теплового ъаланса земного шара."

Passing on to the values of $\rho\chi$ determined from the data of the oceanic heat balance, we note that as a rule, they yield larger magnitudes of evaporation. Robinson's review contains values of $\rho\chi$ obtained in six investigations in which the values of the oceanic radiation balance were determined by means of calculation methods. The mean coefficient derived from these data is equal to $(2.4 \pm 0.4) \times 10^{-6}$ g cm^{-3}. This value differs little from that used when constructing the maps of evaporation from the oceans in "Атлас теплового баланса земного шара."

For determination of the product $\rho\chi$ from the heat balance, great importance attaches to the fact that during recent years, various authors have made calculations of the radiation balance of the oceans that have given rather close results.

Thus, the values of radiation balance found by Albrecht (1960, 1961) are smaller than the data from "Атлас теплового баланса земного шара," (1963) for the Atlantic Ocean by 9%, for the Indian and Pacific Oceans by 3%, and for the world ocean by 5%. According to Privett (1960), the radiation balance of the oceans of the Southern Hemisphere is 8% greater than the data from the atlas mentioned. The radiation balance of the northern part of the Pacific Ocean found by Wyrtki (1965) is 4% less than the atlas data. According to the data of Samoilenko (1966), the value of the radiation balance of the Pacific Ocean is 13% less than the values from the atlas. The value of the radiation balance of the Indian Ocean (to 50° S), according to the data of Mani et al. (1967), is also 13% less than the atlas data.

In all the cases of mapping evaporation from the oceans by use of material on the radiation balance, data on the oceanic radiation regime obtained by means of calculation methods have been used. During recent years, numerous direct measurements of radiation balance have been taken by various expeditions, and on the basis of their data, the means of the radiation balance relating to the latitudinal zones of the ocean were determined (Strokina, 1968). Having compared the value obtained in this way for the oceanic radiation balance in the zone from 50° N to 50° S with a similar value from "Атлас теплового баланса земного шара," Strokina found that the first value is less than the second one by 1%. In this situation, it is evident that calculation of evaporation by estimating the value $\rho\chi$ from measured values of the radiation balance gives results that are close to the estimates based on calculated values of the radiation balance.

Turning to the question of possible errors associated with various methods of determining evaporation, we note that for the evaluation of evaporation from single oceans or from the whole world ocean, systematic errors, which are not excluded by averaging, have major importance.

When calculating evaporation without the use of data on the radiation balance, a fundamental error is associated with the difficulty of determining the mean of the coefficient χ from Eq. (3.7) for the world ocean. The values of this coefficient found in current investigations relate either to short time periods or to restricted water bodies. For these reasons, they might differ from typical values for the world ocean, averaged in time and space.

At the same time, when using Eq. (3.7) without consideration of the relation between evaporation and the radiation balance, the value of evaporation may be substantially affected by systematic errors in measurements of the water-surface temperature and several other factors considered in the paper of Budyko and Gandin (1966).

Equation (3.6) shows that the role of errors in temperature measurement becomes significantly reduced when determining evaporation from the radiation balance. In this case, the accuracy of evaporation values being calculated corresponds approximately to that of the data of the oceanic radiation balance. As shown by results of many investigations, existing calculation methods permit determining the means of the radiation balance at the land surface with errors not exceeding 10%. Although the problem of the accuracy of calculation of the oceanic radiation balance is less clear, it can be considered that probable errors in such calculations are not very large, since the application of various methods for calculating the radiation balance leads to similar results. Besides, the available materials on direct measurements of the oceanic radiation balance are in good agreement with the results of the corresponding calculations (Albrecht, 1949; Strokina, 1967b, 1968). Worthy of attention is the close dependence between measured and calculated values of the oceanic radiation balance in different geographical regions and seasons, found in the papers of Strokina. A very high coefficient of correlation, approximately equal to 0.95, between measured and calculated values of the radiation balance shows that random and systematic errors of measurements and calculations cannot be very great.

It was mentioned above that the latest maps of precipitation on the oceans, constructed by different methods, give rather close values of precipitation for individual oceans or for the whole world ocean. Since the means of the radiation balance for individual oceans and the world ocean determined by various authors differ little from one another, the values of evaporation from the oceans found on the basis of the radiation balance turn out to be close.

One can compare the available data on total precipitation and evaporation for the world ocean. Let us take into account the fact that the annual sum of precipitation on the world ocean, according to the data of Kuznetsova and Sharova (1964), is 114 cm. The sum of evaporation from the world ocean, according to "Атлас теплового баланса земного шара," amounts to 126 cm. The difference between these values, corresponding to run-off, turns out equal to 12 cm, which lies within the range of the above-stated estimates of this value (10-13 cm). Such agreement permits us to suggest that the errors in determination of both precipitation and evaporation, according to the available maps, are rather small. It is possible that in determining precipitation from observational data, compensation of comparatively small errors takes place, associated with underestimation of precipitation by the instruments used and with different intensities of precipitation on land and oceans.

Thus, among the above-stated five independent methods for determination of components of the ocean water balance, four (observation of precipitation, calculation of precipitation, calculation of evaporation on the basis of the calculated radiation balance, calculation of evaporation on the basis of the measured radiation balance) yield matching results. Calculation of evaporation without consideration of data of the radiation balance gives smaller values, which are, presumably, less accurate.

Using the world map of precipitation designed by Kuznetsova and Sharova and the world map of evaporation from "Атлас теилового баланса земного шара," we shall give the values of components of the oceanic water balance (Table 26).

As indicated earlier, the difference between evaporation from the world ocean surface and precipitation equals the value of river run-off from the continents into the ocean. For individual oceans, this difference equals the sum of river run-off and the horizontal water transfer from one ocean to another due to circulation processes. It is difficult to determine the value of this transfer by means of direct methods, since it represents a small difference between two values: the inflow and outflow of water, both of which are determined with significant error. It is slightly easier to evaluate water

TABLE 26

WATER BALANCE OF THE OCEANS

Ocean	Precipitation (cm yr^{-1})	Evaporation (cm yr^{-1})	Run-off (cm yr^{-1})
Atlantic	89	124	23
Pacific	133	132	7
Indian	117	132	8
World Ocean	114	126	12

exchange between oceans as a residual component of the water balance of each ocean, though in this case also, the accuracy of determining the appropriate values is not high.

The values of river run-off into each ocean in Table 26 are taken from the data of Zubenok (1956), these values being increased by 20% in order to bring into agreement total precipitation, evaporation, and run-off relating to the whole world ocean.

Although this table does not include data on the water balance of the Arctic Ocean (their accuracy is lower than that for other oceans), these data have been taken into consideration in determining the components of the water balance for the whole world ocean.

As seen from this table, the sum of precipitation and run-off for the Atlantic Ocean is less than evaporation. Hence, it follows that water from other oceans, the Arctic Ocean included, where evaporation is noticeably less than the sum of precipitation and run-off, comes into the Atlantic Ocean.

In the Indian Ocean, the sum of precipitation and run-off is slightly less than evaporation, while for the Pacific Ocean, the sum of precipitation and run-off is greater than evaporation, which corresponds to a transfer of water surplus to other oceans. It can be thought that further development of meteorological observations on the oceans will permit us in the future to make these evaluations of components of the oceanic water balance more exact.

Accepting the above values of precipitation and evaporation for land and oceans, we find that for the whole earth, the value of precipitation for the year, which is equal to the value of evaporation, amounts to 102 cm. We must note that this value is appreciably larger than similar values found in most earlier investigations (Wüst, 1936; Möller, 1951; and others).

Using the maps of precipitation designed by Kuznetsova and Sharova and the maps of evaporation from "Атлас теплового баланса земного шара," one can determine the components of the water balance of the latitudinal zones of the earth.

The relation of the water-balance components to latitude is presented in Fig. 77. It is apparent from this figure that in different latitudinal zones, the income of water vapor into the atmosphere from evaporation may be greater or less than the outgo as precipitation. In this condition, the source of water vapor for the atmosphere is mainly the belts of high pressure, where evaporation noticeably exceeds precipitation. Removal of this water-vapor surplus occurs in a zone near the Equator and also in middle and high latitudes, where precipitation is greater than evaporation.

It is evident that the value f, which is equal to the difference between precipitation and evaporation, is also equal to the difference between the income and outgo of water vapor in the atmosphere.

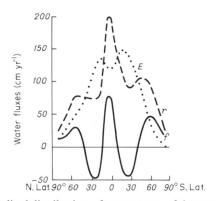

Fig. 77   Mean latitudinal distribution of components of the water balance of the earth.

The large values of component f give an idea of the importance of the water-vapor transfer in the atmosphere for the precipitation regime of different regions. At the same time, it would be wrong to suggest that the effect of water-vapor transfer in the atmosphere on formation of precipitation in different latitudinal zones is determined by the value of the component f. The problem of interdependence among the principal components of the atmospheric water balance, namely, precipitation, evaporation, and horizontal transfer of water vapor, is related to the study of water exchange in the geographical envelope of the earth.

Water exchange

The first investigations of water exchange were aimed at evaluation of the effect of horizontal water-vapor transfer on the amount of precipitation falling onto land.

The authors of these studies (Brückner, 1901; and others) suggested (though sometimes with certain reservations) that in each land region, precipitation is formed from a quantity of water vapor brought in from outside and not exceeding the difference between precipitation and evaporation.

Since the total amount of precipitation on land is usually much greater than this difference, these authors implied the existence of a multiple internal water exchange. In other words, they postulated that the water vapor brought from outside into a certain region of land falls in this region in the form of precipitation, and only then [following evaporation] is it carried away further by the atmospheric circulation.

Another point of view was offered in an investigation on water exchange, in which the quantitative theory of this phenomenon was worked out (Kashin and Pogosian, 1950; Budyko and Drozdov, 1950; and others).

We shall set forth here in brief the derivation of the principal equations of water exchange [refer to Budyko and Drozdov (1953)].

Let us consider the transfer of water vapor in the atmosphere above a certain territory whose linear scale equals l. The flow of water vapor brought by air currents into the given territory can be assumed equal to wu, where w is the mean water content of the atmosphere on the windward portion of the contour of the territory under consideration, and u is the mean speed of the air stream transferring water vapor across the territory. Along a stream line, the water content of the atmosphere varies in accordance with the difference between the water outgo as precipitation and the gain from evaporation.

It is evident that the flux of water vapor carried away from the given territory by air currents equals $wu - (r - E)l$, where r is the total precipitation, E is the total evaporation for the time period under examination, and l is the linear scale of the territory.

The total flux of water vapor transported above the chosen territory is composed of two fluxes—the flux of external (advective) water vapor formed by evaporation outside the given territory, and the flux of local water vapor formed by local evaporation.

The initial flow at the windward contour of the region equals wu and at the lee contour (coming out of the territory) $wu - r_a l$, where r_a is the sum of precipitation formed from the external (advective) water vapor. The second flux is equal to zero at the windward contour, and at the lee contour (coming out from the given territory) is equal to $(E - r_M)l$, where r_M is the precipitation falling from water vapor of local origin.

Thus, on the average, above the territory under consideration, there is the flux of external water vapor, equal to $wu - \frac{1}{2}r_a l$, and the flux of local vapor, $\frac{1}{2}(E - r_M)l$, yielding in sum the total flux, $wu - \frac{1}{2}(r - E)l$. It must be remembered that $r_a + r_M = r$. Since the molecules of water vapor of local and external origin are completely mixed in the atmosphere in the process of turbulent exchange, it is evident that the relationship between the sums of precipitation formed from the local and external water vapor is equal to that between the corresponding quantities of vapor molecules in the atmosphere.

In other words, we can consider that

$$\frac{r_a}{r_M} = \frac{wu - \frac{1}{2}r_a l}{\frac{1}{2}(E - r_M)l}.$$

(3.8)

From this the two following formulas can be derived:

$$r_a = r\,\frac{1}{1 + (El/2wu)},$$

(3.9)

$$r_M = r\,\frac{1}{1 + (2wu/El)}.$$

(3.10)

From Eq. (3.8), we can also determine the value of the water-exchange coefficient β, which is equal to the ratio of the total precipitation to the amount of precipitation of external (advective) origin:

$$\beta = \frac{r}{r_a} = 1 + \frac{El}{2wu}.$$

(3.11)

With the use of the formulas obtained, we can analyze the relationships of the water-exchange characteristics with the principal factors affecting water exchange. Thus, particularly, it follows from Eq. (3.11) that the water-exchange coefficient depends on the factors of water-vapor balance in the atmosphere, and does not depend directly on the value of river run-off. We also note the dependence of external precipitation, local precipitation, and the water-exchange coefficient on the scale of the given territory, from Eqs. (3.9–3.11). With an increase in scale l, the sums of local precipitation and the water-exchange coefficient also increase, and the total precipitation formed by water vapor of external origin decreases. In this case, the actual dependence of the water-exchange coefficient on scale for not too small territories is not linear; with an increase of territory, the effect of curvature of the trajectory of the air particles slightly lowers the mean velocity of water-vapor transfer u.

To estimate the effect of water-vapor transfer in the atmosphere on the formation of precipitation, we give here calculations of the water-exchange components for the European territory of the USSR (Table 27).

The material in Table 27 shows that precipitation formed from local water vapor makes up a very small fraction of the total amount of precipitation. For the whole year, as well as for single months, the water-transfer coefficient but little exceeds unity, which indicates the erroneous character of the concept about multiple internal water turnover.

Actually, even on so extensive a territory of land as the European part of

TABLE 27

ANNUAL CYCLE OF COMPONENTS OF THE WATER EXCHANGE IN THE EUROPEAN PART OF THE USSR

	Jan.	Feb.	Mar.	Apr.	May	June	July	Aug.	Sept.	Oct.	Nov.	Dec.	Year
E (mm month^{-1})	5	5	10	36	50	54	50	39	22	11	7	5	294
w (mm)	4	4	6	9	15	20	23	22	16	12	8	5	12
$\bar{u}$ (m sec^{-1})	7.7	7.8	7.8	7.2	6.6	6.2	5.8	6.3	6.9	7.5	7.7	7.6	7.1
β	1.07	1.08	1.09	1.24	1.22	1.19	1.17	1.12	1.08	1.05	1.05	1.06	1.12
r (mm month^{-1})	27	23	24	28	38	55	63	59	51	49	38	32	487
r_a (mm month^{-1})	25	21	22	23	31	46	54	53	47	47	36	30	435
r_M (mm month^{-1})	2	2	2	5	7	9	9	6	4	2	2	2	52

242

the USSR, only a very small portion (about 12%) of the total amount of precipitation falls a second time as a result of using vapor from local evaporation. The main portion of the precipitation falling onto a limited territory of land is formed from water vapor brought from outside. Even on the most extensive continents, where the relative role of local evaporation is the greatest, as calculations show, the main portion of precipitation is formed from water vapor of external origin, not local.

4. The Thermal Regime of the Earth

Possessing material on the heat balance at the earth's surface and of the atmosphere, it is possible to explain a number of regularities relating to the thermal regime of the earth.

As the data of meteorological observations show, the mean temperature of the air near the earth's surface is approximately 15°C. The distribution of mean annual temperature by latitude in the Northern Hemisphere is presented in Fig. 78 (curve T). It can be seen from this figure that the difference between the annual mean temperatures near the Equator and the pole exceeds 40°.

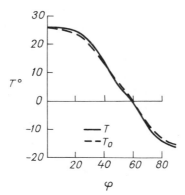

Fig. 78   Mean latitudinal distribution of temperature. T_0 is the calculated temperature, T is the measured temperature.

Let us see how the atmosphere influences the mean temperature of the earth's surface. Without an atmosphere, the mean temperature of the earth's surface will be determined by the conditions of radiative equilibrium, that is, the long-wave emission from the earth's surface will equal the short-wave radiation absorbed. We present this condition in the form of the relation

$$\delta\sigma T^4 = \frac{1}{4} S_0(1 - \alpha_p),\qquad (3.12)$$

where δ is the coefficient characterizing the difference between the properties of the radiating surface and a black body, σ is the Stefan–Boltzmann constant, T is the surface temperature, S_0 is the solar constant, and α_p is the mean albedo of the earth.

Assuming that $\delta = 0.95$, $\sigma = 8.14 \times 10^{-11}\,\mathrm{cal\,cm^{-2}\,min^{-1}}$, and $S_0 = 1.95$ $\mathrm{cal\,cm^{-2}\,min^{-1}}$, we find from Eq. (3.12) that for $\alpha_p = 0.33$, the mean temperature of the earth is equal to $255°\mathrm{K}$ or $-18°\mathrm{C}$. Thus, at the same albedo value, the atmosphere increases the mean temperature of the earth by approximately $33°$. This rise in temperature is associated with the "greenhouse" effect, that is, with the greater transparency of the atmosphere for short-wave radiation compared to long-wave.

It must be noted that such an evaluation has a conditional character: without the atmosphere, the planetary albedo could not be equal to the now existing value, which was assumed as 0.33. Under contemporary conditions, the mean albedo of the earth's surface is 0.14. It might be considered that before the atmosphere appeared, the albedo of the earth was less than this value and possibly differed little from the albedo of the moon, which equals 0.07. At the latter albedo value, the mean temperature of the earth's surface would be equal to approximately $3°\mathrm{C}$.

In order to estimate the effect of incoming solar radiation and albedo on the mean temperature near the earth's surface under actual conditions, it is necessary to know the dependence of the long-wave emission at the outer boundary of the atmosphere on the distribution of temperature. Such a dependence can be established in two ways.

The first way involves building a theoretical model of the vertical distribution of radiative fluxes, temperature, and humidity.

The other method of establishing the dependence on temperature of emission at the outer boundary of the atmosphere is based on the empirical comparison of data of long-wave emission, obtained as a result of observations and calculations, with the factors affecting it.

Such a method was used in studies (Budyko, 1968, 1969), in which for this purpose the results of calculation of the monthly means of the outgoing emission, made when preparing the maps for "Атлас теплового баланса земного шара" (1963), were used.

This material included data on outgoing emission at 260 points, uniformly situated on the land and oceans of the world. Since the calculations of outgoing emission were made for each month, we had in all 3120 values of monthly means of outgoing radiation.

Comparing these data with various elements of the meteorological regime, we succeeded in establishing the fact that the monthly means of outgoing emission, in general, depend on the temperature of the air near the earth's surface, and on cloudiness.

This dependence was expressed in the form of the empirical formula

$$I_s = a + bT - (a_1 + b_1 T)n, \qquad (3.13)$$

where I_s is the outgoing emission in kcal cm^{-2} month^{-1}, T is the temperature in degrees Celsius, n is the cloudiness in fractions of a unit, and the dimensional coefficients are $a = 14.0$, $b = 0.14$, $a_1 = 3.0$, and $b_1 = 0.10$.

The mean deviation of the values of outgoing emission, according to the results of calculation with the use of Eq. (3.13) for each month, turned out to be rather small—less than 5%. This corroborates the conclusion about the comparatively small effect of all other factors, the peculiarities of vertical temperature distribution included, on outgoing emission.

It should be indicated that this conclusion was obtained for values of outgoing emission averaged over long periods of time and relating to geographical regions of considerable area. Physical explanation of this conclusion implies that the outgoing emission is, in general, formed in the troposphere, where deviations of temperature from its mean vertical distribution are usually small in comparison with the spatial variation of temperature or its variations during the annual march.

Equation (3.13) can be compared with the results of several theoretical investigations, among which the work of Manabe and Wetherald (1967) is worthy of special attention. This paper established the dependence of outgoing emission on temperature and cloudiness in an atmosphere in radiative-convective equilibrium. This dependence was presented in the form of a graph, whose curves approximately correspond to the formula (with the same dimensions of terms as above)

$$I_s = 14 + 0.14T - 1.6n. \qquad (3.14)$$

It is apparent that Eqs. (3.13) and (3.14), derived by independent methods, coincide for conditions of absence of cloudiness. Consideration of the influence of cloudiness in these formulas is different, it being assumed for the first formula that the effect of cloudiness on emission varies with the variation in temperature and that for extensive cloudiness the effect of temperature near the earth's surface on emission turns out to be relatively weak.

It might be considered that such a dependence is better grounded than is the separate consideration of the effects of cloudiness and temperature on emission in Eq. (3.14).

To check the formulas relating outgoing long-wave emission with meteorological factors, it is necessary to use the condition of equality of outgoing emission for the whole globe with the amount of absorbed radiation,

$$Q_{sp}(1 - \alpha_{sp}) = I_{sp}, \qquad (3.15)$$

where the values Q_{sp}, α_{sp}, and I_{sp} relate to the planet as a whole.

Taking into consideration that the mean Q_s for the globe is equal to 20.8 kcal cm^{-2} month^{-1}, the mean temperature at the level of the earth's surface is 15°, and the mean cloudiness is 0.50, we find that when Eq. (3.13) is used, the condition of Eq. (3.15) is fulfilled at $\alpha_{sp} = 0.33$. Such a value of the planetary albedo agrees with the evaluations obtained by means of independent methods in a number of contemporary investigations (refer to Chapter II), which confirms the correctness of Eq. (3.13).

From Eqs. (3.13) and (3.15), we derive a formula for the mean temperature of the earth,

$$T_p = \frac{1}{b - b_1 n} [Q_{sp}(1 - \alpha_{sp}) - a + a_1 n]. \qquad (3.16)$$

This formula is fulfilled within the range of the actual variation in monthly mean temperatures at the level of the earth's surface, its accuracy depending on the accuracy of Eq. (3.13). It must be borne in mind that in accordance with the structure of Eq. (3.16), the accuracy of the temperature calculation at large values of cloudiness (with n approaching unity) decreases noticeably in comparison with calculations for conditions of small and moderate cloudiness. Although this restricts the possibility of using Eq. (3.16), it might still be possible to draw some conclusions from it about the effect of cloudiness on the thermal regime of the lower layers of the air.

For this purpose, it is necessary to take into account the dependence of albedo on cloudiness. This dependence has the form

$$\alpha_s = \alpha_{s_n} n + \alpha_{s_0} (1 - n), \qquad (3.17)$$

where α_{s_n} and α_{s_0} represent albedos of the earth–atmosphere system with complete cloudiness and cloudless sky, respectively.

From Eqs. (3.16) and (3.17) follows the formula

$$T_p = \frac{1}{b - b_1 n} \{Q_{sp}[1 - \alpha_{s_n p} n - \alpha_{s_0 p}(1 - n)] - a + a_1 n\}. \qquad (3.18)$$

Assuming, in accordance with the procedure used for the construction of maps in "Атлас теплового баланса земного шара," that

$$\alpha_{s_0 p} = 0.66\alpha + 0.10, \qquad (3.19)$$

where α is the albedo of the earth's surface, we find as the mean for the Northern Hemisphere that $\alpha_{s_0 p}$ is equal to 0.20. Then, from Eq. (3.17), we obtain that at $\alpha_{sp} = 0.33$ and $n = 0.50$, the mean $\alpha_{s_n p} = 0.46$.

Taking into consideration the values derived here for $\alpha_{s_0 p}$ and $\alpha_{s_n p}$, we find from Eq. (3.18) that for the mean planetary value Q_s, the effect of cloudiness on temperature is comparatively small and probably lies within the limits of accuracy of the calculations.

In individual latitudinal zones of the earth, the thermal regime is substantially influenced by horizontal redistribution of heat in the atmosphere and the hydrosphere.

The problem of the quantitative accounting of the effect of the horizontal redistribution of heat on the thermal regime of the atmosphere is very complicated. The results of analyzing this problem in studies of the theory of climate have shown that for the correct numerical model of the thermal regime, it is necessary to take into account all the forms of horizontal heat transfer in the atmosphere and the hydrosphere that are comparable in value with absorbed solar radiation. They include transport of heat by mean motion and by macroturbulence in the atmosphere and hydrosphere, and the redistribution of heat involved in phase transformations of water. Since a full accounting of all these forms of heat transfer has not yet been attained in existing theoretical schemes, it is difficult to determine the characteristics of horizontal redistribution of heat in the geographical envelope of the earth by means of the methods of dynamic meteorology. To cope with this question, it is possible to use material on the components of the heat balance of the earth–atmosphere system.

The equation of heat balance of the earth–atmosphere system has the form

$$Q_s(1 - \alpha_s) - I_s = C + B_s, \qquad (3.20)$$

where C equals $F_s + L(E - r)$, the sum of heat income caused by horizontal movements in the atmosphere and hydrosphere.

For mean annual conditions, the term B_s, characterizing the accumulation or loss of heat for a given time period, equals zero, and the total income of heat owing to horizontal motion in the atmosphere and hydrosphere, C, equals the value of the radiation balance of the earth–atmosphere system. Since the values of this balance can be determined either from observational data or by calculation methods, it is evident that simultaneously the values of horizontal redistribution of heat can also be found.

It might be suggested that the values of C are in some way connected with the horizontal distribution of mean tropospheric temperature. Taking into consideration the fact that deviations of air temperature from the mean vertical distributions in the troposphere are small compared to the geographical variability of temperature, we may consider that the mean air temperature in the troposphere is closely connected with the temperature at the level of the earth's surface. This assumption is completely corroborated when comparing the mean monthly temperatures at the level of the earth's surface and at the height of the 500-mbar surface in different geographical regions and different seasons of the year.

Thus, reasons exist for postulating the existence of a relation between horizontal heat transfer and the distribution of temperature near the earth's surface.

Let us examine the relation between these values for mean annual conditions of the latitudinal zones of the Northern Hemisphere. For this purpose, we will calculate the radiation balance by the formula

$$R_s = Q_s(1 - \alpha_s) - I_s. \tag{3.21}$$

In this case, the albedo for latitudes 0–60° will be determined from Eqs. (3.17) and (3.19), and for polar latitudes (where Eq. (3.19) is not sufficiently accurate), we will use albedo values obtained from observations made from satellites (Raschke *et al.*, 1968).

It is obvious that meridional heat transfer is carried out in the form of heat transfer from warmer regions to colder. We may therefore consider that it depends on the value $T - T_p$, where T_p is the mean planetary temperature of the lower layer of air.

To study this dependence, we compare the derived values of R_s with the corresponding values of $T - T_p$, which is done in Fig. 79. It is apparent

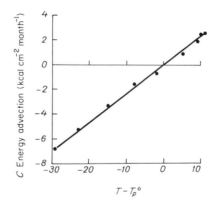

Fig. 79   Dependence of horizontal heat transfer on temperature difference.

from this graph that there is a distinct relation between the values under consideration, which can be presented in the form of the empirical formula

$$Q_s(1 - \alpha_s) - I_s = \gamma(T - T_p), \tag{3.22}$$

where $\gamma = 0.235$ kcal cm^{-2} month^{-1} degree^{-1}.

The existence of such a dependence means that for mean annual conditions, the intensity of the meridional exchange in different latitudes does not differ very much.

From Eqs. (3.13) and (3.22), we find that

$$T = \frac{Q_s(1 - \alpha_s) - a + a_1 n + \gamma T_p}{\gamma + b - b_1 n}. \tag{3.23}$$

With the use of this formula, we can calculate mean annual temperatures in different latitudes. The results of such a calculation, depicted as line T_0, were presented in Fig. 78, along with line T, characterizing measured temperatures. It is apparent that the measured and calculated temperatures agree well.

It must be kept in mind that this agreement was obtained by using a model containing only one empirical parameter depending on the distribution of temperature—the coefficient γ, which is considered independent of latitude. Besides, in this model, all the principal components of the heat balance of the earth-atmosphere system are taken into consideration.

We note that a dependence similar to Eq. (3.22) can also be established for mean conditions of single months. In this case, for the determination of the horizontal redistribution of heat, one must use Eq. (3.20) and take into account the values of term B_s, which basically characterizes the changes in heat content of the oceans in the annual cycle. The comparison of the values of C with the differences $T - T_p$ for single months shows that there is a relation between them that is similar to that for the mean annual values, this relation being broken only in summer months in low latitudes.

It becomes clear as a result of analyzing the relations between these values that the coefficient γ in Eq. (3.22) varies slightly during the annual cycle, reaching its maximum in winter and its minimum in summer. This variation is probably to be explained by the annual cycle in the intensity of meridional circulation in the atmosphere and the hydrosphere.

From Eqs. (3.16) and (3.23), it is possible to draw some conclusions about the effect of climate-forming factors on the mean temperature near the earth's surface and on the temperature of the latitudinal zones.

Variations in solar radiation by 1% change the mean temperature, at cloudiness equal to 0.50 and with the existing earth albedo, by approximately 1.5°. This evaluation is almost twice as great as that of the corresponding effect without the atmosphere. Thus, the radiative properties of the atmosphere considerably intensify the effect of variations in radiation on the thermal regime of the earth's surface.

A change in albedo by 0.01 changes the mean temperature by 2.3°. Consequently, the thermal regime depends substantially on variations in albedo, if this variation is not caused by conditions of cloudiness. As indicated above, the effect of cloudiness on the thermal regime, associated with albedo variations, is, to a considerable extent, compensated by corresponding variations in outgoing long-wave emission.

The influence of changes in radiation and albedo in individual zones of latitude on the temperature, under constant mean planetary conditions, is much less significant. In this case, for middle latitudes, a change in radiation of 1% changes the temperature by 0.5°, and a change in albedo of 0.01 changes it by 0.6°. Circulation in the atmosphere and hydrosphere significantly decreases the effect of local changes in climate-forming factors on the thermal regime.

The material set forth in this section points to the possibility of explaining a number of regularities in the thermal regime of the earth by the method of analyzing its heat balance. Another way of investigating these regularities is associated with development of a general theory of climate, which makes it possible to establish the dependence of the temperature field directly on the climate-forming factors. It is worth mention that in many contemporary works on the theory of climate, data on the heat balance are widely used. The first use of material on the heat balance was in calculating the distribution of temperature in the atmosphere in work of Rakipova (1957; and elsewhere). Later, the world maps of heat-balance components prepared by the members of the Main Geophysical Observatory were used in the papers of Malkus (1962), Adem (1964; and elsewhere), and other authors investigating different individual problems of the theory of climate. The materials on the heat balance were widely applied in studies of Smagorinsky and Manabe and their collaborators, the object of which was to work out a planetary theory of climate (Manabe et al., 1965; Manabe and Byran, 1969; and others).

It was demonstrated in the works of these authors that the methods of theoretical meteorology permit calculation of the mean latitudinal distributions of the principal components of the heat and water balances of the earth's surface and atmosphere that are close to the distributions found from the material of climatological investigations.

The latest paper of this group of authors (Holloway and Manabe, 1971) is particularly interesting because it presents the first world maps of the components of the heat and water balance constructed by means of theoretical methods. These maps turned out similar to those presented in this chapter, constructed by empirical methods.

This result is indicative of great progress in the contemporary theory of climate. It represents one more example of the high reliability of the material obtained in the empirical investigations of the heat and moisture balance, and points to the possibility of a significant convergence of the methods of theoretical meteorology and climatology in studying the transformations of energy in the geographical envelope of the earth.

REFERENCES

Айзенштат Б. А., Зуев М. В. (1961). Радиационный режим, тепловой баланс и микроклимат горной долины. Труды САНИГМИ, вып. 6(21).
Aizenshtat, B. A., and Zuev, M. V. (1961). Radiation regime, heat balance, and micro-climate of a mountain valley. *Tr. Tashkent. Sredneaziatskii Nauch. Issled. Gidrome-teorol. Inst.* **6** (21), 3–40, 1961.
Айзенштат Б. А. [и. др.] (1953). Изменение теплового баланса деятельной поверхности при орошении. Труды ГГО, вып. 39 (101).
Aizenshtat, B. A., Kyrillova, T. V., Laikhtman, D. L., *et al.* (1953). Modification of the heat balance of the active surface by irrigation. *Tr. Gl. Geofiz. Observ.* **39** (101).
Архипова Е. Г. (1960). Межгодовые изменения теплового баланса северной части Атлантического океана за последнее десятилетие. Труды ГОИН, вып. 54.
Arkhipova, E. G. (1960). Interannual changes of the heat balance in the northern part of the Atlantic Ocean during the last decade. *Tr. Gos. Okeanogr. Inst.* **54**, 35–60. MGA 13E-232; U.S. Weather Bur., WB/T No. 42. U.S. Weather Bur., Washington, D.C., 1961.
Атлас теплового баланса земного шара. (1963). Под ред. М. И. Будыко. Междуве-домственный геофизический комитет, М.
"Atlas Teplovogo Balansa Zemnogo Shara (Atlas of the Heat Balance of the Earth)" (M. I. Budyko, ed.). Akad. Nauk SSSR, Prezidium. Mezhduvedomstvennyi Geofiz. Komitet, 1963; Guide to the "Atlas of the Heat Balance of the Earth." U.S. Weather Bur., WB/T No. 106. U.S. Weather Bur., Washington, D.C., 1964.
Барашкова Е. П. [и др.]. (1961). Радиационный режим территории СССР. Гидро-метеоиздат, Л.
Barashkova, E. P., Gaevskii, V. L., D'iachenko, L. N., Lugina, K. M., and Pivovarova, Z. I. (1961). "Radiatsionnyi Rezhim Territorii SSSR (Radiation Regime of the USSR)." Gidrometeoizdat, Leningrad. MGA 14.7-17.
Берлянд Т. Г. (1961). Распределение солнечной радиации на континентах. Гидро-метеоиздат, Л.
Berliand, T. G. (1961). Raspredelenia Solnechnoi Radiatsii na Kontinentakh (Distribution of Solar Radiation on the Continents)." Gidrometeoizdat, Leningrad. MGA 17.4-1.
Берлянд Т. Г. (1968). Междусуточная изменчивость солнечной радиации в северном полушарии. Труды ГГО, вып. 233.
Berliand, T. G. (1968). Interdiurnal variability of solar radiation in the Northern Hemi-sphere. *Tr. Gl. Geofiz. Observ.* **233**, 3–16. MGA 20.6-275.
Бирюкова Л. А. (1956). Некоторые особенности суточного хода суммарной радиации и радиационного баланса в разных климатических областях СССР. Труды ГГО, вып. 66.
Biriukova, L. A. (1956). Some characteristics of the daily march of incoming solar radiation and the radiation budget in different climatic regions of the USSR. *Tr. Gl. Geofiz. Observ.* **66**, 10–16. MGA 10:1618.
Борзенкова И. И. (1965). О некоторых закономерностях изменения составляющих радиационного и теплового балансов в горных районах. Труды ГГО, вып. 179.
Borzenkova, I. I. (1965). Some regular variations of radiation and heat-balance com-ponents in mountainous regions. *Tr. Gl. Geofiz. Observ.* **179**, 186–198. MGA 17.6-276.
Будыко М. И. (1956). Тепловой баланс земной поверхности. Гидрометеоиздат, Л.
Budyko, M. I. (1956). "Teplovoi Balans Zemnoi Poverkhnosti." Gidrometeoizdat, Lenin-grad; "Heat Balance of the Earth's Surface," translated by N. Stepanova. U.S. Weather Bur., Washington, D.C., 1958. MGA 8.5-20, 13E-286.

Будыко М. И. (1968). О радиационных факторах изменений климата. Изв. АН СССР, сер. геогр., № 5.

Budyko, M. I. (1968). On the radiation factors of climatic change. *Izv. Akad. Nauk SSSR Ser. Geogr.* **No. 5**, 36–42.

Будыко М. И. (1969). Изменения климата. Гидрометеоиздат, Л.

Budyko, M. I. (1969). "Izmeneniia Klimata (Changes of Climate)." Gidrometeoizdat, Leningrad. *Sov. Geogr. Rev. Transl.* **10**, 429–457 (1969). MGA 21.4-323.

Будыко М. И., Берлянд Т. Г., Зубенок Л. И. (1954). Тепловой баланс поверхности Земли. Изв. АН СССР, сер. геогр., № 3.

Budyko, M. I., Berliand, T. G., and Zubenok, L. I. (1954). Heat balance of the surface of the earth. *Izv. Akad. Nauk SSSR Ser. Geogr.* No. 3, 17–41. MGA 7H-61.

Будыко М. И., Гандин Л. С. (1966). Об определении турбулентного теплообмена между океаном и атмосферой. Метеорология и гидрология, № 11.

Budyko, M. I., and Gandin, L. S. (1966). On determination of the turbulent heat exchange between ocean and atmosphere. *Meteorol. Gidrol.* No. 11, 15–25. MGA 18.4-436.

Будыко М. И., Дроздов О. А. (1950). О влагообороте на ограниченной территории суши. Сб. «Вопросы гидрометеорологической эффективности полезащитного лесоразведения». Гидрометеоиздат, Л.

Budyko, M. I., and Drozdov, O. A. (1950). On the water circulation in a limited land area. *In* "Voprosy Gidrometeorologicheskoi Effektivnosti Polezashchitnogo Lesorazvedeniia (Problems of the Hydrometeorological Effectiveness of Shelter Belts)." (N. A. Bagrov, ed.). Gidrometeoizdat, Leningrad.

Будыко М. И., Дроздов О. А. (1953). Закономерности влагооборота в атмосфере. Изв. АН СССР, сер. геогр., № 4.

Budyko, M. I., and Drozdov, O. A. (1953). Characteristics of the moisture circulation in the atmosphere. *Izv. Akad. Nauk SSSR Ser. Geogr.* No. 4, 5–14.

Будыко М. И., Дроздов О. А. (1966). О применении осреднения в климатологических исследованиях. Метеорология и гидрология, № 10.

Budyko, M. I., and Drozdov, O. A. (1966). The use of averaging in climatological investigations. *Meteorol. Gidrol.* No. 10, 3–6. MGA 18.8-89.

Будыко М. И., Ефимова Н. А. (1964). Изменчивость радиационных факторов теплового баланса земной поверхности. Метеорология и гидрология, № 4.

Budyko, M. I., and Efimova, N. A. (1964). The variability of radiative factors in the heat balance at the earth's surface. *Meteorol. Gidrol.* No. 4, 9–15. MGA 16.4-334.

Будыко М. И. [и др.]. (1962). Тепловой баланс поверхности Земли. Изв. АН СССР, сер. геогр., № 1.

Budyko, M. I., Efimova, N. A., Zubenok, L. I., and Strokina, L. A. (1962). The heat balance of the surface of the earth. *Izv. Akad. Nauk. SSSR Ser. Geogr.* No. 1, 6–16; *Sov. Geogr. Rev. Transl.* **3**, No. 5, 3–16 (1962). MGA 14.9-629.

Будыко М. И., Каган Р. Л., Строкина Л. А. (1966). Об аномалиях членов теплового баланса океана. Метеорология и гидрология, № 1.

Budyko, M. I., Kagan, R. L., and Strokina, L. A. (1966). Anomalies of the components of the heat balance of the ocean. *Meteorol. Gidrol.* No. 1, 24–28. MGA 17.6-318.

Будыко М. И., Строкина Л. А. (1970). Водный баланс океанов. Метеорология и гидрология, № 4.

Budyko, M. I., and Strokina, L. A. (1970). The water balance of the oceans. *Meteorol. Gidrol.* No. 4, 49–58. MGA 22.2-477.

Будыко М. И., Юдин М. И. (1946). Условия термического равновесия в атмосфере. ДАН СССР, т. 53, № 7.

Budyko, M. I., and Iudin, M. I. (1946). Conditions of thermal equilibrium in the atmosphere. *Dokl. Akad. Nauk SSSR* **53**, No. 7.

Будыко М. И., Юдин М. И. (1948). Тепловой обмен поверхности земли с атмосферой и равновесный градиеинт температуры. Метеорология и гидрология, № 1.

Budyko, M. I., and Iudin, M. I. (1948). Heat exchange of the surface of the earth with the atmosphere and the equilibrium gradient of temperature. *Meteorol. Gidrol.* No. 1.

Веремейчикова Е. А. (1962). Особенности теплового баланса высокогорья Восточного Памира. Геофизический бюллетень Междуведомственного геофизического комитета при Президиуме АН СССР, № 11.

Veremeichikova, E. A. (1962). Properties of the heat balance of the high mountains of the eastern Pamirs. *Akad. Nauk SSSR, Geofiz. Biull. Mezhduvedomstvennogo Geofiz. Komitete*, No. 11.

Винников К. Я. (1965). Уходящее излучение системы земля—атмосфера. Труды ГГО, вып. 168.

Vinnikov, I. Ia. (1965). Outgoing radiation of the system earth-atmosphere. *Tr. Gl. Geofiz. Observ.* **168**, 123–140. MGA 16.12-324.

Волошина А. П. (1961). Актинометрические и общеметеорологические наблюдения в седловине Эльбруса. Вестн. ЛГУ, сер. геол. и геогр., вып. 1.

Voloshina, A. P. (1961). Actinometric and general meteorological observations in the col of Elbrus. *Vestn. Leningrad. Gos. Univ. Ser. Geol. Geogr.* **1**.

Гаврилова М. К. (1959). Радиационный баланс Арктики. Труды ГГО, вып. 92.

Gavrilova, M. K. (1959). The radiation balance of the Arctic. *Tr. Gl. Geofiz. Observ.* **92**, 3–26. MGA 12.9-26.

Гаврилова М. К. (1963). Радиационный климат Арктики. Гидрометеоиздат, Л.

Gavrilova, M. K. (1963). "Radiatsionnyi Klimat Arktiki." Gidrometeoizdat, Leningrad; "Radiation Climate of the Arctic." Isr. Program Sci. Transl., Jerusalem, 1966. MGA 16.1-42, 18.11-4.

Гальцов А. П. (1962). Исследования некоторых закономерностей мирового распределения осадков как основы генетико-климатологического районирования земного шара. Труды ВНМС, т. IV. Гидрометеоиздат, Л.

Gal'tsov, A. P. (1962). Investigations of some regularities in the world distribution of precipitation as a basis for establishing genetic-climatologic zones of the Earth. *Tr. Vses. Nauch. Meteorol. Soveshch. 1st, Leningrad, 1961*, **4**, 78–87. Gidrometeoizdat, Leningrad.

Гойса Н. И. (1959). О приведении резулътатов актинометричесрих наблюдений к единому ряду. Труды УкрНИГМИ, вып. 16.

Goisa, N. I. (1959). On reduction of the results of actinometric observations to a single series. *Tr. Ukr. Nauch. Issled. Gidrometeorol. Inst.* **16**, 101–113. MGA 12.8-312.

Гонгодзе Д. Н., Сулаквелидзе Г. К. (1953). Некоторые результаты исследования интенсивности прямой солнечной радиации на склонах Эльбруса. Труды ЦАО, вып. 10.

Gongodze, D. N., and Sulakvelidze, G. K. (1953). Some results of the investigation of the intensity of direct solar radiation on the slopes of Elbrus. *Tr. Tsent. Aerol. Observ.* **10**.

Горленко С. М. (1933). К вопросу об устойчивости реального солнечного кадастра. Бюллетень постоянной актинометрической комиссии, № 1(24).

Gorlenko, S. M. (1933). On the problem of the stability of the actual solar cadastre. *Biul. Postoiannoi Aktinometrich. Komissii* No. 1 (24).

Данилова И. А. (1954). Некоторые черты радиационного климата на северных склонах хребта Терскей-Алатау. Труды Ин-та географии АН СССР, № 60.

Danilova, I. A. (1954). Some features of the radiation climate of the northern slopes of the Terskei-Alatau Range. *Tr. Akad. Nauk SSSR Inst. Geogr.* No. 60.

Дроздов О. А., Берлин И. А. (1953). Годовые суммы осадков. Морской Атлас, т. II, лист 48.

Drozdov, O. A., and Berlin, I. A. (1953). Annual total precipitation. "Morskoi Atlas (Marine Atlas)," Vol. 2 (I. S. Isakov, V. V. Shuleikin, and L. A. Demin, eds.) sheet 48. MGA 11A-6.

Дроздов О. А., Николаенко Г. И. (1964). Радиационный баланс поверхности ледников Средней Азии в период абляции. Сб. «Гляциологические исследования», № 13. Изд. АН СССР, М.

Drozdov, O. A., and Nikolaenko, G. I. (1964). The radiation budget of the surface of glaciers of Middle Asia in the ablation period. *Akad. Nauk SSSR Prezidium Mezhduvedomstvennyi Geofiz. Komitet, Gliatsiolog. Issled.* No. 13, 115–119. MGA 16.7-326.

Дьяченко Л. Н., Кондратьев К. Я. (1965). Распределение длинноволнового баланса атмосферы по земному шару. Труды ГГО, вып. 170.

D'iachenko, L. N., and Kondrat'ev, K. IA. (1965). The global distribution of the long-wave radiation budget of the atmosphere. *Tr. Gl. Geofiz. Observ.* **170**, 192–201. MGA 17.7-263.

Ефимова Н. А. (1956). Аномалии радиационного баланса на территории Европейской части СССР. Труды ГГО, вып. 66.

Efimova, N. A. (1956). Anomalies of the radiation budget in the European area of the USSR. *Tr. Gl. Geofiz. Observ.* **66**, 3–9. MGA 10:1618.

Ефимова Н. А., Строкина Л. А. (1963). Распределение эффективного излучения на поверхности земного шара. Труды ГГО, вып. 139.

Efimova, N. A., and Strokina, L. A. (1963). The distribution of net long-wave radiation at the surface of the globe. *Tr. Gl. Geofiz. Observ.* **139**, 16–26.

Зубенок Л. И. (1956). Водный баланс континентов и океанов. ДАН СССР, т. 108, № 5.

Zubenok, L. I. (1956). The water balance of the continents and oceans. *Dokl. Akad. Nauk SSSR* **108**, No. 5, 829–832. MGA 8.9-258.

Зубенок Л. И. (1968). Об определении суммарного испарения за отдельные годы. Труды ГГО, вып. 233.

Zubenok, L. I. (1968). Determination of evapotranspiration in individual years. *Tr. Gl. Geofiz. Observ.* **233**, 101–109. MGA 20.6-379.

Зуев М. В. (1958). О тепловом балансе долины озера Кара-Куль. Сб. «Современные проблемы метеорологии приземного слоя воздуха». Гидрометеоиздат, Л.

Zuev, M. V. (1958). The heat balance of the Kara-Kul' Lake valley (East Pamirs, Central Asia). *In* "Sovremennye Problemy Meteorologii Prizemnogo Sloia Vozdukha (Contemporary Problems in the Meteorology of the Layer of Air Near the Ground)" (M. I. Budyko, ed.), pp. 61–66. Gidrometeoizdat, Leningrad; Translated by N. A. Zikeev, U.S. Weather Bur., WB/T No. 40. U.S. Weather Bur., Washington, D.C., 1960. MGA 14.2-700.

Казанский А. Б., Колесникова В. Н. (1961). Тепловой баланс поверхности долины реки Сельдары, вблизи языка ледника Федченко. Сб. «Гляциологические исследования», № 6. Изд. АН СССР.

Kazanskii, A. B., and Kolesnikova, V. N. (1961). The heat balance of the surface of the valley of the Sel'dara River near the tongue of the Fedchenko Glacier. *Gliatsiolo-*

gicheskie Issl. Akad. Nauk SSSR, Prezidium Mezhduvedomstvennyi Geofiz. Komitet No. **6**, 104–110. MGA 13.9-406.

Калитин Н. Н. (1921). Радиационные и поляриметрические наблюдения, произведенные в г. Архангельске и Белом море летом 1920 г. Метеорол. вестн., № 1—12.

Kalitin, N. N. (1921). Radiation and polarization observations made in Arkhangel'sk and the White Sea in the summer of 1920. *Vestn. Meteorol.* No. 1–12.

Калитин Н. Н. (1924). Радиационные, поляриметрические и облачные наблюдения, произведенные в августе и сентябре 1921 г. Гидрографической экспедицией Северного Ледовитого океана. Зап. по гидрографии, т. XLVIII.

Kalitin, N. N. (1924). Radiation, polarization and cloud observations made in August and September 1921 by the Hydrographic Expedition to the Arctic Ocean. *Zap. Gidrogr.* **48.**

Калитин Н. Н. (1929). Несколько данных о приходе лучистой энергии для Маточкина Шара. Изв. ГГО, № 4.

Kalitin, N. N. (1929). Data on incoming radiant energy at Matochkin Shar. *Izv. Gl. Geofiz. Observ.* No. 4.

Калитин Н. Н. (1945). Суммы тепла солнечной радиации на территории СССР. Природа, № 2.

Katlitin, N. N. (1945). The total energy of solar radiation in the USSR. *Priroda* No. 2. **No. 2.**

Кароль Б. П. (1962). Некоторые особенности радиационного и теплового балансов Северного Памира в летний период. Труды ВНМС, т. IV. Гидрометеоиздат, Л.

Karol', B. P. (1962). Some features of the radiation and heat balances of the Northern Pamirs in summer. *Tr. Vses. Nauch. Meteorol. Soveshch., 1st, Leningrad, 1961,* **4,** 123–131. Gidrometeoizdat, Leningrad.

Кашин К. И., Погосян Х. П. (1950). О влагообороте в атмосфере. Сб. «Вопросы гидрометеорологической эффективности полезащитного лесоразведения». Гидрометеоиздат, Л.

Kashin, K. L., and Pogosian, Kh. P. (1950). On the circulation of water in the atmosphere. *In* "Voprosy Gidrometeorologicheskoi Effektivnosti Polezashchitnogo Lesorazvedeniia (Problems of the Hydrometeorological Effectiveness of Shelter Belts)" (N. A. Bagrov, ed.). Gidrometeoizdat, Leningrad.

Кузнецова Л. П., Шарова В. Я. (1964). Количество осадков. Год. Физико-географический атлас мира, стр. 42—43.

Kuznetsova, L. P., and Sharova, V. Ia. (1964). Precipitation amount. Year. *Fiz. Geogr. Atlas Mira* pp. 42–43; Physico-geographical atlas of the world. Sov. Geogr. Rev. Transl. **6** (no. 5–6), 3–403 (1965).

Лопухин Е. А. (1957). Некоторые результаты актинометрических наблюдений на Памире. Труды Ташк. ГО, вып. 13.

Lopukhin, E. A. (1957). Some results of actinometric observations in the Pamirs. *Tr. Tashkent. Geofiz. Observ.* **13,** 218–223. MGA 9:1475.

Лопухин Е. А. (1959). Актинометрические наблюдения на Памире в сентябре 1957. Труды САНИГМИ, вып. 2.

Lopukhin, E. A. (1959). Actinometric observations in the Pamirs in September 1957. *Tr. Tashkent. Sredneaziatskii Nauch. Issled. Gidrometeorol. Inst.* No. 2 **(17),** 160–164. MGA 11:1360.

Львович М. И. (1964). Речной сток. Физико-географический атлас мира, стр. 61.

L'vovich, M. I. (1964). Stream Flow. *Fiz. Geogr. Atlas Mira,* sheet 61, Physico-geographical atlas of the world. *Sov. Geogr. Rev. Transl.* **6** (No. 5–6), 3–403 (1965).

Маршунова М. С. (1961). Основные закономерности радиационного баланса подстилающей поверхности и атмосферы в Арктике. Труды ААНИИ, т. 229.

Marshunova, M. S. (1961). The basic regularities in the radiation budget of the underlying surface and the atmosphere in the Arctic. *Tr. Arkt.-Antarkt. Nauch. Issl. Inst.* **229**, 5–53; Res. Mem. RM-5003-PR, pp. 51–131. Rand. Corp., Santa Monica, California, 1966. MGA 18.2-255.

Маршунова М. С., Черниговский Н. Т. (1968). Численные характеристики радиационного режима Советской Арктики. Проблемы Арктики и Антарктики, № 28.

Marshunova, M. S., and Chernigovskii, N. T. (1968). Numerical characteristics of the radiation regime of the Soviet Arctic. *Probl. Arktiki Antarktik* No. 28, 46–57.

Мосидзе Ш. В. (1956). Радиационный и тепловой балансы Тбилиси и его окрестностей. Труды ТбилНИГМИ, вып. 1.

Mosidze, Sh. V. (1956). The radiation and heat budgets of Tbilisi and its environs. *Tr. Tbilisi. Nauch. Issl. Gidrometeorol. Inst.* **1**.

Нездюров Д. Ф. (1909). Актинометрические наблюдения во время поездки к Араратам в 1907 году. Зап. импер. Акад. Наук по физ.-мат. отд., СПб.

Nezdiurov, D. F. (1909). Actinometric observations on the expedition to Ararat in 1907. *Zap. Imp. Akad. Nauk Fiz. Mat. Otdel, St. Peterburg.*

Огнева Т. А. (1955). Некоторые особенности теплового баланса деятельной поверхности. Гидрометеоиздат, Л.

Ogneva, T. A. (1955). "Nekotorye Osobennosti Teplovogo Balansa Deiatel'noi Poverkhnosti (Some Characteristics of the Heat Balance of the Active Surface)." Gidrometeoizdat, Leningrad. MGA 8.7-21.

Пивоварова З. И., Плешкова Т. Т. (1962). О радиационном режиме СССР по материалам наблюдений сети станций. Труды ВНМС, т. IV. Гидрометеоиздат, Л.

Pivovarova, Z. I., and Pleshkova, T. T. (1962). On the radiation regime of the USSR from observational data at network stations. *Tr. Vses. Nauch. Meteorol. Soveshch. 1st, Leningrad, 1961,* **4**, pp. 195–205. Gidrometeoizdat, Leningrad. MGA 14:2321.

Равновесный градиент температуры. (1967). Под ред. М. И. Будыко, М. И. Юдина. Гидрометеоиздат, Л.

"Ravnovesnyi Gradient Temperatury (Equilibrium Gradient of Temperature)" (1967). (M. I. Budyko and M. I. Iudin, ed.). Gidrometeoizdat, Leningrad.

Ракипова Л. Р. (1957). Тепловой режим атмосферы. Гидрометеоиздат, Л.

Rakipova, L. R. (1957). "Teplovoi Rezhim Atmosfery (Thermal Regime of the Atmosphere)." Gidrometeoizdat, Leningrad. MGA 10.9-9.

Русин Н. П. (1961). Метеорологический и радиационный режим Антарктиды. Гидрометеоиздат, Л.

Rusin, N. P. (1961). "Meteorologicheskii i Radiatsionnyi Rezhim Antarktidy." Gidrometeoizdat, Leningrad. MGA 15.5-6; "Meteorological and Radiational Regime of Antarctica" (OTS 64-11097). Isr. Program Sci. Transl., Jerusalem, 1964. MGA 16.8-5.

Русин Н. П., Строкина Л. А., Брагинская Л. Л. (1966). Суммарная солнечная радиация. Радиационный баланс. Атлас Антарктики, т. I, стр. 73—75.

Rusin, N. P., Strokina, L. A., and Braginskaia, L. L. (1966). Summarnaia Solnechnaia Radiatsiia. Radiatsionnyi Balans (Total solar radiation; radiation budget). *Atlas Antarktiki* **1**, 73–75.

Рухадзе И. А. (1960). Рассеянная радиация на ст. Казбеги. Сб. работ Тбил. гидрометобсерватории, вып. 1.

Rukhadze, I. A. (1960). Diffuse radiation at the Kazbek mountain meteorological station. *Sb. Rab. Tbilis. Gidrometeorol. Observ.* No. 1, 69–74. MGA 13.8-660.

Самойленко В. С. (1966). Теплооборот и влагооборот в Тихом океане. В книге «Тихий океан», т. I. Метеорологические условия над Тихим океаном. Изд. «Наука», М.

Samoilenko, V. S. (1966). Heat- and water-turnover in the Pacific Ocean. *In* "Akademiia Nauk. SSSR, Institut Okeanologii, Tikhii Okean," Vol. 1, "Meteorologicheskie Usloviia nad Tikhim Okeanom" (V. S. Samsilenko, ed.). Izdat. Nauka, Moscow. MGA 18.8-7.

Строкина Л. А. (1963). Теплообмен поверхности океана с нижележащими слоями воды. Метеорология и гидрология, № 1.

Strokina, L. A. (1963). Heat exchange of the ocean surface with the underlying water layers. *Meteorol. Gidrol.* No. 1, 25–30. MGA 14.9–419.

Строкина Л. А. (1966). Затрата тепла на испарение. Турбулентный теплообмен вод с атмосферой. Атлас Антарктики, т. I, стр. 109.

Strokina, L. A. (1966). Zatrata Tepla na Isparenie. Turbulentnyi Teploobmen Vod s Atmosferoi (Expenditure of heat for evaporation; Sensible-heat exchange between the water and atmosphere). *Atlas Antarktiki* 1, 109.

Строкина Л. А. (1967a). Определение изменения теплосодержания океанов. Труды ГГО, вып. 209.

Strokina, L. A. (1967a). Determination of variation in the heat content of the oceans. *Tr. Gl. Geofiz. Observ.* 209, 58–69. MGA 19.10-726.

Строкина Л. А. (1967б). О сравнении рассчитанных и наблюденных величин радиационного баланса океанов. Труды ГГО, вып. 193.

Strokina, L. A. (1967b). Comparison of computed and observed values of the radiation budget of the oceans. *Tr. Gl. Geofiz. Observ.* 193, 44–46. MGA 19.9-368.

Строкина Л. А. (1968). Изучение радиационного режима океанов. Метеорология и гидрология, № 10.

Strokina, L. A. (1968). Study of the radiation regime of the oceans. *Meteorol. Gidrol.* No. 10, 77–83. MGA 20.7-295.

Строкина Л. А. (1969). Изменение теплосодержания океанов южного полушария. Труды ГГО, вып. 249.

Strokina, L. A. (1969). Variation in the heat content of the oceans of the Southern Hemisphere. *Tr. Gl. Geofiz. Observ.* 249, 58–64. MGA 21.12-737.

Тарнижевский Б. В. (1959). О точности определения средних месячных и годовых сумм радиации. Труды ГГО, вып. 96.

Tarnizhevskii, B. V. (1959). Accuracy in the determination of average monthly and yearly totals of radiation. *Tr. Gl. Geofiz. Observ.* 96, 101–106. MGA 12:638.

Цуцкиридзе Я. А. (1960). Солнечный кадастр территории Армении. Труды Тбил-НИГМИ, вып. 7.

Tsutskiridze, Ia. A. (1960). The solar cadastre of the territory of Armenia. *Tr. Tbilis. Nauch. Issl. Gidrometeorol. Inst.* 7.

Шихлинский Э. М. (1960). Радиационный баланс Азербайджана. Труды Геогр. о-ва АзССР, Баку.

Shikhlinskii, E. M. (1960). The radiation budget of Azerbaidzhan. *Tr. Geograf. Obshchestvo Azerb. SSR.*

Шихлинский Э. М. (1968). Радиационный и тепловой балансы. В книге «Климат Азербайджана». Под ред. А. А. Мадатзаде и Э. М. Шихлинского. Изд. АН АзССР, Баку.

Shikhlinskii, E. M. (1968). Radiation and heat balances. *In* "Klimat Azerbaidzhana" (A. A. Madatzade and E. M. Shikhlinskii, eds.). Izdat. Akad. Nauk Azerb. SSR, Baku.

Шулейкин В. В. (1935). Элементы теплового режима Карского моря. Труды Таймырской гидрографической экспедиции, ч. 2.

Shuleikin, V. V. (1935). Elements of the thermal regime of the Kara Sea. *Tr. Taimyrskii Gidrograf. Ekspeditsiia* Pt. 2.

Adem, J. (1964). On the physical basis for numerical prediction of monthly and seasonal temperatures in the troposphere-ocean-continent system. *Mon. Weather Rev.*, **92**, No. 3.

Albrecht, F. (1949). Über die Wärme- und Wasserbilanz der Erde. *Ann. Meteorol.* **2**, Pt. 5/6.

Albrecht, F. (1951). Monatskarten des Niederschlages im Indischen und Stillen Ozeans. *Ber. Deut. Wetterdienstes US-Zone* No. 29.

Albrecht, F. (1960). Jahreskarten des Wärme- und Wasserhaushaltes der Ozeane. *Ber. Deut. Wetterdienstes* **9**, No. 66.

Albrecht, F. (1961). Der jährliche Gang der Kompenenten des Wärme- und Wasserhaushaltes der Ozeane. *Ber. Deut. Wetterdienstes* **11**, No. 79.

Alessandri, C. (1909). Messungen der Intensität der Sonnenstrahlung auf dem Monte Rose. *Meteorol. Z.* **26**, Pt. 2.

Alt, E. (1929). Der Stand des meteorologischen Strahlungsproblems. *Meteorol. Z.* **46**, Pt. 12.

Baur, F., und Philipps, H. (1934). Der Würmehaushalt der Lufthülle der Nordhalbkugel . . ., 1. *Gerlands Beitr. Geophys.* **42**, 160–207.

Baur, F., und Philipps, H. (1935). Der Würmehaushalt der Lufthülle der Nordhalbkugel . . ., 2. *Gerlands Beitr. Geophys.* **45**, 82–132.

Brückner, E. (1901). Die Herkunft der Regens, *Gäa, Natur und Leben*, Leipzig and Cologne, **36**.

Dines, W. H. (1917). The heat balance of the atmosphere. *Quart. J. Roy. Meteorol. Soc.*, **43**, No. 151.

Dirmhirn, I. (1951). Untersuchungen der Himmelstrahlung in den Ostalpen mit besonderer Berücksichtigung ihrer Höhenabhängigkeit. *Arch. Meteorol. Geophys. Bioklimat.* **2**, Pt. 4.

Dorno, C. (1925). Klimatologie des Hochgebirges. *Verh. Klimat. Tagung in Davos.* Basel.

Dove, H. (1848). "Temperaturtafeln nebst Bemerkungen über die Verbreitung der Wärme auf der Oberfläche der Erde und ihre jährliche periodischen Veränderungen." G. Reimer, Berlin.

Götz, W. (1926). "Das Strahlungsklima von Arosa." J. Springer, Berlin.

Hand, I. (1953). Distribution of solar energy over the United States. *Heat. Vent.* **50**, No. 7.

Holloway, J. L., Jr., and Manabe, S. (1971). Simulation of climate by global general circulation model: 1. Hydrologic cycle and heat balance. *Mon. Weather Rev.* **99** No. 5, 335–370, 1971.

Houghton, H. G. (1954). On the annual heat balance of the northern hemisphere. *J. Meteorol.* **11**, No. 1.

Humboldt, A. von (1817). Des lignes isothermes et de la distribution de la chaleur sur le globe. *Mém. phys. chim. Soc.* d'Arcneil, **3**, 462–602.

Jacobs, W. C. (1951). The energy exchange between sea and atmosphere and some of its consequences. *Bull. Scripps Inst. Oceanogr.* **6**, No. 2.

Kaemtz, L. (1831–1836). "Lehrbuch der Meteorologie." Gebauer, Halle.

Lettau, H. (1954). Study of the mass, momentum and energy budget of the atmosphere. *Arch. Meteorol., Geophys. Bioklimat. Ser. A*, **7**.

Liljequist, G. (1957). "Energy Exchange of an Antarctic Snow Field." *Norweg.-Brit.-Swed. Antarct. Exped., 1949–1952, Sci. Res.*, **2**, Pt. 1, Norsk Polarinstituut, Oslo.

Loewe, F. (1956). Études de glaciologie en Terre Adelie 1951–1952. "Expéditions Polaires Françaises." Paris.

London, J. (1957). A study of the atmospheric heat balance. Final Rep., Contract No. AF 19(122)—165, New York Univ., New York.

Malkus, J. (1962). Climatology of energy exchange and the global heat and water budgets. "The Sea," (M. N. Hill, Ed.), Vol. 1. Wiley (Interscience), New York.

Manabe, S., and Bryan, K. (1969). Climate and the ocean circulation. *Mon. Weather Rev.* 97, No. 11.

Manabe, S., Smagorinsky, J., and Strikler, R. F. (1965). Simulated climatology of general circulation model with a hydrologic cycle. *Mon. Weather Rev.* 93, No. 12.

Manabe, S., and Wetherald, R. T. (1967). Thermal equilibrium of the atmosphere with a given distribution of relative humidity. *J. Atmos. Sci.* 24, No. 3.

Mani, A., Chacko, O., Krishnamurthy, V., and Desikan, V. (1967). Distribution of global and net radiation over the Indian Ocean and its environments. *Arch. Meteorol. Geophys. Bioklimat. Ser. B* 15, Pt. 1–2.

Meinardus, W. (1934). Eine neue Niederschlagskarte der Erde. *Pettermanns Geogr. Mitt.* 80, Pt. 1–2.

Möller, F. (1951). Vierteljahreskarten des Niederschlags für die ganze Erde. *Pettermanns Geogr. Mitteil.* 95, Pt. 1.

Mörikofer, W. (1935). Klimatologische Einflüße des Hochgebirges. *Verh. Deut. Ges. Inn. Med.* 47.

Mosby, H. (1932). Sunshine and radiation. The Norwegian North Polar expedition with the "Maud," 1918–1925. *Sci. Results* Ia, No. 7.

Oltman, R. E. (1968). Reconnaissance investigations of the discharge and water quality of the Amazon river. *U.S. Geol. Survey Circ.* 552.

Pflugbeil, C., and Steinborn, E. (1963). Zur Klimatologie des Nordatlantischen Ozeans. *Deut. Wetterdienst. Seewetteramt. Einzelveröffentlichungen*, No. 39.

Privett, D. W. (1960). The exchange of energy between the atmosphere and the oceans of the southern hemisphere. *Geophys. Mem.* No. 104.

Raschke, E., Möller, F., and Bandeen, W. (1968). The radiation balance of the earth-atmosphere system over both polar regions obtained from radiation measurements of the Nimbus II meteorological satellite. *Sver. Meteorolo. Hydrolo. Inst. Medd. Ser. B* No. 28.

Robinson, G. D. (1966). Another look at some problems of the air-sea interface. *Quart. J. Roy. Meteorol. Soc.* 92, No. 394.

Roden, G. I. (1959). On the heat and salt balance of the California current region. *J. Mar. Res.*, 18, No. 1.

Sauberer, F. (1938). Strahlungsmessungen auf dem Hohen Sonnblick. *Meteorol. Z.* 55, Pt. 12.

Sauberer, F. (1954). Zur Abschätzung der Gegenstrahlung in den Ostalpen. *Wetter Leben* 6, No. 3-4.

Sauberer, F. (1955). Zur Abschätzung der Globalstrahlung in verschiedenen Höhenstufen der Ostalpen. *Wetter Leben* 7 No. 1-2.

Sauberer, F., and Dirmhirn, I. (1951). Untersuchungen über die Strahlungsverhältnisse auf Alpengletschern. *Arch. Meteorol. Geophys. Bioklimat. Ser. B*, 3 248–260.

Sauberer, F., and Dirmhirn, I. (1958). Das Strahlungsklima. Klimatographie von Österreich. Österreichische Akademie Wissenschaft. *Denkschr. Gesamtakad.* 3.

Schmidt, W. (1921). Wird die Atmosphäre durch Konvektion von der Erdoberfläche her erwärmt? *Meteorol. Z.* 38, Pt. 9.

Schott, G. (1926). "Geographie des Atlantischen Ozeans." C. Boysen, Hamburg.

Schott, G. (1935). "Geographie des Indischen und Stillen Ozeans." C. Boysen, Hamburg.

Steinhauser, F. (1939). Die Zunahme der Intensität der direkten Sonnenstrahlung mit der Höhe in Alpengebiet und die Verteilung der ,,Trübung" in den unteren Luftschichten. *Meteorol. Z.* 56, Pt. 5.

Steinhauser, F. (1951). Über die Abbhängigkeit den Sonne- und Himmelstrahlung von der Höhe in der Ostalpen. *Ann. Meteorol.* Pt. 1–16.

Tucker, G. B. (1961). Precipitation over the North Atlantic Ocean. *Quart. J. Roy. Meteorol. Soc.* **87**, No. 372.

Vonder Haar, T. H., and Suomi, V. E. (1969). Satellite observations of the Earth's radiation budget. *Science* **163**, 667–669.

Wegener, K. (1939). Ergänzungen für Eismitte. Deutschen Grönland-Exped. A. Wegener 1929 und 1930/31. *Wiss. Ergebn.* **4**, Pt. 2.

Westman, I. (1903). Mesures de l'intensité de la radiation solaire faites en 1899 et en 1900 à la station d'hivernage suédoise à la baie de Treurenberg, Spitzberg. Miss. scient. pour la mesure d'un arc de méridien au Spitzberg, entreprises en 1899–1902, Book II, Sect. VIII, B. Radiation Solaire, Stockholm.

Wüst, G. (1936). Oberflächensalzgehalt, Verdunstung und Niederschlag auf dem Weltmeere, *Länderkundliche Forsch. Festschr. Norbert Krebs.*

Wyrtki, K. (1965). The average annual heat balance of the North Pacific Ocean and its relation to ocean circulation. *J. Geoph. Res.* **70**, No. 18.

Ångström, A. (1933). On the total radiation from sun and sky at Sveanor. *Geogr. Ann.* **15**, Pt. 2–3.

Ångström, K. (1901). "L'intensité de la radiation solaire à differentes altitudes. Recherches faites à Ténériffe 1895 et 1896." *Acta Nova Regiae Soc. Sci. Upsaliensis*, Ser. 3, **20**, No. 3. Uppsala.

IV

Polar Ice and Climate

1. Polar Ice as a Factor of Climate

Polar ice

In the contemporary epoch, ice surrounds both poles of the globe. In the Northern Hemisphere, permanent ice cover takes up more than two thirds of the surface of the Arctic Ocean, and also covers Greenland and several other islands and continental regions in high latitudes. Its total area in the Arctic is about 12 million km², sea ice occupying approximately 10 million km² and land ice 2 million km².

Polar sea ice is an enormous lens, in the center of which mean ice thickness reaches 3–4 m, decreasing towards its periphery. As this ice consists of a great many individual ice fields, it is constantly moving under the action of air and sea currents, which leads to fluctuations in the boundaries of the ice cover.

In moving ice, contraction of the ice fields often occurs, which results in formation of hummocks—a conglomeration of ice, the thickness of which far exceeds the mean thickness of ice cover. But hummocks amount to a comparatively small part of the total area of the Arctic sea ice.

In summer months, the ice thickness diminishes as a result of thawing, which occurs mainly at the upper surface of the ice. In the cold season, ice becomes thicker as a result of freezing of sea water at the lower surface of the ice. Seasonal variation in thickness of sea ice accompanies the variation in the total area of ice cover, which reaches its maximum in March and its minimum in August. Figure 80 presents the mean boundaries of sea ice in these months (Ice Atlas of the Northern Hemisphere, 1946).

261

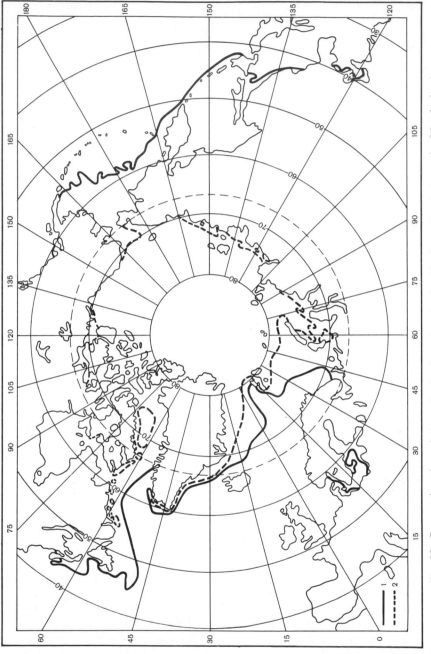

Fig. 80 Present location of the polar ice boundary in the Northern Hemisphere. 1—March, 2—August.

Paleoclimatic studies have shown that in the past the sea-ice cover has varied significantly. During the Quaternary period (that is, for the last million years), ice cover on the seas repeatedly spread to middle latitudes, in correspondence to the periods of development of large-scale continental glaciations. The hypothetical boundary of permanent sea ice and also the boundary of glaciation on land at the period of the greatest (Riss) glaciation, according to the data of Markov (1960), are presented in Fig. 81. In the intervals between the glacial epochs, the sea-ice cover receded towards the north, and during the warmest interglacial epochs, it possibly disappeared completely.

In pre-Quaternary time, there was a warm climate during several hundred million years, and no ice cover existed in high latitudes.

As is known from paleogeographical data and historical sources, the position of the ice cover in the Arctic during the last millennia has also been subject to noticeable variations. During the periods of warming, the sea ice

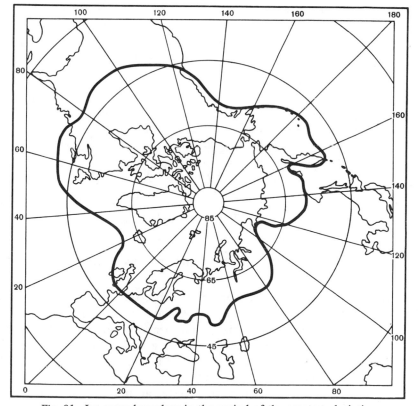

Fig. 81 Ice-cover boundary in the period of the greatest glaciation.

receded far to the north and the glaciated area on land shrank significantly. The last period of such a warming was observed about a thousand years ago, when the Norsemen reached Greenland by ice-free seas and established colonies there on territories that had been freed of ice by the receding glaciers. Several centuries later, a new fall in temperature broke the connection of these colonies with Scandinavia, which, together with the advances of the glaciers on land, led to the end of the colonies.

The problem of the interrelation of the regime of polar ice and climatic conditions in the Arctic is very important. Solution of this problem is necessary for working out a general theory of climate.

At the same time, determination of the relations between climatic conditions and the regime of polar ice is necessary for developing methods for predicting changes in ice cover. They are taken into account in providing polar navigation with meteorological probabilities, and in other descriptive works on the Arctic.

Data on the thermal regime of the Central Arctic in the contemporary epoch are presented in Fig. 82, where curve T_{80} is the annual march of air

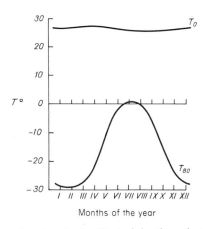

Fig. 82   Thermal regime in the Central Arctic and at the Equator.

temperature at 80° N latitude. For comparison, the annual march of the mean latitudinal air temperature at the Equator is also given (curve T_0). As is seen in Fig. 82, the air temperature near the earth's surface in the Central Arctic is lower than the air temperature near the Equator by 27° in summer and 55° in winter. The mean annual temperature at 80° N latitude is lower than the temperature near the Equator by 42°.

It is obvious that the low temperatures of the air in the polar zone are the main cause of the formation of polar ice. Less clear is the question of the extent to which polar ice influences the thermal regime in high latitudes, furthering the fall in temperature in these latitudes.

The idea that the ice cover is a substantial factor influencing the thermal regime was set forth in the works of Brooks (Brooks, 1950; and elsewhere). He pointed out that the high albedo of ice cover significantly diminishes the absorption of solar radiation at a surface covered by snow and ice. Therefore, he believed that the ice cover in the high latitudes lowers the Arctic temperature by several tens of degrees.

This suggestion, however, was not substantiated in Brooks' works by calculations based on the methods of physical climatology, which were but little developed at the time when Brooks was carrying out his research. For this reason, Brooks' views on the genesis of the climate of the Arctic were not generally accepted, and until recently, the influence of polar ice on the climate of high latitudes was not taken into consideration in works on the theory of climate.

The importance of ice cover as a factor in the formation of climate can be established on the basis of the following simple considerations (Budyko, 1969).

Let us consider the heat balance of the earth–atmosphere system (that is, the heat balance of a vertical column embracing the atmosphere, the hydrosphere, and the upper layers of the lithosphere). The income of heat to this system occurs in the form of absorbed solar radiation, to which is added the income of heat owing to the change of heat content of matter contained in the column and the income of heat as a result of horizontal motion in the atmosphere and hydrosphere. The algebraic sum of these components of the heat balance equals the value of long-wave radiation into space.

Assuming a solar constant equal to 1.92 cal cm^{-2} min^{-1},* we find that in June at $80°$ N latitude 31.0 kcal cm^{-2} month^{-1}, and at the Equator 23.5 kcal cm^{-2} month^{-1} reach the upper boundary of the denser layers of the atmosphere.

At the Equator as well as in the Central Arctic, changes in the heat content of the earth–atmosphere system in June are small in comparison with the income of solar radiation. The cause of this is the fact that this component of the heat balance reaches appreciable values only with substantial changes in ocean temperature in the annual cycle. Meanwhile, the temperature of ocean water changes little, either near the Equator (because of the lack of significant annual variation in the mean altitude of the sun) or in the central region of the Arctic Ocean (because of the isolating influence of sea ice on the heat exchange of ocean with atmosphere).

---

* This is the conditional solar constant, which corresponds to the flux of short-wave radiation on the outer boundary of the troposphere.

Taking this conclusion into account and considering the fact that the horizontal flux of heat in the atmosphere and hydrosphere is directed from Equator to pole, we can easily see that with the albedo in all latitudes being the same, the long-wave radiation to space at 80° N latitude in June must be much greater than it is near the Equator. It has been found in modern investigations (see Chapter III, Section 4) that radiation emission into space, which is closely connected with the mean temperature near the earth's surface, increases with the rise of this temperature.

Thus, if the albedo of the earth–atmosphere system is the same at the Equator and in high latitudes, the air temperature near the earth's surface in June in high latitudes must be higher than the temperature near the Equator, which in reality is not observed.

The only explanation of this paradox lies in a significant difference in the albedo of the earth–atmosphere system with and without ice cover. Such a difference was defined with the help of material from direct experimental observations in the works of Raschke et al. (1968) and other authors, who constructed maps of albedo according to data of measurements taken from satellites.

As is seen from the data in the paper mentioned, the mean value of albedo at 80° N latitude turns out to be 0.62, while the mean albedo for regions free of ice equals only 0.30. Taking these albedo values into account, we find that in June, the absorbed radiation at the Equator amounts to 16.4 kcal cm^{-2} month^{-1}, and at 80° N latitude 11.8 kcal cm^{-2} month^{-1}.

Thus, the air temperature at the Equator in summer is higher than it is at the pole because the albedo of the earth–atmosphere system in the Central Arctic is much greater than it is in the lower latitudes.

One might ask the question: How would the thermal regime of the Arctic change without polar ice, if the albedo in high latitudes did not differ much from that of low latitudes? It should be pointed out that the thermal regime of the Arctic in this case ought to depend not only on the quantity of radiation absorbed, which is determined by the new value of albedo, but also on other factors connected with the disappearance of the ice cover.

In particular, the meridional heat exchange in the atmosphere and hydrosphere could change significantly under those conditions. The water temperature in the Arctic Ocean with an ice-free regime would change noticeably during the annual cycle, which would lead to a substantial redistribution of heat in the earth–atmosphere system during the course of the year.

It is evident that for answering the question posed, we need to determine the components of the Arctic heat balance with and without ice, and to estimate the effect of changes in these components on the thermal regime. In this way, the importance of the ice cover as a factor in the genesis of the Arctic climate can be explained.

Study of the thermal balance of the Arctic permits us also to solve the reverse problem, that is, to investigate the dependence of parameters of the ice cover on climatic factors.

The working out of these problems makes it possible to answer the question about the stability of the existing polar ice and the climatic regime associated with it.

The heat balance of the Arctic

The problem of studying the heat balance of the Arctic includes investigation of the heat balance at the earth's surface and of the heat balance of the atmosphere, or the earth–atmosphere system, embracing the atmosphere, the hydrosphere, and the upper layers of the lithosphere.

In the first section of Chapter III is given material characterizing the radiation regime of the northern polar zone. Determination of all the components of the heat balance for Arctic conditions involves considerable difficulties, which have been overcome only in recent years. As a result of the observations made at the drifting stations, "Северный Полюс," the investigation of the Arctic heat balance has accelerated, a large contribution to this work being made by the staff of the Arctic and Antarctic Institute (Leningrad).

Accumulation of observational material relating to the radiation and heat balances permitted the determination of the norms of the components of these balances in a number of Arctic regions. These norms were found by means of direct generalization of the observational data, as well as by calculations made by formulas that permitted determination of the balance components from observations of the basic meteorological elements. Such calculations became possible after testing these formulas for Arctic conditions by observational data on the components of the heat balance and, in necessary cases, making their coefficients more precise.

One of the first studies of the heat balance of the Arctic was carried out by Iakovlev (1958). The results of further calculations relating to the heat balance of the earth's surface and the atmosphere in the Arctic are presented in works of Doronin (1963), Nazintsev (1964), Fletcher (1965, 1966), Untersteiner (1966), Badgley (1966), Vowinkel and Orvig (1964, 1966, and elsewhere), and others. Such calculations were also made in works of the author (Budyko, 1961, 1962, 1966) dedicated to the genesis of Arctic climate.

It might be noted that in the above-mentioned papers, all the basic components of the heat balance for the different Arctic regions were determined. Although quantitative values of the components of the balance determined by individual authors are a little different, they are in good agreement with respect to general regularities.

Let us consider the material on the heat balance of the Central Arctic, which correspond to the mean conditions for the 80° parallel.

In Fig. 83 are given values of the elements of the radiation regime at the ice surface in this region in the different months of the year. Curve Q defines the variation of incoming short-wave radiation, $Q(1 - \alpha)$ absorbed radiation, and R the radiation balance. This figure shows that in the summer months, a considerable amount of solar radiation reaches the ice surface, which is explained by the long duration of the polar day and also by downward scattering of a fraction of the radiation reflected from the ice and snow surfaces.

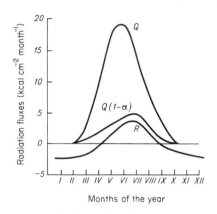

Fig. 83 Radiation regime in the Central Arctic.

The amount of absorbed radiation $Q(1 - \alpha)$ depends on the albedo value α, which was determined for Arctic conditions at the drifting polar stations as well as by measurements from aircraft (Koptev, 1964; Marshunova and Chernigovskii, 1965, 1968; and elsewhere).

According to the available observational data, we may consider the albedo of the Central Arctic in spring and autumn to be about 0.80; in summer, it decreases to 0.70 in the period of most active melting. Such albedos of the earth's surface, which far exceed albedos in the absence of ice and snow, diminish absorbed radiation to a small fraction of the incoming short-wave radiation.

The radiation balance R, equal to the difference between the absorbed short-wave radiation and the net long-wave emission, has a small positive value in summer months. At this time, it is noticeably less than the radiation balance observed in lower latitudes, where ice cover is absent.

In winter, with solar radiation absent, the radiation balance is determined by the value of the net long-wave radiation and is negative. The annual sum of the radiation balance turns out to be equal to a small negative value.*

This result confirms the earlier conclusion (Budyko, 1956) that the radiation regime of polar regions with permanent ice cover differs radically from that of polar regions without ice cover. One of the chief peculiarities of this regime is that the annual sums of the radiation balance are small in absolute magnitude and often negative, as opposed to comparatively large positive values in all other regions of the globe.

In this connection, it should be borne in mind that even if relative accuracy of determining certain heat-balance components is low, the absolute errors in estimating components of the balance cannot amount to any great value, because all these components are small in comparison with the main components of the heat balance at the earth's surface in other geographical regions, and also in comparison with the heat balance of the atmosphere in the Arctic.

Difficulties that arise in estimating the heat balance at the surface of the central regions of the Arctic Ocean are to some extent connected with the fact that this surface is not homogeneous. Part of it is occupied by ice of different thicknesses, and part by leads, in which the ocean water remains open. As we have no accurate data, there are very different estimates of the area occupied by leads. Thus, in Hare's review (Hare, 1968), it is noted that this area is considered by different authors to be from 2 to 12%. Using calculations of the ocean heat balance, Badgley (1966) and Untersteiner (1966) deduced that the area of leads in winter must be less than 1%.

The importance of the problem concerning the area of leads lies in the fact that in the cold season, the ocean loses much heat from their surface. Calculations of the heat exchange in the leads, performed by Doronin (1963) and Badgley (1966), show that at their surface, the loss of heat per year as a result of turbulent sensible-heat exchange and evaporation can exceed 100 and even 200 kcal cm^{-2}. It is necessary to add the outgo of radiative energy to this value because the large net long-wave emission from the surface of the leads is not compensated by increased quantities of absorbed short-wave radiation resulting from low values of water albedo.

Taking into consideration the fact that the ocean rapidly loses heat in the leads, it is possible, however, to consider that their importance for the heat exchange of the Central Arctic as a whole is rather limited. This conclusion

---

* Such an estimate is probably more accurate than that of Gavrilova (1963) (Chapter III of this book), who found the radiation balance of the Central Arctic equal to a small positive value. (The cause of this discrepancy is the smallness of the absolute value of the annual radiation balance in the Arctic in comparison with the sum of the absolute values of its monthly values.)

follows from estimates of the heat balance components of the whole Arctic Ocean zone occupied by permanent ice.

The quantity of heat brought to this zone by currents is relatively small. Thus, according to the data of Leonov (1947), for example, it equals approximately 2.2 kcal cm^{-2} yr^{-1}; Badgley (1966) considers it to be 1.6 kcal cm^{-2} yr^{-1}. To this value, one should add the latent heat of fusion of ice taken out of the Arctic every year by currents. Antonov (1968) points out that the quantity of this ice is estimated by different authors to be from 900 to 3000 km^3 yr^{-1}, the most probable value being close to 1900 km^3 yr^{-1}. The latter value corresponds to an additional income of heat to the Central Arctic equal to 1.6 kcal cm^2 yr^{-1}.

Thus, as a result of the oceanic circulation, the Central Arctic receives 3–4 kcal cm^{-2} yr^{-1}. Almost all of this value is off-set by the negative value of the radiation balance at the surface of the ice.

As a result, the sum of the rest of the components of the oceanic heat balance, including the turbulent sensible-heat flux and the conversion of heat for evaporation, should equal a value of approximately 0–1 kcal cm^{-2} yr^{-1}. This value can be compared with a similar value for ice fields.

According to Doronin's data (1963), the annual sum of the heat converted in evaporation of the ice fields amounts to 3.2 kcal cm^{-2} yr^{-1}, and the income of heat owing to the exchange of sensible heat to approximately 2.7 kcal cm^{-2} yr^{-1}.

The difference between these values, amounting to 0.5 kcal cm^{-2} yr^{-1}, is close to the estimate given above for the heat income for the Central Arctic as a whole. Thus, it turns out that the heat exchange at the surface of the leads does not play a great role in the heat balance of the central regions of the Arctic Ocean. It follows that in the cold season, the leads take up a very small part of the total area of the Central Arctic.

The annual march of the components of the heat balance of an ice field is given in Fig. 84. This figure presents, along with values of the radiation balance R, values of the sensible-heat flux P and the latent-heat flux LE, the last values being presented according to the data of Doronin given above.

The values of the radiation balance portrayed in this figure are considered positive when they express an income of heat, and the values of the sensible and latent heat fluxes are considered positive when they express an outgo from the surface of the ice.

The sum of the annual values of the heat-exchange components shown is equal to the outgo of heat, which is compensated by the inflow of heat through the lower boundary of the ice, equal to the income of heat resulting from ocean-current activity (without taking into account removal of ice). Although the value of heat outgo at the surface of the ice fields determined on the basis of heat-balance calculations agrees with the above-mentioned

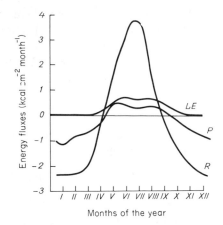

Fig. 84   Heat balance of the surface of an ice field.

estimates of heat transfer accomplished by currents, one should not over-estimate the importance of such an agreement. We may consider that the relative error of determining all the components of the heat balance is rather large and probably comparable with the outgo of heat through leads, which cannot be equal to zero.

Let us proceed now to the problem of the heat balance of the earth–atmosphere system in the Central Arctic.

The values of the components of the radiation balance of this system are presented in Fig. 85, where line Q_s depicts the annual march of radiation

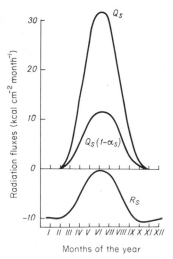

Fig. 85   Radiation balance of the earth–atmosphere system in the Central Arctic.

incident on the external boundary of the atmosphere at a solar constant equal to 1.92 cal cm^{-2} min^{-1}. The line $Q_s(1 - \alpha_s)$ represents the absorbed radiation, which has been calculated with albedo $\alpha_s = 0.62$ in accordance with the mean value obtained by satellite [refer to Raschke *et al.* (1968)].

The value of the radiation balance of the system R_s is determined by the formula

$$R_s = Q_s(1 - \alpha_s) - I_s, \tag{4.1}$$

where I_s is the long-wave radiation emitted to space, which is calculated by the formula (refer to Chapter III, Section 4)

$$I_s = a + bT - (a_1 + b_1T)n, \tag{4.2}$$

where T is the temperature at the earth's surface in degrees Celsius, n is the cloudiness in fractions of a unit, and a, b, a_1, and b_1 are empirical coefficients.

As seen from Fig. 85, the radiation balance of the earth–atmosphere system in the Arctic is negative during the whole year, including summer months, when the income of radiation to the external limit of the atmosphere is rather large. This is explained by the high albedo of the earth–atmosphere system in regions with a permanent ice cover. The annual value of the radiation balance, which equals -80.9 kcal cm^{-2}, is compensated by the inflow of heat from lower latitudes through horizontal heat transfer in the hydrosphere and atmosphere, including the redistribution of the latent heat of vaporization.

The above estimate shows that heat transfer owing to marine currents makes up a negligible part of the value of the radiation balance. The heat of condensation exceeds the expenditure of heat for evaporation in the Central Arctic by an amount that is also comparatively small, not more than a few kilocalories per square centimeter per year.

Thus, the negative radiation balance of the earth–atmosphere system in the Arctic is basically compensated by meridional [sensible] heat transfer in the atmosphere, which is especially essential in the winter months.

On the basis of the data given above, we can draw some conclusions concerning regularities of the energy balance of the Central Arctic.

Because of the high albedo of polar ice, the radiation balance of the earth–atmosphere system even in summer does not reach positive values, and in this season a certain quantity of heat is spent in warming and melting ice. In this situation, the expenditure of heat energy is compensated by the advective income of [sensible] heat from lower latitudes, where summer air temperatures are markedly higher than these in the Central Arctic.

In wintertime, without any income of solar heat, the outgo of energy by emission to space is only to a small extent compensated by an income of heat resulting from the cooling of the ice cover and the accretion of new ice onto it. As noted above, this outgo is in general covered by the large influx of heat from lower latitudes due to the atmospheric circulation.

Thus, over the course of the entire year, and especially in the winter months, the thermal regime of the Arctic essentially depends on the transport of heat from extrapolar latitudes.

2. Interrelation of Climatic Factors and Ice Cover

The influence of climatic conditions on ice cover

The formation and destruction of ice on the ocean surface is closely connected with the conditions of the thermal energy balance.

Ice cover appears when, as a result of cooling, the temperature of the upper layer of water reaches the freezing point. For mean conditions of salinity of ocean water, this temperature is $-1.8°$.

Increase in the thickness of ice occurs when the temperature of its upper surface comes to be lower than that of water at the lower boundary of the ice cover. Under these conditions, freezing occurs on the lower boundary of the ice, the rate of which is determined by the heat balance at this surface. If the income of heat from the ocean to the lower surface of the ice is small, then the rate of freezing equals the value of the heat flux from the lower ice surface to its upper surface divided by the latent heat of fusion.

The value of the vertical heat flux in the ice depends on the difference between temperatures on its upper and lower surfaces, on its heat conductivity, and on its thickness (together with the snow cover on it).

The temperature at the surface of the ice (or at the surface of snow, if it is present) depends on conditions of the heat balance. At comparatively small values of the vertical heat flux between ice and atmosphere, this temperature is usually close to the temperature of the lower layer of air. As the temperature of the lower surface of the ice is usually constant, and the thermal conductivity of ice varies comparatively little, the rate of freezing in general turns out to depend on air temperature and ice thickness. In these circumstances, rate of freezing increases with a fall in air temperature and decreases with a growth in ice thickness.

The dependence of the thickness of ice cover on the factors mentioned was established nearly a century ago by Weinprecht on the basis of observations made in the Arctic. This problem was then theoretically investigated by Stefan, who used the equation of heat conduction in solids for this purpose. Stefan ascertained that at a constant difference between the temperatures at the upper and lower surfaces of ice, the ice thickness is proportional to the square root of the product of the difference mentioned and the length of time of ice accretion. Later, for calculation of the rates of freezing, various empirical formulas were offered. They permitted a more accurate determination of ice thickness than the schematic solution of Stefan.

One such formula, suggested by Zubov (1945), was used for constructing tables that established the relationship between the value of ice accretion and its initial thickness and the mean daily temperature of the air (Table 28).

Zubov pointed out that the value of ice accretion is influenced not only by air temperature but also by circulation conditions in the ocean. An additional heat flux to the lower surface of the ice, associated with horizontal heat transport from low latitudes to high, can substantially retard ice accretion.

TABLE 28

Ice Growth (cm day^{-1})

Initial thickness (cm)	Temperature (degrees)							
	-5	-10	-15	-20	-25	-30	-35	-40
0	0.8	1.6	2.4	3.2	3.8	4.7	5.5	6.3
10	0.6	1.1	1.7	2.3	2.9	3.4	4.0	4.6
20	0.4	0.9	1.3	1.8	2.2	2.6	3.1	3.5
30	0.4	0.7	1.1	1.5	1.8	2.2	2.6	3.0
40	0.3	0.6	0.9	1.2	1.5	1.8	2.1	2.4
50	0.3	0.5	0.8	1.1	1.3	1.6	1.9	2.1
75	0.2	0.4	0.6	0.8	1.2	1.4	1.6	1.8
100	0.2	0.3	0.5	0.6	0.8	1.0	1.1	1.0
150	0.1	0.2	0.3	0.5	0.6	0.7	0.8	0.9
200	0.1	0.2	0.3	0.4	0.4	0.5	0.6	0.7

The rate of accretion depends also on the thickness of snow cover on the ice surface, because the low heat conductivity of snow decreases the heat flux between the lower surface of the ice and the atmosphere.

Empirical formulas for calculating the freezing rate usually take into account only the mean effect of the factors mentioned, which limits their accuracy.

In the mass balance of polar sea ice, an increase of the mass of water in the solid phase is determined by the freezing process and, to a lesser extent, by the fall of solid precipitation. In this balance, the outgo of mass depends on the melting process, on evaporation from the ice surface, and on the outflow of ice into lower latitudes.

Melting of ice generally occurs on its surface, when the temperature of this surface reaches the freezing point. Because the salinity of the upper layers of ice decreases during the process of melting, the temperature at which melting takes place approximates zero.

The rate of ice melting is defined by conditions of the heat balance at the ice surface [refer to Budyko (1962)]. The equation of this balance can be presented in the form

$$R = LE + P + A + lh\rho_1, \tag{4.3}$$

where R is the radiation balance, L is the latent heat of vaporization, E is evaporation from the ice surface, P is the turbulent flux of sensible heat between the ice surface and the atmosphere, A is the heat flux from the ice surface to the lower layers of the ice, l is the latent heat of fusion of ice, h is the change in ice thickness due to melting, and ρ_1 is the ice density.

The dependence of the first three components of the heat balance on meteorological factors can be presented in the following form:

$$R = Q(1 - \alpha) - I_0 - 4\delta\sigma T^3(T_w - T), \tag{4.4}$$

$$LE = L\rho\chi u(q_s - q), \tag{4.5}$$

$$P = \rho c_p \chi u(T_w - T), \tag{4.6}$$

where Q is the total short-wave radiation, α is the albedo of ice, I_0 is the net long-wave radiation, calculated according to the air temperature, δ is the coefficient characterizing the difference between the properties of the radiating surface and those of a black body, σ is the Stefan–Boltzmann constant, T is the air temperature, T_w is the ice-surface temperature, χ is a coefficient of proportionality, ρ is the air density, u is the wind speed, q_s is the specific humidity of saturated air at temperature T_w, q is the specific humidity of the air, and c_p is the heat capacity of the air at constant pressure.

From Eqs. (4.3–4.6), we determine

$$h = \frac{1}{\rho_1 l}[Q(1 - \alpha) - I_0 - L\rho\chi u(q_s - q)$$
$$-(\rho\chi c_p u + 4\delta\sigma T^3)(T_w - T) - A]. \tag{4.7}$$

In applying this formula to calculate ice melting, one may use some simplifications. Since the relative humidity of the air above ice does not change very much on the average, and the difference between temperatures of the ice surface and air are usually small, then we may, without material damage to the accuracy of the calculation, consider that $L\rho\chi u(q_s - q) = L\rho\chi u q_s \eta$, where the coefficient η is approximately equal to 0.1. Taking into account the fact that the value of A in the melting period is relatively small, it is possible to employ an approximate estimate of it in accordance with the change in the mean temperature of the ice, taking into account the value of its effective heat capacity.

Using Eq. (4.7), it is possible to evaluate which factors influence ice melting the most. Such calculations show that the rate of melting depends primarily on changes in solar radiation Q and air temperature T. It follows from these calculations that the total amount of melting per year in the Central Arctic amounts to several tens of centimeters. This value, which is in good conformity with the observational data, is markedly greater than the loss of ice mass by evaporation, which in this region is equal, according to available data, to a few centimeters a year.

Compared to evaporation, the transport of ice into lower latitudes has a more important influence on the ice balance in the Central Arctic. As noted above, the quantity of ice carried by ocean currents annually from the high latitudes amounts to approximately 2000 km³, which corresponds to an annual decrease in thickness of the ice cover of approximately 20 cm.

Employing the methods stated above, we can calculate for any region the annual march in thickness of the ice that is in equilibrium with the climatic conditions of the given region. Let us assume in this case that changes in ice thickness are mainly determined by the freezing and melting processes, and use the method of successive approximations (Budyko, 1962).

In accordance with the principle of this method, we assume for the beginning of the calculation period an arbitrary ice thickness, and then calculate for every subsequent month the rate of freezing (or melting) in accordance with the climatic conditions. Let us continue with this calculation for an array of successive years until the total annual values of melting turn out to be equal to the annual values of freezing. The ice thicknesses obtained in this way for each month will correspond to the climatic regime of the given region.

Using such a calculation method shows that it gives satisfactory results in determining the changes in ice thickness in the annual cycle. The absolute values of ice thickness computed by this method do not always correspond to observations and, particularly for the Central Arctic, often prove to be larger than the observed values of the ice thickness. The cause of this discrepancy lies in the effect of drift of ice fields on the ice balance in the high latitudes. As a result of this effect, ice is carried out of the Central Arctic area until it reaches a thickness corresponding to the climatic conditions of the particular region.

In the work of Zubenok (1963), the above-stated method was applied to calculating the mean boundaries of permanent polar ice in different months of the year. The result of this calculation proved to agree well with the observational data.

The method mentioned has been used also for studying the effect of anomalies of meteorological elements on the thickness and area of ice cover. In this way, changes of ice thickness with various air-temperature anomalies have been calculated (Budyko, 1966).

In Fig. 86 are given the results of calculating changes in thickness of the ice in the Central Arctic with a positive temperature anomaly in the three summer months (June–August) equal to 2° (Fig. 86a), and with a positive anomaly in the six cold months (November–April) equal to 10° (Fig. 86b). Curve 1 characterizes the changes of the greatest, curve 2 of the smallest, ice thicknesses in the annual cycle. It is seen from this figure that a comparatively small anomaly in summer temperature reduces ice thickness much more strongly than the far greater temperature anomaly in the cold months.

With a positive anomaly of summer temperatures equal to 4°, ice of four meters thickness under mean climatic conditions for the Central Arctic disappears completely in four years (Fig. 86c). Thus, at an increase of 4° in the summer temperature in the Arctic, the ice of many years over most of the Arctic Ocean turns into one-year ice.

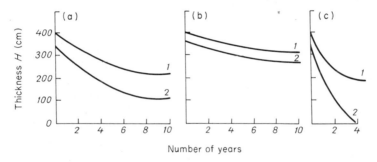

Fig. 86 Effect of temperature anomalies on ice cover (see text). (a) Summer, 2°; (b) Winter, 10°; (c) Summer, 4°.

It is clear, however, that this evaluation of the temperature anomaly at which Arctic ice of many years growth is destroyed is maximal. Since, with reduction of ice area, the amount of radiation absorbed at the open ocean surface increases considerably, then after partial destruction of the ice, a further rise in temperature might occur, which in its turn will intensify the melting of the ice.

In order to clarify what anomaly of the meteorological regime is sufficient for complete destruction of many-year ice, it is necessary to evaluate how ice influences the thermal regime in the Arctic.

The effect of ice cover on climate

It was noted at the beginning of this chapter that the thermal regime of the high latitudes depends substantially on the effect of ice cover on the absorption of solar radiation.

Let us give a simple example, illustrating what influence snow and ice cover can produce on the climate of the earth as a whole. Let us imagine a hypothetical earth, without any clouds, the surface of which is entirely covered with snow and ice. Under such conditions, the albedo of the earth is noticeably increased compared to the value existing now, and this will influence the temperature of the air. The "effective" temperature of the earth, corresponding to its long-wave emission, is proportional to $(1 - \alpha_s)^{1/4}$ (where α_s is the albedo). Therefore, as albedo changes from a value α_s' to a value α_s'', the absolute value of the "effective" temperature changes as $[(1 - \alpha_s'')/(1 - \alpha_s')]^{1/4}$. Considering the present-day albedo of the earth equal to 0.33 and the albedo of dry snow cover equal to 0.80, we find that for a snow-covered earth the mean "effective" temperature must be reduced by approximately 75°.

One might think that the reduction of mean air temperature near the earth's surface will be greater than the value given. At present, the mean temperature of the lower layers of air is considerably increased all over the earth's surface by the "greenhouse" effect, which is associated with the absorption of long-wave radiation by water vapor and carbon dioxide in the atmosphere. At very low temperatures, this effect is not important, and also the formation of dense clouds that change the radiation fluxes appreciably becomes impossible. Under these conditions, the atmosphere becomes more or less transparent for both long-wave and short-wave radiation.

The mean temperature of the earth's surface with a transparent atmosphere is determined by the simple formula $[S_0(1 - \alpha_s)/4\sigma]^{1/4}$, where S_0 is the solar constant, and σ is the Stefan–Boltzmann constant. It follows from this formula that at $\alpha_s = 0.80$, the mean temperature of the earth is 186°K or -87°C.

Thus, if snow and ice covered the whole surface of the earth even for a short period of time, its mean temperature (equal now to $+15$°C) would be reduced by approximately 100°. This estimate shows what an enormous effect snow cover can exert on the thermal regime.

Turning to the problem of the influence of the existing ice cover on the thermal regime of the Arctic, we note that this influence is easily evaluated for the hypothetical case in which, along with the disappearance of the ice cover, only the albedo of the earth–atmosphere system changes, but the values of the horizontal heat fluxes in the atmosphere and hydrosphere remain the same.

Under such conditions, the difference $T - T'$ between the mean annual temperatures with and without ice can be calculated by the equation

$$Q_s(1 - \alpha_s') - Q_s(1 - \alpha_s) = I_s(T') - I_s(T), \qquad (4.8)$$

where α_s and α_s' are the albedos of the earth–atmosphere system with and without ice.

Taking into account the fact that at 80° N latitude the mean annual value of Q_s equals 11.0 kcal cm^{-2} month^{-1}, and assuming $\alpha_s' = 0.30$, $\alpha_s = 0.62$, we determine from Eqs. (4.2) and (4.8) that $T' - T = 44°$.

Thus, the disappearance of polar ice under existing conditions of horizontal heat exchange might raise the temperature in the Arctic by more than 40°.

It is evident, however, that polar ice has a considerable effect not only on the albedo but also on the meridional heat exchange in the atmosphere and hydrosphere. A quantitative picture of such an effect can be presented in the following way.

The income of heat in the hydrosphere of the Central Arctic that is caused by the meridional heat exchange, without ice, probably would increase in comparison with existing conditions. As pointed out above, this income at present is insignificant, because the ice-covered ocean cannot give out any noticeable amount of heat for heating the atmosphere in winter. Heat-balance investigations show that in high latitudes in winter, ice-free oceans give out into the atmosphere a great amount of heat, which is reimbursed by the horizontal heat exchange in the hydrosphere. The value of the corresponding heat flux depends on the activity of the currents, the thermal regime of the atmosphere, and the meridional temperature gradient in the upper layers of the ocean water.

Polar ice being present, the meridional temperature gradient in the upper layers of the ocean water in the high latitudes is small, which corresponds to the smallness of the meridional heat income through the activity of currents.

Polar ice being absent, this temperature gradient must increase. In these conditions, the temperature of the surface water in winter can approximate the freezing point only on the coldest regions of the polar basin, while in the zone connecting this basin with the Atlantic Ocean, the water temperature would be noticeably higher than now. Accordingly, the meridional gradient of the temperature of surface water will increase along with the associated heat transfer by ocean currents.

As the inflow of heat in the hydrosphere increases, in the absence of ice, the flow of heat in the atmosphere to high latitudes should become substantially reduced, as a consequence of the increased temperature of the air in the Arctic and the weakening of the intensity of macroturbulent exchange resulting from the reduced meridional gradient of temperature.

The reduction of heat inflow in the atmosphere into high latitudes must exceed in absolute value the increase of heat inflow in the hydrosphere, without which the latitudinal distribution of temperature will not correspond with the distribution of absorbed radiation.

Quantitative interpretation of the influence of ice cover on the thermal regime of the Arctic, including consideration of the effect of changes in the meridional heat exchange, involves great difficulties, which up to now have been only partially overcome. The first calculation of this kind, carried out in the early 1960s (Budyko, 1961), had the following content.

For evaluating the influence of polar ice on the thermal regime of the high latitudes, the annual march of temperature that would take place in the upper layer of water and lower layer of air in the Central Arctic regions without ice cover was calculated.

For this purpose, a joint solution of the equation of the heat balance at the ocean surface was used,

$$R = LE + P + A,$$ (4.9)

(where A is the heat flux from the ocean surface to the deeper layers), together with an equation characterizing the transformation of air masses on the earth's surface. This is expressed in the form

$$T_1 - T = \nu(T_1 - T_w),$$ (4.10)

where T_1 is the mean air temperature at the periphery of the Arctic Ocean, T_w and T are the mean temperatures of water surface and the air over the ocean, and ν is a coefficient depending on the relation of the linear scale of the ocean to the speed of air-mass movement.

Taking into consideration the relationship between the components of the heat balance and various meteorological elements, Eq. (4.9) was presented in the following form:

$$Q(1 - \alpha) - \delta\sigma T^4(K - Nq)(1 - cn) - 4\delta\sigma T^3(T_w - T)$$
$$= L\rho\chi u(q_s - q) + c_p\rho\chi u(T_w - T) + \beta(T_w - \bar{T}_w),$$ (4.11)

where n is the cloudiness in fractions of a unit, $\bar{T}_w$ is the mean annual temperature of the water, and K, N, c, and β are numerical coefficients.

From Eqs. (4.10) and (4.11), we can first determine the mean annual temperature of water and air for the ice-free ocean and then the temperature in different months, if the air temperature T_1 at the periphery of the ocean is known.

With such a calculation, the albedo value was considered equal to 0.10, which corresponds to the conditions of an ice-free water surface in high latitudes. Because, with the reduction of albedo, diffuse radiation also decreases, then according to observational data, the values of total short-wave radiation appearing in Eq. (4.11) were assumed equal to 80% of the [presently] observed values of radiation in the Central Arctic.

In connection with the small variation in the mean values of relative humidity over the oceans, the absolute humidity was considered to be proportional to the saturation humidity at the temperature of the water surface. Other meteorological parameters entering into the calculation (cloudiness and wind speed) were accepted as corresponding to the mean conditions of the regime now existing.

Because, with an ice-free regime, the temperature at the periphery of the ocean is greatly changed, to calculate this change we may assume that the meridional heat flux between the Equator and the periphery of the Arctic Ocean is proportional to the flux of heat between the periphery of the ocean and its central regions. Considering the meridional heat fluxes proportional to the meridional temperature gradients, we obtain

$$T_0 - T_1 = \varepsilon(T_1 - T), \qquad (4.12)$$

where T_0 is the mean latitudinal temperature at the Equator, and ε is a coefficient of proportionality.

Supposing that the air temperature near the Equator changes little with changes in the ice regime of the Arctic, we can use Eq. (4.12) along with Eqs. (4.10) and (4.11) for calculating the thermal regime of the Arctic Ocean without ice.

As a result of this calculation, it was found that the water and air temperatures for the ice-free regime in the Arctic remain positive during the entire year. It follows that, in principle, there is a possibility of the existence of an ice-free regime in the Arctic of the contemporary epoch.

In recent papers of the author (Budyko, 1962, 1966, 1968, 1969, and others) were suggested some other models for estimating the effect of polar ice on the thermal conditions of the Arctic. The results of applying these models confirmed the conclusion about the possibility of existence of two climatic regimes in high latitudes, associated with the presence or absence of polar ice. Along with this, it was established that both of these regimes are unstable. Because of this, ice cover might appear and disappear with the slightest changes in the climate-forming factors, and even without such changes as a result of oscillating processes in the system of atmosphere–ocean–polar ice.

In these works, it was noted that the possibility of the existence of an ice-free regime in the Arctic of the contemporary epoch was foreseen by Lomonosov, who wrote in one of his investigations: "If we consider the Arctic Ocean, which for half a year is almost constantly illuminated by the sun's rays (though by indirect ones), we cannot help believing that it is considerably warmed by them. And however greatly cooled it may become in winter in the long absence of solar heat, the winter cooling cannot exceed the summer warming" (Lomonosov, 1763). From this, Lomonosov drew the conclusion that the central part of the Arctic Ocean, unexplored at that time, must be free of ice. The above calculations show that this idea of Lomonosov had a certain basis.

After publication of the first calculations of the effect of polar ice on the Arctic climate, this problem attracted the attention of several authors in different countries.

Among the Soviet works on this problem, we must mention the studies of Rakipova (1962, 1966), in which the methods of the general theory of climate were used to evaluate the effect of polar ice on climate. In these studies, mean latitudinal temperatures of the air in the cold season at different levels of the troposphere and the lower stratosphere were determined with the contemporary ice regime and without any ice in the Arctic. Rakipova's calculations corroborate the possibility of an ice-free regime in the contemporary epoch.

In the paper of Doronin (1968), it was pointed out that after ice melts, a surface layer of fresh water with stable stratification appears. The vertical heat exchange in this layer is substantially weakened, which makes it easier for the ice cover to be restored in the cold season.

When the upper water layers are mixed, the changes in water temperature in the annual cycle extend to great depths. As the thickness of the water layer in which the annual variation of temperature occurs increases, the probability of restoration of ice cover in the cold season becomes smaller.

In the USA a study of the effect of polar ice on climate was organized by the Rand Corporation, which drew into these investigations several American and Canadian universities.

This corporation held the first international meeting on this problem, which took place in Los Angeles in 1966, with the participation of Soviet, American, Canadian, and Norwegian scientists. The principal results of the investigations made by the Rand Corporation were reported by Fletcher (1966), who cited data on Arctic heat-balance calculations with and without polar ice. Fletcher pointed out that from data on the heat balance of the Arctic Ocean, we can reach a conclusion about the possibility of the existence of an ice-free regime, though this conclusion should be tested by accounting for the effect of changes in atmospheric circulation on the heat balance in the absence of polar ice.

Fletcher expressed the suggestion that the climate of the high latitudes in an ice-free regime would be characterized by a cool summer and a mild winter with copious precipitation, which finally could lead to the development of glaciation in high and middle latitudes.

In the works of Donn and Shaw (1966), an analysis of the heat balance of the Arctic Ocean was also carried out, which resulted in corroboration of the conclusion about the possibility of existence of ice-free conditions in this ocean.

We report some results of calculating the effect of polar ice on climate, based on more general assumptions than those in the investigations carried out earlier (Budyko, 1969).

The equation of the heat balance of the earth–atmosphere system has the form

$$Q_s(1 - \alpha_s) = I_s + C + B_s, \tag{4.13}$$

where C is the heat inflow due to horizontal movement in the atmosphere and hydrosphere and includes the inflow of heat associated with the phase transformations of water, and B_s is the change of heat content in the earth–atmosphere system over the period of time under consideration. This depends mainly on the change in heat content of the upper layers of ocean water.

For the mean latitudinal distribution of the meteorological elements and for mean annual conditions, a relationship between horizontal heat flux and temperature distribution can be expressed by a simple formula (refer to Chapter III, Section 4),

$$C = \gamma(T - T_p), \tag{4.14}$$

where T is the mean latitudinal temperature near the earth's surface, T_p is the mean temperature of the hemisphere, and γ is a coefficient of proportionality, values of which are expressed below in kcal cm^{-2} month^{-1} degree^{-1}.

Further investigations showed that Eq. (4.14) is also satisfied for conditions of individual seasons, the coefficient γ that characterizes the meridional heat exchange being increased in the cold season and decreased in summer.

From Eqs. (4.2), (4.13), and (4.14), we get the formula

$$\gamma = \frac{Q_s(1 - \alpha_s) - a - bT + (a_1 + b_1T)n - B_s}{T - T_p}. \tag{4.15}$$

Using data on temperature, radiation, albedo, and cloudiness for the Central Arctic (80° N latitude), we determined by this formula the value of the coefficient γ, which equals 0.15 in summer (June–August) and 0.24 in winter (December–February). It is evident that the change of this coefficient during the annual cycle is connected with the change in the meridional temperature gradient, on which the intensity of heat exchange between high and low latitudes depends.

From the same equations, we can obtain formulas for the mean temperature near the earth's surface in summer and winter (the values of parameters for these seasons are marked by the appropriate indices: L for summer, Z for winter)

$$T_L = \frac{Q_{sL}(1 - \alpha_s) + \gamma_L T_{pL} - B_s - a + a_1 n_L}{b - b_1 n_L + \gamma_L},\tag{4.16}$$

$$T_Z = \frac{\gamma_Z T_{pZ} + B_s - a + a_1 n_Z}{b - b_1 n_Z + \gamma_Z}.\tag{4.17}$$

We can add to Eqs. (4.16) and (4.17) the equations of the heat balance at the earth's surface,

$$Q_L(1 - \alpha) - \delta\sigma T_L{}^3(K - Nq_L)(1 - cn_L)$$
$$- (4\delta\sigma T_L{}^3 + c_p\rho\chi u_L)(T_{wL} - T_L) - L\rho\chi u_L(q_{sL} - q_L) = B_s \tag{4.18}$$

and

$$- \delta\sigma T_Z{}^3(K - Nq_Z)(1 - cn_Z) - (4\delta\sigma T_Z{}^3 + c_p\rho\chi u_Z)$$
$$\times (T_{wZ} - T_Z) - L\rho\chi u_Z(q_{sZ} - q_Z) = -B_s, \tag{4.19}$$

and a formula connecting the changes in heat content in the upper layers of the ocean with the annual amplitude of temperature (Budyko, 1962),

$$B_s = \mu(T_{wL} - T_{wZ}).\tag{4.20}$$

Using Eqs. (4.16–4.20), we can calculate water and air temperature for the ice-free regime in the Central Arctic. For this calculation, let us consider that humidity is proportional to the absolute humidity of saturated air at the temperature of the evaporating surface.

Let us assume that the thermal regime of the Arctic under ice-free conditions during the whole year will be close to the regime that is observed now in summertime. Then we may consider the value of the coefficient γ and also the values of cloudiness and wind speed for winter months to be close to the contemporary summer conditions.

Let us assume also that heat exchange between the Northern and Southern Hemispheres has little influence on the thermal conditions of high latitudes in the Northern Hemisphere (or that the thermal regime of both hemispheres changes similarly).

The water and air temperatures for the Central Arctic computed under these assumptions are given in Table 29.

As is seen from this table, the winter air temperature in the Central Arctic with the ice-free regime is some degrees lower than the contemporary summer temperature, and the summer temperature is several degrees higher. This relatively small difference permits us to consider that the above assumption about the parameters is admissible.

TABLE 29

THERMAL REGIME OF THE CENTRAL ARCTIC
UNDER ICE-FREE CONDITIONS

	Summer	Winter
Water temperature	+4.3°	−0.8°
Air temperature	+5.8°	−5.4°

The results of the calculation corroborate the possibility of an ice-free regime in the Central Arctic, because the water temperature in winter turns out to be higher than the freezing point of salt water, approximately −1.8°. In addition, the results mentioned suggest a great instability of the ice-free regime, as the water temperature in winter exceeds the freezing point by only 1°.

For correct interpretation of the results of this calculation (and also of other thermal-regime calculations for ice-free conditions in the Arctic), one should bear in mind that the probable error of even the most accurately calculated temperature cannot be less than several degrees. Therefore, we can get unambiguous conclusions from these calculations only in cases when the lowest water temperatures found in them are higher or lower than the freezing point by a value exceeding several degrees.

It is evident that these cases will correspond to the conditions of stable existence of one of the two possible regimes in the Central Arctic. If the ice-free regime in the Arctic is really possible but comparatively unstable, then an appropriate conclusion can be obtained only as a probable consequence of the calculation and not as a unique result of it.

The consequence mentioned refers to the case when the lowest water temperature in the ice-free regime proves to be close to the freezing point or differs from it by a value less than the errors in calculation. Under such conditions, the existence of an unstable ice-free regime is very probable, because the calculated value of temperature relates to mean conditions, on which in fact are superimposed continual fluctuations in the thermal regime due to oscillating processes in the atmosphere and ocean. If the mean level of the lowest water temperatures for ice-free conditions actually lies slightly higher than the freezing point, then with negative anomalies of temperature or radiation, the formation of ice becomes possible. If the mean level of these temperatures is slightly lower than the freezing point, then under long positive anomalies of the elements mentioned, destruction of the ice and temporary restoration of the ice-free regime is possible.

It should be noted that the values of water and air temperatures obtained in the above calculation for the ice-free regime are slightly underestimated. The reason for this lies in the absence of an accounting in the model used of the additional influx of heat in the hydrosphere of the high latitudes that appears under ice-free conditions only. One might think, however, that even with the heat influx mentioned being considered, the water temperature in winter in the Arctic will not much exceed the freezing point. Thus, the ice-free regime in the high latitudes in the contemporary epoch will probably be unstable.

The problem of stability of the existing polar ice is of great importance, since the disappearance of this ice must lead to abrupt changes in climatic conditions over extensive areas. As seen from the above calculation, the mean annual air temperature in the Central Arctic under the ice-free regime increases by approximately 15° in comparison with current conditions. The temperature in the cold season will increase considerably, while that in summer months will be raised only by a few degrees.

Without doubt, a similar rise in temperature will spread in a somewhat weakened form to the peripheral regions of the Arctic and also to middle and even tropical latitudes.

Together with the general rise in temperature under the ice-free regime, the meridional temperature gradients will decrease, especially in winter. This must substantially influence the circulation of the atmosphere and the turnover of water.

Some evaluations of the water-circulation conditions with a considerable warming in the high latitudes, which were made by Drozdov (1966), show that in this case a considerable redistribution of the amounts of atmospheric precipitation occurs. In some coastal regions, the amounts of precipitation increase compared to existing conditions; in many interior regions, the amounts of precipitation decrease.

The consequences of the melting of glaciers on land also has considerable importance, because it would lead to a marked rise in ocean level and to flooding of many populated areas.

Thus, the disappearance of polar ice will be connected with immense changes in the climatic conditions on our planet, some of these changes being favorable for man's activities and some unfavorable.

REFERENCES

Антонов В. С. (1968). Возможная причина пульсаций водообмена между Северным Ледовитым и Атлантическим океанами. Проблемы Арктики и Антарктики, № 29.
Antonov, V. S. (1968). Possible reasons for pulsations in water exchange between the Arctic and Atlantic Oceans. *Prob. Arktiki Antarktiki* No. 29, 13–18. MGA 21.2-751.
Будыко М. И. (1956). Тепловой баланс земной поверхности. Гидрометеоиздат, Л.
Budyko, M. I. (1956). "Teplovoi Balans Zemnoi Poverkhnosti." Gidrometeoizdat, Leningrad; "The Heat Balance of the Earth's Surface," translated by N. A. Stepanova. U.S. Weather Bur., Washington, 1958. MGA 13E-286.

Будыко М. И. (1961). О термической зональности Земли. Метеорология и гидрология, № 11.

Budyko, M. I. (1961). On the thermal zonality of the Earth. *Meteorol. Gidrol.* No. 11, 7–14. MGA 13:794.

Будыко М. И. (1962). Полярные льды и климат. Изв. АН ССР, сер. геогр., № 6.

Budyko, M. I. (1962). Polar ice and climate. *Izv. Akad. Nauk SSSR Ser. Geogr.* No. 6, 3–10. MGA 14.10–297; Res. Mem. RM-5003-PR, 1966, pp. 9–23. Rand Corp., Santa Monica, California, 1966. MGA 17.10-321.

Будыко М. И. (1966). Возможности изменения климата при воздействии на полярные льды. Сб. «Современные проблемы климатологии». Гидрометеоиздат, Л.

Budyko, M. I. (1966). The possibility of changing the climate by action on the polar ice. *In* "Sovremennye Problemy Klimatologii (Contemporary Problems of Climatology)" (M. I. Budyko, ed.), pp. 347–357. Gidrometeoizdat, Leningrad. MGA 18.12-170; Possibility of climate-changing by modification of polar ice. JPRS 43,482. U.S. Joint Publ. Res. Service, 1967. MGA 20.5-182.

Будыко, М. И. (1968). О происхождении ледниковых эпох. Метеорология и гидрология, № 11.

Budyko, M. I. (1968). On the origin of glacial epochs. *Meteorol. Gidrol.* No. 11. 3-12. MGA 20.11-383.

Будыко М. И. (1969). Полярные льды и климат. Гидрометеоиздат, Л.

Budyko, M. I. (1969). "Poliarnye L'dy i Klimat (Polar Ice and Climate)." Gidrometeoizdat, Leningrad. MGA 22.3-609.

Гаврилова М. К. (1963). Радиационный климат Арктики. Гидрометеоиздат, Л.

Gavrilova, M. K. (1963). "Radiatsionnyi Klimat Arktiki." Gidrometeoizdat, Leningrad; "Radiation Climate of the Arctic." Isr. Program Sci. Transl., Jerusalem, 1966. MGA 16.1-42, 18.11-4.

Доронин Ю. П. (1963). О тепловом балансе Центральной Арктики. Труды ААНИИ, № 253.

Doronin, Iu. P. (1963). On the heat balance of the Central Arctic. *Tr. Arkt. Antarkt. Nauch. Issled. Inst.* **253**, 178–184; Res. Mem. RM-5003-PR, 193–205. Rand Corp., Santa Monica, California, 1966. MGA 18.2-283.

Доронин Ю. П. (1968). К проблеме уничтожения арктического льда. Проблемы Арктики и Антарктики, т. 28.

Doronin, Iu. P. (1968). On the problem of the destruction of the Arctic ice. *Probl. Arktiki Antarktiki* **28**.

Дроздов О. А. (1966). Об изменениях осадков северного полушария при изменении температуры полярного бассейна. Труды ГГО, вып. 198.

Drozdov, O. A. (1966). On changes in precipitation in the Northern Hemisphere as related to changes in temperature in the Polar Basin. *Tr. Gl. Geofiz. Observ.* **198**, 3–16. MGA 18.1-244.

Зубенок Л. И. (1963). Влияние аномалий температуры на ледяной покров Арктики. Метеорология и гидрология, № 6.

Zubenok, L. I. (1963). The influence of temperature anomalies on the ice cover of the Arctic. *Meteorol. Gidrol.* No. 6, 25–30.

Зубов Н. Н. (1945). Льды Арктики. Главсевморпуть.

Zubov, N. N. (1945). "L'dy Arktiki (The Ice of the Arctic)." Izdat. Glavsevmorput', Moscow. MGA 13E-65.

Коптев А. П. (1964). Альбедо снежно-ледяного покрова моря. Проблемы Арктики и Антарктики, № 15.

Koptev, A. P. (1964). Albedo of the snow-ice cover of the sea. *Probl. Arktiki Antarktiki* No. 15, 25–36. MGA 16.9-410, 19.2-204.

Леонов А. К. (1947). Опыт количественного учета водной массы, тепла и солей, вносимых Атлантическим и Тихоокеанским течениями в Арктический бассейн. Метеорология и гидрология, № 5.

Leonov, A. K. (1947). An experiment in quantitative calculation of water masses, heat, and salt brought by Atlantic and Pacific currents into the Arctic Basin. *Meteorol. Gidrol.* No. 5.

Ломоносов М. В. (1763). Краткое описание разных путешествий по северным морям. (Полное собр. соч., т. VI. Изд. АН СССР, 1952.)

Lomonosov, M. V. (1763). A short description of different voyages in the Northern Seas, 1763. "Polnoe Sobrannye Sochenenie," Vol. 6. (Reprint: *Izdat. Akad. Nauk SSSR*, 1952.)

Марков К. К. (1960). Палеогеография. Изд. МГУ, М.

Markov, K. K. (1960). "Paleogeografii (Paleogeography)." Izdat. Mosk. Gosudarst. Univer., Moscow.

Маршунова М. С. и Черниговский Н. Т. (1965). Климат советской Арктики (радиационный режим). Гидрометеоиздат, Л.

Marshunova, M. S., and Chernigovskii, N. T. (1965). "Klimat Sovetskoi Arktiki: Radiatsionnyi Rezhim (Climate of the Soviet Arctic: Radiation Regime)." Gidrometeoizdat, Leningrad. MGA 18.1-11 [Chernigovkii and Marshunova].

Маршунова М. С. и Черниговский Н. Т. (1968). Численные характериетики радиационного режима Советской Арктики. Проблемы Арктики и Антарктики, № 28.

Marshunova, M. S., and Chernigovskii, N. T. (1968). Numerical characteristics of the radiation regime in the Soviet Arctic. *Probl. Arktiki Antarktiki* No. 28, 46–57 (cf. Res. Mem. RM-5233-NSF, pp. 279–297. Rand Corp., Santa Monica, California, 1966. MGA 18.7-365).

Назинцев Ю. Л. (1964). Тепловой баланс поверхности многолетнего ледяного покрова в Центральной Арктике. Труды ААНИИ, т. 267.

Nazintsev, Iu. L. (1964). The heat balance of the surface of many-year ice cover in the Central Arctic. *Tr. Arkti. Antarkt. Nauch. Issled. Ints.* **267.**

Ракипова Л. Р. (1962). Изменение климата при воздействии на льды Арктики. Метеорология и гидрология, № 9.

Rakipova, L. R. (1962). Changing the climate by action on the ice of the Arctic Basin. *Meteorol. Gidrol.* No. 9, 28–30. MGA 14:600.

Ракипова Л. Р. (1966). Изменения зонального распределения температуры атмосферы в результате активных воздействий на климат. Сб. «Современные проблемы климатологии». Гидрометеоиздат, Л.

Rakipova, L. R. (1966). Variation in the zonal distribution of temperature as a result of climate modification. In "Sovremennye Problemy Klimatologii (Contemporary Problems of Climatology)" (M. I. Budyko, ed.), pp. 358–383. Gidrometeoizdat, Leningrad. MGA 18.12-175.

Яковлев Г. Н. (1958). Тепловой баланс ледяного покрова Центральной Арктики. Проблемы Арктики, № 5.

Iakovlev, G. N. (1958). Heat balance of the ice cover of the Central Arctic. *Probl. Arktiki* No. 5.

Badgley, F. I. (1966). Heat budget at the surface of the Arctic Ocean. *Proc. Symp. Arctic Heat Budget and Atmos. Circ.* Lake Arrowhead, Calif., 1966 (J. O. Fletcher, ed.). Rep. RM-5223-NSF, Rand Corp., Santa Monica, California, pp. 267–277.

Brooks, C. E. P. (1950). "Climate Through the Ages," rev. ed., Ernest Benn, London. (Русский перевод: Брукс. Климат прошлого. ИЛ, М., 1952.)

Donn, W. L., and Shaw, M. (1966). The heat budgets of an ice-free and ice-covered Arctic Ocean. *J. Geoph. Res.* **71**, No. 4.

Fletcher, J. O. (1965). The heat budget of the Arctic Basin and its relation to climate. Rep. R-444-PR, Rand Corp., Santa Monica, California.

Fletcher, J. O. (1966). The Arctic heat budget and atmospheric circulation. *Proc. Symp. Arctic Heat Budget and Atmos. Circ.* Lake Arrowhead, Calif., 1966 (J. O. Fletcher, ed.). Rep. RM-5223-NSF, Rand Corp., Santa Monica, California, pp. 23–43.

Hare, F. K. (1968). The Arctic. *Quart. J. Roy. Meteorol. Soc.* **94**, No. 402.

"Ice Atlas of the Northern Hemisphere." U.S. Hydrographic Office, Publ. No. 550, Washington, 1946.

Raschke, E., Möller, F., and Bandeen, W. (1968). The radiation balance of the earth-atmosphere system over both polar regions obtained from radiation measurements of the Nimbus II meteorological satellite. *Sver. Meteorol. Hydrol. Inst. Medd. Ser. B*, No. 28.

Untersteiner, N. (1966). Calculating thermal regime and mass budget of sea ice. *Proc. Symp. Arctic Heat Budget and Atmos. Cir.* Lake Arrowhead, Calif., 1966 (J. O. Fletcher, ed.). Rep. RM-5223-NSF, Rand Corp., Santa Monica, California, pp. 203–213.

Vowinkel, E., and Orvig, S. (1964). Energy balance of the Arctic. *Arch. f. Meteorol. Geophys. Bioklimatol. Ser. B*, **13**, Pt. 3–4.

Vowinkel, E., and Orvig, S. (1966). Possible changes in the radiation budget over the Polar Ocean. *Proc. Symp. Arctic Heat Budget Atmos. Circ.* Lake Arrowhead, Calif., 1966 (J. O. Fletcher, ed.). Rep. RM-5223-NSF, Rand Corp., Santa Monica, California, pp. 299–303.

V

Climatic Change

1. Introduction

Studies on climatic change in the contemporary period and the geological past contain a large body of data on climatic conditions at various periods of time and in different geographical regions. Fewer results have been obtained on the reasons for climatic change. Although many authors have been interested in this problem, it has not so far been worked out sufficiently, apparently because the descriptive methods that prevailed in the past are not effective in explaining the causal mechanism of the processes being studied.

In this chapter, we will consider the possibility of applying materials on energy balance to study the problem of the reasons for change and fluctuation in climate. Such a mode of investigation was used in the studies of Humphreys (1929), Wexler (1953), Bernard (1964), Flohn (1964), Mitchell (1965), and other authors.

Let us first consider empirical data on climatic conditions of the past. There are three basic sources of such data.

The most exact climatic data cover the period of instrumental meteorological observations. Since instrumental observations began on a mass scale only in the second half of the 19th century, the period covered is equal to about one century.

Certain data on climatic conditions over a period of several thousand years can be obtained from materials of noninstrumental observations reflected in various historical sources.

Finally, data on the climate of more remote eras, extending over hundreds of millions of years, are furnished by paleogeographic studies in which the relationship between meteorological factors and the life activities of animals and plants, as well as hydrological processes, processes of lithogenesis, and so forth, are used as clues to past climatic conditions.

The interpretation of data on the physical conditions of remote eras for an explanation of past climates is fraught with great difficulties, some of which are crucial. They involve, in particular, the need for using the principle of uniformitarianism, which in this case calls for the assumption that the relationships between climate and other natural phenomena in the past were the same as exist at the present time. Although this approach is open to argument, the great diversity of natural processes that are functions of climate make possible independent testing of the results of climatic reconstruction on the basis of various paleogeographic indices. The more general regularities of past climates can therefore be accepted as reliable, even though some particular results may be open to question and may require additional investigation.

An important additional source of information on past climates is furnished by paleotemperature data obtained through analysis of the isotopic composition of organic residues [see Bowen (1966) and others]. An evaluation of the precision of these data and the question of their practical interpretation involve certain difficulties, which are gradually being overcome as the methods of paleotemperature analysis are improved.

The principal results of the empirical study of past climates can be presented in the form of the following conclusions:

1. Climatic conditions that prevailed over the last few hundred million years differed markedly from those of the present. Throughout this entire segment of time, except for the relatively brief Quaternary period, the difference in temperatures between low and high latitudes was relatively small, with low-latitude temperatures roughly at present levels and temperatures in the middle and high latitudes substantially higher than those observed at the present time.

2. The evolution of the present contrast between the temperatures at the Equator and those at the poles began about 70 million years ago, at the beginning of the Tertiary period. That process went rather slowly, and by the beginning of the Quaternary (about a million years ago), the difference of temperatures at high and low latitudes was still substantially less than the present difference.

3. In the Quaternary period, temperature dropped sharply in the high latitudes in conjunction with the beginning of polar glaciation. Glaciation in the Northern Hemisphere was subjected to considerable fluctuation, in the course of which it increased several times, reaching the middle latitudes, and

then retreated again to the higher latitudes. The last advance of the ice sheet in Eurasia (the Würm stage) ended about 10,000 years ago, and since then the permanent ice cover in the Northern Hemisphere has been limited largely to the Arctic Ocean and to islands in the higher latitudes (besides mountain regions).

4. In the last 10,000 years, thermal conditions in higher and middle latitudes have continued to change. This has been connected with substantial fluctuations in the area covered by polar ice.

5. In the last century, a period for which instrumental data are available, climatic fluctuations continued. The first half of the 20th century witnessed a warming trend that was particularly evident in the 1920s and 1930s. This trend ceased in the 1940s and was followed by a cooling trend, which has not yet reached the magnitude of the preceding warming trend. Present changes in climate are most evident in the middle and especially in the higher latitudes of the Northern Hemisphere.

In an attempt to explain the foregoing regularities of climatic change, several hypotheses have been proposed which link climatic change with a variety of terrestrial and cosmic factors [see reviews by Flohn (1964), Mitchell (1965), Sellers (1965), and others]. Most of these hypotheses have not been confirmed by quantitative calculations or observational data, and the grounds on which they were advanced have been challenged. As a result, there is at the present time no generally accepted view on the causes of climatic change and fluctuation.

Without attempting to evaluate the numerous proposals regarding the factors that cause climatic change, we will try to distinguish causes whose influence on climatic change is more or less self-evident. If these causes turn out to be sufficient to explain the aforementioned regularities of climatic change, this would reduce the need for recourse to additional hypotheses for an interpretation of this phenomenon.

We know that the earth's climate is determined by solar radiation received at the outer boundary of the atmosphere and by the structure of the underlying surface. The formerly widespread view that atmospheric circulation is also a climate-forming factor is unacceptable, as we have repeatedly noted, because the motion of atmospheric air is one of the elements of climate and not an external causative factor.

In recognizing that, for a given chemical composition of the atmosphere, the radiation of the sun and the structure of the underlying surface are the principal climate-forming factors, we must explain the meaning of the term "structure of the underlying surface."

It is evident that climatic genesis in the broad sense covers not only processes of the atmosphere but also physical processes in the hydrosphere and the entire complex of hydrometeorological processes at the earth's surface, including glaciation, if it takes place.

By the underlying surface as a climate-forming factor, we thus mean the structure of relief, that is, form of the earth's surface, that determines the area of seas and oceans and their depths, and the area of continents and their heights. Changes in the underlying surface associated, say, with glaciation may be treated as a climate-forming factor in a particular period, but in the general sense, such changes should also be considered as one of the elements of climate produced by the two basic causal factors—the influx of radiation and the structure of relief.

Let us now see to what extent we can explain the basic regularities of climatic change on the basis of changes in climate-forming factors. We will start with the period of instrumental observations, for which we have the most detailed climatic data.

2. Contemporary Climatic Changes

As has been established in the work of Rubinshtein (1946 and elsewhere), Lamb (1966 and elsewhere), and many other authors, climatic changes during the period of instrumental observations have not been uniform for various parts of the earth and for different seasons of the year, and thus present a rather complicated picture. If we want to explain the general regularities of climatic change, we would be best advised to use data on meteorological conditions relating to large areas. With this aim in mind, Willett and Mitchell [see Mitchell (1961, 1963)] averaged temperature data for many stations situated in various regions. These data served as the basis for conclusions about changes in the mean temperature of the earth's surface from year to year.

Such analysis can be performed more precisely by the use of air-temperature anomaly maps, rather than the observational data of individual stations. These maps, which have been prepared at the Main Geophysical Observatory, shed light on the distribution of mean monthly temperature anomalies for every month from 1881 to 1960 in the Northern Hemisphere, except in the equatorial zone, where observational data in the early years are inadequate for the construction of anomaly maps.

Figure 87 shows the secular course of yearly air-temperature anomalies in the zone between 17 and 90° N latitude, as calculated from the anomaly maps with the assistance of L. P. Spirina. Curve 1 represents the unsmoothed anomaly values, and curve 2, the anomalies averaged by 10-year moving periods.

The figure shows that the warming period beginning at the end of the 19th

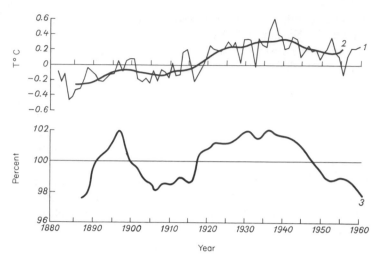

Fig. 87 Secular trend of anomalies of air temperature and radiation.

century ended about 1940 and gave way to a cooling trend. In this process, the Northern Hemisphere temperature, after having risen by 0.6°C during the warming trend, then dropped by 0.2° by the middle 1950s. A relatively brief warming trend with a smaller amplitude also occurred in the last few years of the 19th century.

A calculation of temperature anomalies in various latitudinal zones showed that the greatest temperature changes occurred in the middle latitudes and especially the higher latitudes. A warming trend in the subtropical and tropical regions was appreciably weaker, and it is therefore not quite clear from the observational data whether a cooling period set in after 1940 in these regions too.

Data on temperature anomalies in different periods of the year show that the mean temperature anomalies at various latitudes vary similarly in all seasons, with the absolute magnitudes of the anomalies in winter exceeding those in other seasons.

The findings presented in Fig. 87 confirm once again the existence of noticeable climatic fluctuations of a planetary character. The causes of these fluctuations have been discussed widely in the literature. Among the various hypotheses proposed in this connection, mention should be made, above all, of the supposition that the earth's thermal regime might be affected by changes in atmospheric transparency for the flux of short-wave radiation because of changes in the amount of atmospheric dust.

Some authors have also related contemporary climatic change to the effect of changes in the amount of carbon dioxide on long-wave radiation, to the instability of solar radiation (solar activity), to autofluctuations of the system consisting of the atmosphere, the oceans and polar ice, and to other factors.

It should be noted that not all of these hypotheses can be tested quantitatively at the present time. We can, however, assess the effect of some of the above-mentioned factors on climatic change. If such an assessment suggests that a particular factor plays a determining role in observed changes of climate, it may indicate indirectly a lesser role for other factors whose effect cannot yet be directly determined.

One of the first hypotheses concerning the causes of climatic fluctuation was stated in the 18th century by Benjamin Franklin, who suggested that a reduction of atmospheric transparency for solar radiation might lead to cooling. This concept was further developed by Humphreys (1929), Wexler (1953), and other investigators.

One of our own papers (Budyko, 1967) contained some results of a study of the effect of changes in atmospheric transparency on the thermal regime, and we will discuss this here in greater detail.

It was first known at the beginning of the 20th century that the mean amount of direct solar radiation reaching the earth's surface under cloudless conditions may vary noticeably from year to year. These changes show up well on curves of the secular march of direct-beam radiation constructed on the basis of observational data from actinometric stations. Such curves show [see Budyko and Pivovarova (1967)] that direct radiation, in addition to changing from year to year, also varies over longer periods, on the order of decades.

Savinov (1913), Kimball (1918), and others have established that sharp reductions of solar radiation occur when the lower layers of the atmosphere are filled with volcanic dust, after volcanic eruptions of an explosive character.

In such cases, the global magnitude of direct radiation may drop by 10–20% over a period of several months. An example appears in Fig. 88, showing changes in the ratio of the mean monthly values of direct radiation under

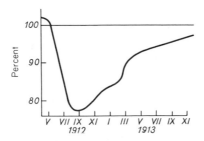

Fig. 88   Changes in radiation after a volcanic eruption.

cloudless skies to the long-term norm after an eruption of Mount Katmai in Alaska. This curve, constructed on the basis of observational data from several European and American actinometric stations, shows that volcanic dust reduced direct radiation by more than 20% in individual months. Similar changes in radiation were observed after the 1883 eruption of Krakatoa (Indonesia). In both cases, anomalous optical phenomena in the atmosphere were observed over huge areas after the volcanic eruptions, confirming the global character of changes in the radiation regime resulting from the dissemination of volcanic dust.

The effect of changes in radiation on the thermal regime after volcanic eruptions was studied in the above-mentioned works of Humphrey, Mitchell, and others, who established that after great eruptions, the earth's mean temperature dropped by a few tenths of a degree.

Of particular interest is a comparison of the secular march of temperatures in the Northern Hemisphere with the secular march of radiation reaching the earth's surface. For this purpose, Pivovarova analyzed actinometric observational data over the period 1880–1965 for a group of European and American stations with the longest observation series, and constructed a mean curve of the secular march of direct radiation under cloudless skies (Pivovarova, 1968). Figure 87 shows the 10-year moving average values of solar radiation during this study period (curve 3).

Figure 87 shows two maxima for solar radiation—a short maximum at the end of the 19th century, and a longer maximum in the first half of the 20th century with highest values in the 1930s.

It might be supposed that the increase in radiation at the end of the 19th century resulted from the clearing of the atmosphere after the spread of volcanic dust from the Krakatoa eruption. The next reduction of radiation would have been the result of eruptions of Mont Pelée and other volcanoes. (The downward trend of the curve begins before these eruptions because of the use of 10-yr moving means.) The rise of radiation during 1915–1920 can apparently be attributed to an increase in transparency after the dust from the Katmai eruption had settled. For a long time afterward, no great explosive eruptions occurred.

Let us now turn to the causes of the decline of radiation observed in the 1940s. A number of authors (Davitaia, 1965; and others) have suggested that this decline was a result of the pollution of the atmosphere by industrial wastes and by dust from nuclear test explosions. The eruptions of Mount Spurr (Alaska) in 1953, Mount Bezymiannyi (Kamchatka) in 1956, and other volcanoes may also have played a role.

If we compare curve 3 with the smoothed curve 2 of the secular march of temperature in Fig. 87, we find certain qualitative similarities between the two. Both curves display two maxima, one at the end of the 19th century and a second and more important maximum in the 1930s. There are, however, differences between the two curves, particularly the more pronounced character of the first maximum in the radiation curve. The similarity between the two curves suggests that changes in radiation produced by the instability of atmospheric transparency represent a significant factor in climatic change. Further clarification of this question requires quantitative calculation of temperature changes resulting from changes in atmospheric transparency for short-wave radiation.

Humphreys (1929) established that global fluctuations in atmospheric transparency are most affected by the relatively fine dust of volcanic eruption that spreads after eruptions of the explosive type and remains for a long time in the lower layers of the stratosphere.

Humphreys and Wexler (1953) suggested that the finest fractions of dust might remain in the atmosphere for many years. This dust has little effect on long-wave radiation, but it does increase the scattering of short-wave radiation, thus increasing the earth's global albedo and reducing the magnitude of radiation absorbed by the earth as a planet.

It should be pointed out that because of the predominant scattering of radiation by dust in the direction of the incident ray (the Mie effect), direct radiation is reduced much more substantially by scattering than is total solar radiation. Since it is changes in total radiation that affect the earth's thermal regime, an evaluation of the effect of volcanic eruptions of climate requires determination of the change in total radiation resulting from the appearance of volcanic dust.

This can be done by the method used by Shifrin and his associates in studies on atmospheric optics (Shifrin and Minin, 1957; Shifrin and Piatovskaia, 1959).

We used their data to determine the ratios of the decline of total short-wave radiation to the decline of direct-beam radiation under average conditions at various latitudes in the presence of a layer of silica dust in the stratosphere. The results of the computation appear in Table 30.

According to Shifrin's findings, the values listed in this table depend relatively little on the particle size of the dust, provided most of the particle diameters lie between 0.02–0.03 and 0.2–0.3 μm.

Let us now estimate how changes in the amount of direct radiation affect the mean temperature of the earth. For this purpose, we will consider the relationship between the earth's mean temperature and incoming solar radiation. Several attempts have been made to relate change in the earth's mean temperature to changes in incoming radiation. The findings of the last few years show that a 1% change in radiation results in a change of 1.2–1.5° in the mean temperature at the earth's surface for a constant albedo (see Chapter III, Section 4).

We will now compare the earth's radiation and thermal regimes over two 30-yr periods: 1888–1917 and 1918–1947. It follows from Fig. 87 that direct-beam radiation in the second period was 2% greater than in the first. Since, on the basis of the data in the table above, the weighted mean ratio of changes in total radiation to changes in direct radiation for the earth as a whole is 0.15, we find that total radiation in the second 30-yr period was 0.3% higher than in the first period. Such an increase in total radiation corresponds to an increase in the mean temperature by roughly 0.4°C. The actual difference of temperature for the two periods, on the basis of curve 1, was 0.33°, which agrees quite well with the computed figure.

TABLE 30

Effect of Dust on the Radiation Regime

Latitude (degrees)	Decline of total radiation / Decline of direct-beam radiation
90	0.24
80	0.23
70	0.22
60	0.21
50	0.19
40	0.18
30	0.16
20	0.14
10	0.13
0	0.13

It is evident that such a computation technique can be used to arrive at temperature changes only under stationary conditions, when correspondence exists between the radiative influx of heat and the thermal regime. But during short-term changes of radiation lasting a few months or years, there can be no such correspondence because of the substantial thermal inertia of the earth's outer envelope caused by heat exchange in the upper layer of the oceans.

Let us discuss the effect of short-term radiation changes on temperature. This effect can be calculated theoretically through the use of the thermal conductivity and heat capacity of ocean water. But since we are interested in only an approximate evaluation of this effect, we will make use of a simpler relationship between temperature and radiation fluctuations that can be established empirically from changes in their magnitudes during the annual march.

We will assume that the rate of change of the earth's temperature is proportional to the difference between the temperature at a given time T and the temperature corresponding to stationary conditions, T_r, that is,

$$\frac{dT}{dt} = -\lambda(T - T_r),\tag{5.1}$$

where λ is a proportionality coefficient.

Designating the temperature at the initial moment of time as T_1, we obtain from Eq. (5.1)

$$T - T_r = (T_1 - T_r)\, e^{-\lambda t}.\tag{5.2}$$

For an approximate evaluation of the magnitude of λ, we will use data on the annual march of solar radiation and temperature for the Northern Hemisphere.

Since the ratio of the magnitude of solar radiation received at the outer boundary of the atmosphere of the Northern Hemisphere during the warm half of the year (April–September) to the mean annual magnitude of radiation is 1.29, we find from the relationship between temperature and radiation changes derived in Section 4 of Chapter III that such a change in radiation in the absence of thermal inertia would raise the temperature by roughly 40°. The observed difference between the mean temperatures of the Northern Hemisphere during the warm half of the year and the entire year is 3.5°. Accordingly, since for $t = \frac{1}{4}$ yr, $T - T_1 = 3.5°$, and since $T_r - T_1 = 40°$, we can derive λ from Eq. (5.2) as being roughly equal to 0.4 yr^{-1}.

Taking this evaluation into account, we now calculate the change in mean temperature that would occur during the year following a volcanic eruption that resulted in a 10% reduction of direct radiation on the average for the year. In this case, the reduction of global radiation would be 1.5%, and the reduction of T_r would be about 2°. From Eq. (5.2), we find that the value representing the temperature change after the eruption would amount to a few tenths of a degree. This value agrees quite well with the magnitude of the mean annual temperature anomaly observed after great volcanic eruptions.

The data presented here indicate that changes in incoming solar radiation caused by the instability of atmospheric transparency have a significant effect on climate and presumably represent the basic cause of contemporary climatic change. This conclusion does not exclude the possibility that other factors may affect climate, but they evidently play a less significant role, when compared with changes in atmospheric transparency.

It should be pointed out, of course, that fluctuations in the earth's mean temperatures are a highly schematic measure of the complex climatic changes that arise as a result of changes in the radiation regime.

When a layer of volcanic dust is present in the atmosphere, direct radiation decreases inversely with the optical mass of the atmosphere, that is, direct radiation decreases with the mean elevation of the sun. This means that direct radiation decreases to a greater extent in higher latitudes than in lower latitudes, and more strongly in winter than in summer. This effect is even more pronounced in total solar radiation because the ratio of the decrease of total radiation to the decrease of direct radiation also increases inversely with the mean elevation of the sun.

This regularity is one of the factors that produce a greater lowering of temperature after volcanic eruptions at high latitudes than at low.

The above-mentioned data on temperature anomalies show that during the general warming trend in the first half of the 20th century, the differences between temperatures in the high and low latitudes declined by 2°, or by several per cent of the existing mean meridional temperature gradient.

This change in temperature field significantly affected the circulation in the atmosphere and hydrosphere, and the circulatory changes in turn had an effect on the temperature field and were reflected in such climatic elements as the circulation of water and the regime of atmospheric precipitation. There are grounds for assuming, in particular, that the reduction of the meridional temperature gradients in the 1920s and 1930s weakened the zonal circulation in the middle latitudes, thus affecting precipitation in Eastern Europe and producing a drop in the level of the Caspian Sea.

In addition to the effect of the instability of atmospheric transparency, changes in climate and in its individual elements undoubtedly depend also on autofluctuating processes in the atmosphere and hydrosphere.

The simplest example of such an autofluctuating process is the change of level of a body of water without an outlet. Budyko and Iudin (1960) have shown that the level of water in an inland basin cannot remain stable even in the absence of climatic change if its shoreline is vertical, that is, if its area is not a function of its level. The instability is related to the fact that the sum of the annual fluctuations of the components of the water balance of such a water body increases without limit with time, in view of the random character of these fluctuations.

Since, however, natural water bodies have sloping shorelines, the changes of area with fluctuations in level tend to stabilize these fluctuations. The above-mentioned study established that if the successive annual fluctuations of the Caspian Sea level were independent of one another, the total amplitude of these fluctuations could be explained as the sum of the annual random changes in the sea level. In that case changes of the Caspian Sea level would represent an example of a purely autofluctuating process.

Drozdov and Pokrovskaia (1961) noted that the successive annual fluctuations in the level of the Caspian Sea are not independent of one another.

Their interconnection suggests that a large part of the amplitude of fluctuations in level can be explained by external factors (that is, general climatic fluctuations), even though a substantial part of this amplitude is a result of the autofluctuating process.

Far more complicated autofluctuating processes take place in the atmosphere occan–polar ice system. Models of these processes were first examined by Shuleikin (1941 and elsewhere). The study of these processes by statistical methods provides the basis for many long-range and extra-long-range weather forecasting methods.

Changes of such external climate-forming factors as the input of solar radiation presumably substantially affect the autofluctuating processes in the atmosphere and the hydrosphere. As a result, the regularities of climatic fluctuations turn out to be rather complicated, as was pointed out at the beginning of this chapter.

3. Climates of the Past

The Quaternary glaciations

The Quaternary period, beginning about a million years ago, was marked by the appearance of major glaciations that expanded during the glacial epochs to cover a substantial part of the earth's surface and retreated during interglacial times.

According to the latest data (Markov, 1960; and others), the ice sheet on land and sea in the Northern Hemisphere reached an average latitude of 56° N and, in some lowland areas, even 40° N latitude.

Although only a small part of the ice sheet has been preserved in our time compared with the epoch of its maximum extent, even the present glaciation in the Antarctic and in Greenland suggests the tremendous size that an ice sheet can attain on continents.

An explanation of the causes of the appearance and disappearance of this ice sheet is of crucial significance in explaining climatic change in Quaternary times.

In the preceding section, we noted that contemporary climatic change is explained to a large extent by fluctuations of atmospheric transparency resulting from changes of volcanic activity. Moreover, it can be shown that while contemporary changes in volcanic activity produce fluctuations in total solar radiation of a few tenths of one per cent and fluctuations in global temperature of several tenths of a degree, the corresponding changes in radiation and temperature in the past reached much larger values.

It is obvious that the number of volcanic eruptions during a given time interval will tend to vary from a constant mean level of volcanic activity for purely statistical reasons, and the difference will tend to increase with the length of time under discussion. We also know that the level of volcanic activity in different geological epochs changed substantially with changes in the intensity of tectonic processes.

Since fluctuations of volcanic activity produced by tectonic factors are distinguished by long time scales, a calculation of the effect of the associated radiation changes on the earth's thermal regime must also consider changes in the earth's albedo resulting from increases or decreases of the area occupied by ice cover on land and water.

Measurements by meteorological satellites have shown that the albedo of the earth–atmosphere system in ice-covered areas is much greater than the albedo in ice-free regions, so that a change in glaciated area will tend to enhance the effect of radiation fluctuations on the thermal regime.

In order to evaluate the influence of radiation changes on the temperature of latitudinal zones in view of the above-mentioned effect, we will make use of one of the numerical models of the mean latitudinal distribution of temperature. Since we are interested only in the distribution of temperature near the earth's surface, we can replace the available models, requiring cumbersome computations, with the simpler scheme stated in Chapters III and IV.

We will use the heat-balance equation relating to the earth–atmosphere system in the form

$$Q_s(1 - \alpha_s) - I_s = C, \qquad (5.3)$$

where Q_s is the solar radiation reaching the outer boundary of the atmosphere, α_s is the albedo of the earth–atmosphere system, I_s is the long-wave radiation at the outer boundary of the atmosphere, and C is the outgo of heat resulting from circulation of the atmosphere and hydrosphere, including the redistribution of heat through the phase transformations of water.

Let us consider that the value of the long-wave emission at the outer boundary of the atmosphere, expressed in kcal cm^{-2} month^{-1}, is determined from the following formula (see Section 4, Chapter III):

$$I_s = a + bT - (a_1 + b_1 T)n, \qquad (5.4)$$

where T is the temperature at the level of the earth's surface in degrees Celsius, n is the cloudiness in fractions of a unit, and a, b, a_1, and b_1 are dimensional coefficients. Let us assume that

$$C = \gamma(T - T_p), \qquad (5.5)$$

where $\gamma = 0.235$ kcal cm^{-2} month^{-1} deg^{-1}, T is the mean annual temperature at a particular latitude, and T_p is the mean planetary temperature.

Taking into account that for the earth as a whole, $C = 0$, we can derive the following equations from Eqs. (5.3–5.5):

$$T = \frac{Q_s(1 - \alpha_s) - a + a_1 n + \gamma T_p}{\gamma + b - b_1 n},$$ (5.6)

and

$$T_p = \frac{Q_{sp}(1 - \alpha_{sp}) - a + a_1 n}{b - b_1 n},$$ (5.7)

where Q_{sp} and α_{sp} relate to the planet as a whole.

In Section 4 of Chapter III, we used Eqs. (5.6) and (5.7) to calculate the mean annual latitudinal temperatures for the present climatic conditions of the Northern Hemisphere. Figure 89 shows the results of a similar calculation, which was made with an additional assumption—it ignores the effect on temperature of deviations of mean latitudinal values of cloudiness from the mean global value of 0.50.

Such an assumption can be made because of the conclusion in Section 4 of Chapter III that cloudiness has a negligible effect on mean temperatures near the ground over a rather wide range of conditions. This inference, obtained on the basis of the relationship between albedo and cloudiness, means that the effect of cloudiness on absorbed short-wave radiation is often roughly compensated by its effect on outgoing long-wave radiation.

The results of calculation of the mean latitudinal temperature distribution appear in curve T_0 in Fig. 89. The results agree quite well with the observed temperatures at different latitudes, shown in curve T. This permits us to use

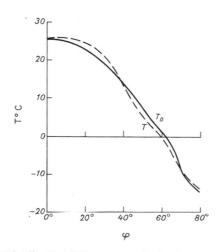

Fig. 89 Distribution of the mean latitudinal temperature.

this model for evaluation of the effect of radiation changes on the thermal regime and glaciation of the earth.

The present permanent ice cover on water and land areas of the Arctic reaches, on the average, 72° N latitude. We will assume that with a decrease of solar radiation the surface of the ice sheet will expand with the increase in size of the area with a temperature equal to or less than the −10°C now observed at 72°N latitude. This assumption can be tested on the basis of data on the mean elevation of the snow line (that is, the limit of permanent snow cover) in different latitudes. Data given by Kalesnik (1947) together with the size of the vertical temperature gradient in mountains suggest that the mean annual temperature at the elevation of the mean latitudinal position of the snow line is approximately constant within middle latitudes and is roughly equal to −10°.

On the basis of observational data, we will assume that the albedo over the area covered by ice is 0.62. The value of the albedo along the margins of the ice cover is 0.50, according to available data.

These albedo values suggest that with a change in the ice-covered area, the mean albedo of the earth changes by a magnitude of $\Delta\alpha = 0.30s$, where the coefficient 0.30 is the difference between albedo with and without an ice cover, and $s = lq$ (where l is the ratio of the change in the ice-covered area to the total area of the Northern Hemisphere, and q is the ratio of mean radiation in the zone of change of ice area to the mean radiation for the entire hemisphere).

It should be noted that when the ice sheet expands into lower latitudes, the values of albedo of ice-covered areas may vary somewhat from the values stated here.

Several studies have established the fact that the albedo of the earth–atmosphere system is a function of the angle of incidence of the sun's rays, and decreases with an increase of the angle. Calculations by Shifrin et al. (1964) have shown that this relationship is relatively weak for the large values of the albedo typical of ice-covered areas. It is somewhat more significant in the case of ice-free areas, especially in the absence of cloud cover.

A consideration of the effect of this relationship on the mean difference between albedo values with and without ice cover, based on data given by Shifrin et al., suggests that this difference diminishes by several hundredths in low latitudes, in comparison with high latitudes.

In addition, the observed mean albedo in higher latitudes refers mainly to the reflective capacity of areas covered with sea ice, since the glaciated land area in the Arctic is relatively small. According to satellite data (Raschke et al., 1968), the albedo over the Greenland ice sheet is substantially higher than the mean high-latitude albedo, and reaches 0.7–0.8. It can therefore be assumed that an advance of the ice sheet into lower latitudes will produce a slight increase in the mean albedo of the ice-covered area because of the development of large-scale continental glaciation.

Since these two effects tend to cancel each other out in affecting the difference between the albedos with and without ice cover, we will use the above-mentioned value of that difference on the assumption that it is evidently not overstated.

To take account of the effect of the change in glaciated area on the earth's mean annual temperature, we will use the following formula, derived from Eqs. (5.3) and (5.4) with $\Delta\alpha = 0.30s$:

$$\Delta T_p = \frac{Q_{sp}}{b - b_1 n}\left[\frac{\Delta Q_{sp}}{Q_{sp}}(1 - \alpha_{sp} - 0.30s) - 0.30s\right], \qquad (5.8)$$

where ΔT_p is the change that occurs in the earth's temperature when mean radiation Q_{sp} changes by the increment ΔQ_{sp}.

From Eqs. (5.3–5.6) and (5.8) we can derive a formula for the temperature at a particular latitude:

$$T = \left\{Q_s(1 - \alpha_s)\left(1 + \frac{\Delta Q_{sp}}{Q_{sp}}\right) - a + a_1 n + \gamma T_p'\right.$$

$$\left. + \frac{\gamma Q_{sp}}{b - b_1 n}\left[\frac{\Delta Q_{sp}}{Q_{sp}}(1 - \alpha_{sp} - 0.30s) - 0.30s\right]\right\}:(\gamma + b - b_1 n), \quad (5.9)$$

where T_p' is the existing mean temperature of the earth.

By using this formula and the values of Q_s and s corresponding to given latitudes, we can calculate the position of the limit of glaciation for different values of $\Delta Q_{sp}/Q_{sp}$. Equation (5.9) also can be used to compute the temperature distributions at various latitudes corresponding to these values. The results appear in Fig. 90, where the curves $T_{1.0}$ and $T_{1.5}$ correspond to tem-

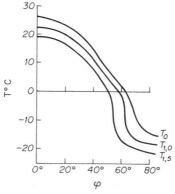

Fig. 90   Dependence of temperature distribution on radiation.

perature distributions when incoming radiation is reduced by 1.0% and 1.5%. The calculation ignores heat exchange between the Northern and Southern Hemispheres, which is permissible in the case of similar changes in the thermal state of both hemispheres.

Figure 91 shows the values of the mean global temperature T_p, and the mean latitude ϕ_0 to which glaciation extends, depending on relative changes in radiation during its gradual reduction. The figure shows that the influence of radiation changes on the thermal state becomes stronger as a result of expanding glaciation, so that the relationship becomes nonlinear.

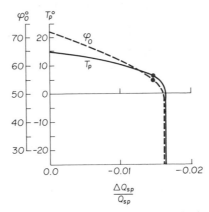

Fig. 91 Dependence of the planetary temperature and the boundary of glaciation on radiation.

While a 1% change in radiation with constant albedo lowers the mean temperature by 1.2–1.5°, a 1% change in radiation with a correspondingly changing albedo will lower the mean temperature by 5°, and a 1.5% change in radiation will lower the temperature by 9°. These reductions of temperature are accompanied by a southward advance of glaciation by 8–18° of latitude, a distance corresponding roughly to the advance of Quaternary glaciation. When radiation is reduced by 1.6%, the ice sheet reaches a mean latitude, about 50° N, after which it begins to advance southward all the way to the Equator as a result of autodevelopment. This is associated with a sharp decline of global temperature, down to several tens of degrees below zero.

The conclusion that the earth would be completely covered by an ice sheet after the ice reaches a critical latitude follows from the calculation of the magnitude of the radiation decrease needed to insure a further southward advance of the ice toward the Equator. The calculation shows that if, as a result of a decline of radiation, the ice sheet were to occupy the entire surface from the pole to the critical latitude, it would continue to advance toward the Equator at the same lowered radiation value and, having reached still lower latitudes, it would continue to advance southward at the now existing magnitudes of radiation, and even at values exceeding the contemporary level.

A similar conclusion based on other considerations was reached by Öpik (1953), who thought, however, that glaciation of the earth would require a substantial reduction of the solar constant. The possibility of the stable existence of complete glaciation of the earth at the contemporary income of radiation was suggested in our previous work (Budyko, 1962, 1966).

Of interest is a comparison of the above-stated conclusions concerning the unstable character of the contemporary climate of the earth (Budyko, 1968) with the results of Sellers' investigation (1969), in which the equation of heat balance of the earth–atmosphere system was also used to construct a model of the mean latitudinal distribution of air temperature.

Sellers calculated in his work the effect of polar ice on the thermal state for various values of albedo difference with and without ice.

It follows from these calculations that for the considered case of the albedo increase of 0.30 that results from the effect of the ice sheets near both poles, the air temperature in the Central Arctic would decrease by 13° and in lower latitudes by 2°. These values agree well with the results of our calculation (see Fig. 92).

Having calculated the value of the decrease in incoming solar radiation that is sufficient for complete glaciation of the earth, Sellers obtained a value equal to 2%, which is also close to the value of 1.6% obtained above.

The good agreement of the basic results of the calculations discussed is interesting, because although the basic idea of the climate models used here is the same, the corresponding calculation schemes, based on many different assumptions, are completely different.

It thus turns out that the contemporary state of glaciation of the earth is highly unstable. Relatively small changes in radiation, of the order of 1–1.5%, would be sufficient to expand the ice cover over land and water areas as far as the middle latitudes. Such radiation changes would be only a few times greater than the fluctuations that were observed as a result of varying volcanic activity over the past century.

In view of the fact that the level of volcanic activity over long periods in the past has changed several fold (Ronov, 1959), the effect of prolonged fluctuations of volcanic activity may be regarded as one of the factors of the spread of glaciation.

This conclusion is supported by the fact that the principal glacial epochs of the Quaternary period corresponded to substantial increases in volcanic activity in several regions of the lower latitudes (Fuchs and Patterson, 1947).

Although we cannot deal here with the many other hypotheses that have been advanced to explain the Quaternary glaciations, we must dwell at least on the widespread view that changes in elements of the earth's orbit and the inclination of the earth's axis had a decisive effect on these glaciations.

This view, advanced by Milankovich (1930 and elsewhere) and others, is shared by many specialists in Quaternary glaciation.

We know that changes in elements of the orbit produce a significant redistribution of the amounts of radiation coming in at various latitudes and in different seasons. Milankovich concluded, on the basis of these changes and by using a model of the latitudinal distribution of temperature, that changes of orbital elements produce significant temperature changes in the middle and high latitudes that might result in glaciation.

It must be pointed out that Milankovich's model of temperature distribution neglected the horizontal transfer of heat in the atmosphere and hydrosphere, so that it overstated the effect on the thermal state of latitudinal zones produced by changes in radiation in a particular latitudinal zone.

On the other hand, the above statement about the great instability of the thermal regime in the presence of polar ice cover allows the possibility of large changes in climatic regime with small fluctuations in incoming radiation.

To test the Milankovich hypothesis, we used our computational model to evaluate the changes in the thermal regime and glaciation for the case of the significant change of orbital elements that occurred 22,000 years ago and is usually associated with the last glaciation. In this calculation, we determined the southward advance of the ice sheet that would correspond to changes in the mean annual values of radiation at various latitudes based on data in the Milankovich study for that particular period.

The calculation showed that in this case, the boundary of glaciation would have moved southward by an amount slightly less than 1° of latitude. This value is an entire order of magnitude less than the actual advance of the ice sheet during the last glaciation. Such a result, however, is not sufficient for an evaluation of this hypothesis, since fundamentally the ice sheet is affected by a change in summer sums of radiation, rather than in annual sums. That change during the period in question at latitudes of 65–75° N exceeds the change in annual values by a factor of 2–3.

Using the model provided in Chapter IV of this book, we evaluated the effect of changes in summer values of radiation on the position of the ice cover. The displacements of the ice limit obtained in this calculation turned out close to those observed during the Pleistocene. This enables one to consider that astronomic factors exerted the major influence on the development of Quaternary glaciation (Budyko, 1972).

The climate of pre-Quaternary times

The Quaternary was preceded by the Mesozoic era and the Tertiary period, which together lasted about 200 million years.

Paleogeographic research (Bowen, 1966; Sinitsyn, 1967) has shown that the climate during this time was relatively warm at all latitudes and that no glaciations took place.

A change in climate began in the Tertiary period, which lasted about 70 million years. This involved at first a slow and later a more rapid drop of temperature in high and middle latitudes. Although this temperature drop was not constant and during some stages apparently gave way to a warming trend, a general tendency toward a reduction of temperature predominated, and by the end of the Tertiary period (in the Pliocene), the temperature contrast between the Equator and the poles reached a significant magnitude.

Let us now deal with the question why fluctuations in volcanic activity, which have taken place throughout the history of the earth, did not produce glaciation over the period of hundreds of millions of years preceding the Quaternary.

We know from geological investigations that a gradual rise in the level of the continents took place in pre-Quaternary times. This led to a weakening of the circulation of water in the oceans between low and high latitudes.

It was established even in the 1940s (Budyko, 1949) that the transfer of heat between the Equator and the poles in the hydrosphere amounts to a significant fraction of the corresponding transfer in the atmosphere, so that changes in oceanic circulation are bound to affect the thermal state of the high and middle latitudes.

We can clarify this question by using our computation technique to calculate temperature distribution in the case of the absence of ice in the high latitudes for various intensities of meridional heat exchange.

An evaluation of the polar-ice effect on the thermal regime of high latitudes was provided in the previous chapter.

The effect of polar ice on the thermal state at different latitudes is presented in Fig. 92, where curve T_0 represents the contemporary temperature distribution and curve T_q the temperature distribution in the absence of polar ice. In the latter case, the albedo of the high latitudes is assumed to be equal to the albedo of ice-free ocean areas, and the coefficient γ is taken equal to the value found earlier of 0.235 kcal cm^{-2} month^{-1} deg^{-1}.

It is evident from Fig. 92 that polar ice produces only a slight change in low-latitude temperatures, but significantly reduces the temperature of the high latitudes. As a result, the mean temperature difference between the pole and the Equator is significantly reduced [if ice is absent]. The mean annual temperature in the polar zone in an ice-free situation turns out to be only a few degrees below zero.

It may be assumed, however, that meridional heat transfer in a polar ocean would be greater in an ice-free situation than under contemporary conditions, because the ocean, now isolated from the atmosphere by the ice cover, would give off a substantial amount of heat to the atmosphere through turbulent heat exchange.

If we consider that an ice-free Arctic Ocean would receive an additional amount of heat equal to the mean amount that now reaches the ice-free regions of the high-latitude oceans, then the mean air temperature in the Arctic calculated by our technique, assuming the additional influx of heat, would actually equal a few degrees above zero.

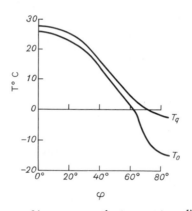

Fig. 92   Influence of ice cover on the temperature distribution.

It is evident that when the mean annual temperature in an ice-free Central Arctic is near the freezing point of water, relatively small anomalies in incoming radiation may lead to a restoration of the ice cover.

The contemporary distribution of land and water on the earth thus makes possible the existence of two climatic states, the first involving the presence of polar ice and a strong thermal contrast between the pole and the Equator, and the second, the absence of ice and a small mean meridional temperature gradient.

Both states are unstable, because relatively small fluctuations in the circulation of the atmosphere and hydrosphere may produce either the freezing of an ice-free polar ocean or the melting of existing polar ice. The probability of a transition from one state to the other increases with the instability of incoming radiation. This climatic characteristic apparently accounted for the principal regularities of climatic change in the Quaternary.

As noted in a previous study (Budyko, 1967), the Arctic basin was joined to the low-latitude oceans in the Mesozoic era and the early Tertiary period by much broader straits than in the Quaternary. This evidently meant that the influx of heat into the Arctic basin by ocean currents exceeded the magnitudes observed in high latitudes under contemporary conditions. If this influx exceeded its contemporary mean for ice-free areas by a factor of 1.5–2, then, according to calculation by the aforementioned formulas, the mean annual temperature in the Arctic reached 10°, thus excluding the possibility of glaciation even with significant anomalies in radiation.

During the Tertiary period, the Arctic basin became gradually more isolated from the tropical oceans. This produced a temperature drop at the pole and brought the temperature distribution closer to the values characteristic of the interglacial epochs in the Quaternary.

Intensive heat exchange in the hydrosphere thus seems to explain satisfactorily the relatively high temperatures in high and middle latitudes during the Mesozoic era and much of the Tertiary period. However, the reasons that the earth's mean temperature during this period was higher than in the contemporary epoch are less clear.

By using Eq. (5.7) and the derived value for the albedo of the polar region, we find that the present ice cover reduces the mean temperature of the earth's surface by approximately 2°C. This magnitude is less than the difference between the temperature of the Mesozoic and early Tertiary as established by paleoclimatic investigations, and the temperature observed at the present time.

Such a discrepancy cannot be explained by changes in the circulation of the hydrosphere, because the mean temperature of the earth's surface is not a function of the intensity of horizontal heat exchange.

It might be conjectured, however, that atmospheric transparency for long-wave radiation in the Mesozoic and early Tertiary was lower than in the contemporary epoch because of a high carbon-dioxide content in the atmosphere. This conjecture agrees with paleographic data and should therefore be tested by the methods of physical climatology.

We know less about climatic regularities in the Paleozoic than in Mesozoic and Cenozoic times. One of the paradoxical aspects of Paleozoic climate was the existence of large glaciations in the lower latitudes, especially the Permian glaciation. All kinds of hypotheses have been advanced to explain this phenomenon, including the idea of a significant displacement of the earth's poles and the movement of continents.

We have pointed out earlier (Budyko, 1961) that the great reflective capacity of ice makes large glaciations possible at any latitude.

This possibility derives, in particular, from the fact that absorbed radiation in an area of large-scale glaciation at the Equator could be the same as the absorbed radiation at an ice-free pole. If we take the albedo for an ice-free Arctic basin as 0.30, we find that the mean annual value of absorbed radiation at latitude 80° equals 7.7 kcal cm^{-2} month^{-1}. The same value of absorbed radiation would be observed at the Equator for an albedo of 0.70, which would be an entirely possible value for albedo in an extensive region of continental glaciation.

The mean latitudinal distribution of temperature with equatorial glaciation can be calculated by the technique given earlier.

We will assume that this glaciation occurred in a latitudinal zone near the Equator covering 5% of the total area of the hemisphere. With an albedo of 0.70 for that zone, the weighted mean value of the albedo of the earth would drop by 0.023, compared with conditions without glaciation.

The latitudinal distribution of the mean annual temperature, as calculated by Eq. (5.9) with the coefficient $\gamma = 0.40$ kcal cm^{-2} month^{-1} deg^{-1}, is shown in Fig. 93. According to the figure, the mean annual temperature in the

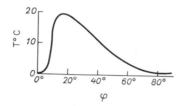

Fig. 93   Temperature distribution with equatorial glaciation.

glaciated zone would be close to 0°C, which suggests the possibility of a stable equatorial ice sheet even on plains lying at sea level. The part of the ice sheet situated above that level would evidently be under negative temperatures.

It should be noted that the temperature at the pole would meanwhile remain positive, so that polar glaciation would not be inevitable.

The possibility that stable large-scale glaciation could exist at low latitudes does not invalidate the hypotheses of continental drift and polar motion during these periods. It simply means that any discussion of these hypotheses, which are highly significant for a proper understanding of the past history of the earth, should not assume that centers of large glaciations must necessarily coincide with the poles.

It was shown above that the effect of individual explosive eruptions on the earth's surface corresponds to a temperature drop of the order of several tenths of a degree. It is easy to understand that the earth's temperature would drop to a much greater extent if many eruptions of an explosive type were to coincide within a short time interval.

It is obvious that such coincidences are not only possible but inevitable over long periods of time. The question concerning the effect of the coincidence of many volcanic eruptions on the temperature will be discussed in Chapter IX, where we will point out that in such cases, the mean temperature near the earth's surface may drop by a value no less than 5–10°.

It must be noted that during a stable climatic regime with a relatively small temperature difference between the poles and the Equator, as existed during Mesozoic and Tertiary times, even such a large short-term reduction in temperature could not lead to glaciation because of the high initial temperatures in the polar latitudes.

It should be pointed out in conclusion that the data presented in this chapter confirm the significant role that the change of relief, volcanic activity, and the position of the earth's surface relative to the sun played in climatic conditions of the past. One gains the impression that these factors may help explain many aspects of climatic change over the last hundreds of millions of years. This does not exclude the possibility that other factors may also have affected climate, especially in the earlier stages of the earth's geological history.

REFERENCES

Будыко М. И. (1949). Тепловой баланс Северного полушария. Труды ГГО, вып. 18.

Budyko, M. I. (1949). Heat balance of the Northern Hemisphere. *Tr. Gl. Geofiz. Observ.* **18.**

Будыко М. И. (1961). О термической зональности Земли. Метеорология и гидрология, №. 11.

Budyko, M. I. (1961). On the thermal zonality of the Earth. *Meteorol. Gidrol.* No. 11, 7–14. MGA 13:794.

Будыко М. И. (1962). Полярные лъды и климат. Изв. АН СССР, сер. геогр., № 6.

Budyko, M. I. (1962). Polar ice and climate. *Izv. Akad. Nauk SSSR Ser. Geogr.* No. 6, 3–10. MGA 14.10-297; Res. Mem. RM-5003-PR, pp. 9–23. Rand Corp., Santa Monica, California, 1966. MGA 17.10-321.

Будыко М. И. (1966). Возможность изменения климата при воздействии на полярные льды. Сб. «Современные проблемы климатологии». Гидрометеоиздат, Л.

Budyko, M. I. (1966). The possibility of changing the climate by action on the polar ice. *In* "Sovremennye Problemy Klimatologii" (Contemporary Problems of Climatology)" (M. I. Budyko, ed.), pp. 347–357. Gidrometeoizdat, Leningrad. MGA 18.12-170; Possibility of climate-changing by modification of polar ice. JPRS 43,482. U.S. Joint Publ. Res. Service Washington, 1967. MGA 20.5-182.

Будыко М. И. (1967). Изменения климата. Метеорология и гидрология, № 11.

Budyko, M. I. (1967). Changes of climate. *Meteorol. Gidrol.* No. 11, 18–27. MGA 19.6-436.

Будыко М. И. (1968). О происхождении ледниковых эпох. Метеорология и гидрология, № 11.

Budyko, M. I. (1968). On the origin of glacial epochs. *Meteorol. Gidrol.* No. 11, 3–12. MGA 20.11-383.

Будыко М. И. (1972). Влияние человека на климат. Гидрометеоиздат, Л.

Budyko, M. I. (1972). "Vliianie Cheloveka na Klimat (The Influence of Man on Climate)."
    Gidrometeoizdat, Leningrad.
Будыко М. И., Пивоварова З. И. (1967). Влияние вулканических извержений на
    приходящую к поверхности Земли солнечную радиацию. Метеорология и гидро-
    логия, № 10.
Budyko, M. I., and Pivovarova, Z. I. (1967). The influence of volcanic eruptions on solar
    radiation reaching the surface of the Earth. *Meteorol. Gidrol.* No.10, 3–7. MGA 19.9-361.
Будыко М. И. и Юдин М. И. (1960). О колебаниях уровня непроточных озер. Метео-
    рология и гидрология, № 8.
Budyko, M. I., and Iudin, M. I. (1960). On the fluctuation in level of lakes without outlets.
    Meteorol. Gidrol. No. 8, 15–19. MGA 12C-26.
Давитая Ф. Ф. (1956). О возможном влиянии запыленности атмосферы на уменьшение
    ледников и потепление климата. Изв. АН СССР, сер. геогр., № 2.
Davitaia, F. F. (1965). Possible influence of atmospheric dust on the recession of glaciers
    and the warming of the climate. *Izv. Akad. Nauk SSSR Ser. Geogr.* No. 2, 3–22. MGA
    16.9-292; JPRS 30,216. U.S. Joint Publ. Res. Serv., Washington, D.C., 1965. MGA
    19.5-169.
Дроздов О. А., Покровс. ая Т. В. (1961). Об оценке роли случайных вариаций водного
    баланса в колебании уровня непроточных озер. Метеорология и гидрология, № 8.
Drozdov, O. A., and Pokrovskaia, T. V. (1961). Assessment of the role of random varia-
    tions in the water balance in the fluctuations of the level of lakes without outlets.
    Meteorol. Gidrol. No. 8, 43–48. MGA 13.11-384.
Калесник С. В. (1947). Основы общего землеведения. Учпедгиз. М.—Л.
Kalesnik, S. V. (1947). "Osnovy Obshchego Zemlevedeniia (Foundations of General
    Geography)." Uchpedgiz, Moscow and Leningrad.
Марков К. К. (1960). Палеогеография. Изд. МГУ, М.
Markov, K. K. (1960). "Paleogeografiia (Paleogeography)." Izdat. Mosk. Gos. Univer.,
    Moscow.
Пивоварова З. И. (1968). Многолетнее изменение интенсивности солнечной радиации
    по наблюдениям актинометрических станций. Труды ГГО, вып. 233.
Pivovarova, Z. I. (1968). Long-term changes in the intensity of solar radiation according to
    observations at actinometric stations. *Tr. Gl. Geofiz. Observ.* **233**, 17–29. MGA 20.6-276.
Ронов А. Б. (1959). К послекембрийской геохимической истории атмосферы и
    гидросферы. Геохимия, № 5.
Ronov, A. B. (1959). On the post-Cambrian geochemical history of the atmosphere and
    hydrosphere. *Geokhimiya* No. 5.
Рубинштейн Е. С. (1946). К проблеме изменений климата. Труды НИУ ГУГМС,
    сер. I, вып. 22.
Rubinshtein, E. S. (1946). "K Probleme Izmenenii Klimata: Nalichie i KHarakter
    Izmenenii Klimata. (The Problem of Climatic Change: and the Character of Climatic
    Change)." Gidrometeoizdat, Leningrad, *Gl. Upr. Gidrometeorol. Sluzhby Nauch. Issled.
    Uchrezhdenii* [1], **22**, 1–83 (1946). MGA 15K-59.
Савинов С. И. (1913). Наибольшие величины напряжения солнечной радиации по
    наблюдениям в Павловске с 1892 г. Изв. АН, сер. 6, т. 7, № 12.
Savinov, S. I. (1913). Maximum values of solar radiation intensity from observations at
    Pavlovsk since 1892. *Izv. Akad. Nauk* [6], **7**, No. 12.
Синицын В. М. (1967). Введение в палеоклиматологию. Изд. «Недра».
Sinitsyn, V. M. (1967). "Vvedenie v Paleoklimatologiiu (Introduction to Paleoclimatology)."
    Izdat. Nedra, Leningrad. MGA 19.9-12.
Страхов Н. М. (1937). Историчская геология, т. I, М.

Strakhov, N. M. (1937). "Istoricheskaia Geologiia (Historical Geology)," Vol. 1, Gos. Uchebno-Pedagog. Inst., Moscow.

Шифрин К. С., Минин И. Н. (1957). К теории негоризонтальной видимости. Труды ГГО, вып. 68.

Shifrin, K. S., and Minin, I. N. (1957). On the theory of slant visibility. *Tr. Gl. Geofiz. Observ.* **68**.

Шифрин К. С., Пятовская Н. П. (1959). Таблицы наклонной дальности видимости и яркости дневного неба. Гидрометеоиздат, Л.

Shifrin, K. S., and Piatovskaia, N. P. (1959). "Tablitsy Naklonnoi Dal'nosti Vidimosti i Iarkosti Dnevnogo Neba (Tables of Slant Visibility and Brightness of the Daytime Sky)." Gidrometeoizdat, Leningrad.

Шифрин К. С., Коломийцев В. Ю., Пятовская Н. П. (1964). Определения потока уходящей коротковолновой радиации с помощью искусственного спутника Земли. Труды ГГО, вып. 166.

Shifrin, K. S., Kolomiitsev, V. Iu., and Piatovskaia, N. P. (1964). Determining the flux of outgoing short-wave radiation by means of satellites. *Tr. Gl. Geofiz. Observ.* **166**, 24–54. MGA 17.4-276.

Шулейкин В. В. (1941). Физика моря. Изд. АН СССР, Л.—М.

Shuleikin, V. V. (1941). "Fizika Moria (Physics of the Sea)." Izdat. Akad. Nauk SSSR, Leningrad and Moscow. MGA 13E-289.

Bernard, E. A. (1964). Regularities of physical paleoclimatology and logical value of paleoclimatological data. *In* "Problems in Paleoclimatology." *Proc. NATO Paleoclimates Conf., 1963*, Univ. of Newcastle on Tyne (A. E. M. Nairn, ed.), Wiley (Interscience), London and New York.

Bowen, R. (1966). "Paleotemperature Analysis." Elsevier, Amsterdam, London, New York.

Flohn, H. (1964). Grundfragen der Paläoklimatologie im Lichte einer theoretischen Klimatologie. *Geol. Rundsch.* **54**.

Fuchs, V. S., and Patterson, T. T. (1947). The relation of volcanicity and orogeny to climate change. *Geol. Mag.* **84**, No. 6.

Humphreys, W. J. (1929). "Physics of the Air," 2nd ed. McGraw-Hill, New York.

Kimball, H. H. (1918). Volcanic eruptions and solar radiation intensities. *Mon. Weather Rev.* **46**, No. 8.

Lamb, H. H. (1966). "The Changing Climate." Methuen, London.

Milankovich, M. (1930). "Mathematische Klimalehre und Astronomische Theorie der Klimaschwankungen." (Handbuch der Klimatologie **1**, Teil A), Gebrüder Borntraeger, Berlin. (Русский перевод: М. Миланкович. Математическая климатология и астрономическая теория колебаний климата. ОНТИ, М., 1938.)

Mitchell, J. M. (1961). Recent secular changes of global temperature. Solar variations, climatic change and related geophysical problems. *Ann. N.Y. Acad. Sci.* **95**, 235–250.

Mitchell, J. M. (1963). On the world-wide pattern of secular temperature change. *In* UNESCO, *Arid Zone Res.* **20**.

Mitchell, J. M. (1965). Theoretical paleoclimatology. *In* "The Quaternary of the United States" (H. E. Wright, Jr., and D. J. Frey, eds.). Princeton Univ. Press, Princeton, New Jersey.

Raschke, E., Möller, F., and Bandeen, W. (1968). The radiation balance of the earth-atmosphere system over both polar regions obtained from radiation measurements of the Nimbus II meteorological satellite. *Sver. Meteorol. Hydrol. Inst. Medd. Ser. B*, No. 28.

Öpik, E. T. (1953). On the causes of paleoclimatic variations and of ice ages in particular. *J. Glaciol.* **2**, No. 13.

Sellers, W. D. (1965). "Physical Climatology." Univ. Chicago Press, Chicago, Illinois.
Sellers, W. D. (1969). A global climatic model based on the energy balance of the earth-atmosphere system. *J. Appl. Meteorol.* **8**, No. 3.
Wexler, H. (1953). Radiation balance of the Earth as a factor of climate changes. *In* "Climatic Change: Evidence, Causes and Effects" (H. Shapley, ed.). Harvard Univ. Press, Cambridge, Massachusetts.

VI

Climatic Factors of Geographical Zonality

1. The Effect of Climatic Conditions on Geographical Processes

The relations of the climatic, hydrologic, soil, exogenous geomorphological, and biological processes have been investigated in many studies, among which we must distinguish those of Grigor'ev (1946, 1954, and elsewhere). It was established in these studies that such relations are based on the exchange of energy and several forms of matter (water, carbon dioxide, nitrogen, and so on) between the atmosphere, hydrosphere, lithosphere, and living organisms.

As we pointed out earlier (Budyko, 1956), the general stock of all categories of organic and mineral matter in the geographic envelope as a whole, as well as the energy supply, changes relatively slowly in time and can be considered practically constant over periods of the order of decades.

The relatively slow variability of the quantity of matter in the geographic envelope is associated with a negligible (compared to the available stocks) intensity of the exchange of matter between the geographic envelope, on the one hand, and the deep layers of the lithosphere or space, on the other hand. The energy supply in the geographic envelope, on the contrary, is maintained approximately at the same level in the presence of an intensive exchange of energy with space, in which the income of absorbed solar radiation equals the outgo of heat energy by long-wave emission from the earth.

The approximate stability of levels of different categories of matter and energy in the geographic envelope as a whole is associated with a substantial and relatively rapid variability of these levels in local sectors of the geographic mantle. Such variability is partially of a periodic character (diurnal and annual periods) and partially aperiodic.

The regularities of changes in the stocks of matter and energy in the geographic envelope are determined, to a considerable extent, by the conditions of climatic energetics, that is, by conditions of the income of solar radiation and its subsequent transformations in the processes of heat exchange, changes in phase states of water, and so on.

Let us consider the general picture of the interrelation between climatic factors and different processes forming the geographic environment.

The dependence of the hydrologic regime of the land upon the climate was established by Voeikov (1884).

The fundamental characteristic of the water regime on the continents is the value of run-off, which varies greatly in space and time. The mean annual sum of run-off equals the difference between precipitation and evaporation from the surface of a river basin, this evaporation depending essentially on precipitation, incoming radiation, and thermal conditions.

At the same time, evaporation (and consequently run-off) depends on the form of relief, vegetation cover, and several other factors. However, as Ol'dekop (1911) established for river basins of large area, the effect of climatic factors on evaporation and run-off is predominant.

The opposite dependence—of climate on the hydrologic regime—also exists, but is much weaker. A change in evaporation from the land surface affects the water circulation in the atmosphere and the amounts of precipitation; however, the dependence of precipitation on local evaporation is comparatively small and becomes noticeable only for changes of evaporation over very extensive areas, of the size of continents. Thus, if significant climatic changes modify the hydrologic regime abruptly, the changes in this regime not associated with climate usually have little effect on climatic conditions.

The relationship between climate and the hydrologic regime of the oceans exhibits quite a different character. While the regime of ocean currents depends substantially on wind, radiation, and thermal conditions at the surface of the oceans, the heat transfer by currents in its turn represents an important climate-forming factor. In the regions of warm and cold marine currents, climatic conditions are sharply different. In some cases, these changes extend over great distances.

Climate is greatly affected by the warming and cooling of the upper layers of ocean water during the annual march in extratropical latitudes. The change in heat content of this water called forth by changes in the meteorological regime itself produces a great influence on atmospheric processes.

In this connection, Shuleikin (1941) pointed out that for an explanation of the formation of climate, it is necessary to examine jointly the physical processes in the atmosphere and oceans as a single complex, which determines the conditions of the hydrometeorologic regime on our planet.

We should note that some elements of the oceanic hydrologic regime that depend on climate affect atmospheric processes very little. These include, for example, the salinity of the surface layer of water, which is closely connected with the difference between precipitation and evaporation. However, practically all the physical processes in the ocean depend to an important degree on climate, under the influence of which the hydrometeorologic regime at the ocean surface takes shape.

Because of the great thermal inertia of oceans and the slow movements of the water masses at considerable depth, many oceanic processes are determined not only by climatic conditions of our epoch but also by conditions of past climates. Thus, in particular, the comparatively low temperatures of deep water are possibly a consequence of the general cooling of the earth that took place during the last glacial epoch.

The effect of climatic conditions on the natural vegetation cover of land is well known. Among the meteorological factors that affect the development of plants, the most important are the thermal regime, radiation regime, and conditions of moisture.

It seems probable that many characteristics of wild plants are determined mainly by climatic conditions to which these plants have become adapted during their long evolution. Such a viewpoint is confirmed, for example, by the close correspondence of the boundaries of geobotanic zones to the distribution of climatic indices characterizing the regimes of heat, radiation, and moisture.

Independent of climatic conditions, the influence on vegetation of such nonclimatic factors as, for example, soil is observed only in small areas, where the zonal distribution of these factors breaks down.

The relations of the animal world of the land to climatic factors have a dual character. On the one hand, all animals have their own limits of climatic conditions that are favorable for their existence. On the other hand, animals are in close connection with the natural vegetation cover by means of various relationships, among which the trophic, that is, the energetic connections, are especially important.

The energy of solar radiation absorbed by autotrophic plants during photosynthesis is then consumed by various living organisms as the foundation of their existence. The transfer of this energy from one organism to another, which is mainly carried out in the process of nutrition, is the basis of many ecological regularities that connect the animal world with natural vegetation. Therefore, the determinant effect of climatic factors on geobotanic zonality frequently extends to the zonality of the animal world.

The effect of hydrometeorologic factors on biologic processes in the ocean is in general analogous to the corresponding effect on land. It can be noted that because of the smaller variability of physical conditions in ocean water, many marine organisms are more sensitive to fluctuations in external conditions and can exist only within a narrow range of changes in the conditions of the external medium.

Although the influence of the activity of living organisms on climate is small in general, in some cases it becomes noticeable. Thus, for example, with a dense cover of vegetation, the transpiration of plants turns out to be a substantial portion of the total evaporation from the land surface, which is associated with a considerable expenditure of energy at the earth's surface. However, because of climatic conditioning of geobotanic zonality, vegetation cover even in this case does not become an independent climate-forming factor.

The vegetation cover has much more greatly affected the evolution of the atmosphere, the chemical composition of which is determined to a considerable extent by its long interaction with photosynthesizing vegetation. Biologic processes have in this way played an important role in the evolution of climates of our planet.

Quite apart stands the question of the effect of man's activities on climate. It will be considered in the last chapter of this book.

The geographic zonality of soils, like geobotanic zonality, is closely connected with climatic conditions, as was noted by Dokuchaev (1900). The reasons for the dependence of soil types on climate are explained, on the one hand, by the great influence of vegetation on soil formation and, on the other hand, by the direct dependence of biological, physical, and chemical processes in the soil on its temperature, humidity, and regime of infiltrating water.

In recent studies, a relationship has been established between surface geomorphological processes and geographic zonality dependent on climatic factors. Such a dependence is natural, since the process of denudation (the outgo of mineral matter of the upper layers of the lithosphere as a result of external factors acting on it) is often determined by the regime of run-off, temperature of the earth's surface, wind regime, and other elements of the hydrometeorologic regime.

It must be indicated that exogenous geomorphologic processes have played a certain role in the evolution of climate, because the changes in the relief of the earth resulting from denudation might have led to substantial changes in the circulation of the atmosphere.

Climatic factors thus play a particular role in the closely connected complex of natural processes that form the geographic milieu of our planet. They produce a great, often a determining, influence on all the basic processes developing within the geographic envelope of the earth. Therefore, study of the interactions between climate and different natural processes makes possible a clarification of general regularities determining the fundamental properties of the geographical medium.

The works of Gerasimov (1945, 1960, and others), Volobuev (1953, and elsewhere), Sochava (1948, 1970, and elsewhere), Kalesnik (1947, 1970, and elsewhere), and other authors have contributed much to the investigation of these interrelations. The results of these studies, together with the afore-mentioned papers of Grigor'ev (1946, 1954), show that for study of all the geographic processes, it is necessary to establish their relations with climatic factors.

It was noted above that the leading role of climatic factors in the complex of geographic processes is explained, to a considerable extent, by the fact that solar energy is practically the unique source of energy for all these processes. Absorption of this energy and transformation of it in the atmosphere, at the earth's surface, and in the hydrosphere are extremely important for all the elements of the geographical environment.

We have already indicated that of the total quantity of solar energy received by the earth as a planet, the main part is absorbed at the earth's surface. As a result, the earth's surface is a main source of energy for the geographical envelope.

Since the interaction of most natural processes in the geographic envelope also reaches its greatest intensity near the level of the earth's surface (where run-off is formed, the process of soil formation is developed, the principal mass of living organic matter is concentrated, and so on), then it is evident that consideration of the transformation of solar energy at the earth's surface must have special importance for explaining the mechanism of interactions among many geographic processes.

Taking this into account, let us discuss the relations of components of the heat balance at the earth's surface to different geographic processes.

2. Interrelation Between the Heat and Water Balances of the Land

We will dwell first on the question of the relationship between the hydrologic regime and the energetic factors of climate.

An important characteristic of the hydrologic regime on land is the norm of run-off—the amount of water running off, on the average, during a year from a unit of land surface in the form of different horizontal flows of water.

An important index of hydrologic conditions is the run-off coefficient—the ratio of the run-off norm to the annual sum of precipitation.

Since the formation of annual run-off depends, to a great extent, on the evaporation process, which simultaneously is one of the basic processes of the transformation of solar energy at the earth's surface, it is evident that the run-off norm and the run-off coefficient are connected in a definite way with the basic components of the heat balance. The study of this connection must contribute to the clarification of regularities determining the features of the hydrologic regime of different geographic zones.

The relationship between the components of the heat and water balances of the land has been established on the basis of the following considerations (Budyko, 1948).

It is obvious that the mean sums of evaporation from the land surface E depend on the amount of precipitation and the income of solar energy, evaporation increasing with an increase in precipitation r and the radiation balance [surplus] R.

With great dryness of the soil, all the water received in the form of precipitation is held back by molecular forces on the soil particles and is finally expended in evaporation. Under such conditions (which, for example, are observed in deserts), the run-off coefficient f/r approaches zero.

Taking into account that the mean dryness of the soil increases with an increase in the radiative income of heat and with a decrease in the amount of precipitation, we can deduce that

$$\frac{f}{r} \to 0 \quad \text{or} \quad \frac{E}{r} \to 1 \quad \text{as } \frac{R}{Lr} \to \infty. \tag{6.1}$$

With a decrease in the ratio R/Lr, which we will refer to as the radiative index of dryness, the values of E/r will diminish (a certain amount of run-off appears), and with sufficiently large total precipitation and sufficiently small income of radiative heat, a state of abundant moisture in the upper layer of the soil will be reached. In this case, the probable maximum heat energy from available resources will be converted in evaporation. The value of this maximum outgo can be evaluated by considering the valve character of the turbulent sensible-heat exchange between the underlying surface and the atmosphere.

In Chapter II of this book, it was pointed out that the eddy heat conductivity of the lower layer of air depends substantially on the direction of the vertical turbulent heat flux. In cases when the turbulent flux is directed from the earth to the atmosphere, a comparatively high intensity of turbulent mixing permits the flux to reach large magnitudes in comparison with the [other] principal components of the radiation and heat balances. With the reverse direction of the turbulent flux, the inversion of the temperature distribution reduces the intensity of exchange considerably, and as a result the turbulent sensible-heat flux turns out to be relatively small.

The action of the valve effect on the turbulent exchange of sensible heat is apparent from the graphs of the annual and diurnal march of the sensible-heat flux presented in Chapter III.

In wintertime in middle latitudes, due to the predominance of inversion conditions in the [vertical] distribution of temperature, the sensible-heat flux is small compared to the maximum values of summer, which are determined by conditions of the daytime superadiabatic distribution of temperature in the air layer near the surface. An analogous regularity is noted in the diurnal march, in comparing the values of the sensible-heat flux for night and day.

Because of the valve effect, the annual sums of turbulent sensible-heat flux turn out to be positive, that is, the mean sensible-heat flux is directed from the earth's surface to the atmosphere in almost all the climatic zones of the continents.

Since the annual sums of the turbulent sensible-heat flux cannot provide a significant input of energy to the earth's surface, we must assume that heat outgo for evaporation is compensated only by the radiation balance. For this reason, the upper limit of increase of the value LE is equal to R.

In other words, we may consider that for conditions of abundant moisture,

$$LE \rightarrow R \qquad \text{at } \frac{R}{Lr} \rightarrow 0. \tag{6.2}$$

Conditions (6.1) and (6.2) determine the form of the function Φ:

$$\frac{E}{r} = \Phi\left(\frac{R}{Lr}\right) \qquad \text{at } \frac{R}{Lr} \rightarrow 0 \quad \text{and at } \quad \frac{R}{Lr} \rightarrow \infty. \tag{6.3}$$

It must be indicated that long ago, Schreiber (1904) and Ol'dekop (1911), on the basis of analyzing materials on precipitation and run-off, called attention to the existence of a certain relationship between the components of the water balance. They expressed it in the following formulas:

$$E = r[1 - \exp(-E_0/r)] \tag{6.4}$$

(Schreiber's equation, modified by Ol'dekop, in which E_0 is the greatest possible value of evaporation under the given conditions) and

$$E = E_0 \tanh (r/E_0) \tag{6.5}$$

(Ol'dekop's equation, in which tanh is the hyperbolic tangent).

It is easy to see that both these formulas will satisfy conditions (6.1) and (6.2), if, according to the considerations expressed, we assume $E_0 = R/L$.

It must be borne in mind that the value of possible evaporation from a given terrain will determine a radiation balance corresponding to conditions of sufficient moisture. The value of radiation balance for conditions of sufficient moisture may differ from the balance values for the same terrain with a deficiency in moisture.

Let us examine the dependence of the radiation balance at the earth's surface on moisture conditions. In most geographical regions with a more or less humid climate, the albedo of the earth's surface varies relatively little with changes in moisture conditions. Since, under conditions of sufficient moisture, the mean difference between the temperatures of the earth's surface and the air are small, it turns out that the values of potential evaporation [potential evapotranspiration] can be calculated by the radiation balance determined for the actual state of the earth's surface.

Another kind of situation is observed under conditions of an arid climate, when, together with moistening of the terrain, there is a change in both the albedo and the temperature of the earth's surface, which, with sufficient moisture, approaches air temperature. It is evident that for determining potential evaporation in this case, it is expedient to use the value of radiation balance found at an albedo equal to that of the moistened surface and at a value of net long-wave radiation calculated from air temperature. This comment should be considered when determining potential evaporation under conditions of a dry climate. At the same time, as will be shown in Section 3 of this chapter, in using the equation of relationship, consideration of the effect of moistening on the radiation balance does not noticeably influence the results of the calculation.

In earlier works, various kinds of factual material were used to test these considerations concerning the character of the dependence of ratio E/r on R/Lr for small and large values of the latter parameter.

As an example, we present here a comparison of values of the radiative dryness index R/Lr with values of the ratio E/r, according to data for river basins of different continents (excluding mountain regions).

In Fig. 94, the dependence of E/r on R/Lr for small values of R/Lr, according to condition (6.2), is shown by line OA, and for large values of R/Lr, according to condition (6.1), by line AB. The points in this figure represent mean values of the ratio E/r obtained from water-balance data by averaging the values of E/r over certain intervals of parameter R/Lr. The experimental points show that actually a smooth transition from line OA to line AB is observed, which, as suggested earlier, shows the limiting condition of the dependence of E/r on R/Lr.

In order to present Eq. (6.3) in an analytical form, one can use formulas analogous to Eqs. (6.4) and (6.5):

$$E = r[1 - \exp(-R/Lr)] \qquad (6.6)$$

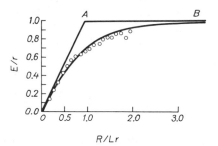

Fig. 94 Dependence of the ratio of evaporation to precipitation upon the radiative index of dryness.

and

$$E = (R/L) \tanh(Lr/R). \qquad (6.7)$$

It is also possible to employ the geometric mean of the right-hand sides of these relations,

$$E = \left[\frac{Rr}{L} \tanh \frac{Lr}{R} \left(1 - \cosh \frac{R}{Lr} + \sinh \frac{R}{Lr} \right) \right]^{1/2} \qquad (6.8)$$

(cosh and sinh are the hyperbolic cosine and sine). This is presented in Fig. 94 by a curve that agrees slightly better with the experimental data than the first two curves. Equation (6.8) establishes the dependence of mean annual evaporation on the radiation balance.

Since the run-off norm equals the difference between the norms of precipitation and evaporation, it is obvious that by means of this formula, one can also determine the run-off from data on precipitation and the radiation balance.

The formulas for run-off and the run-off coefficient following from Eq. (6.8) have the form

$$f = r - \left[\frac{Rr}{L} \tanh \frac{Lr}{R} \left(1 - \cosh \frac{R}{Lr} + \sinh \frac{R}{Lr} \right) \right]^{1/2} \qquad (6.9)$$

and

$$\frac{f}{r} = 1 - \left[\frac{R}{Lr} \tanh \frac{Lr}{R} \left(1 - \cosh \frac{R}{Lr} + \sinh \frac{R}{Lr} \right) \right]^{1/2}. \qquad (6.10)$$

Let us look at the physical meaning of the equation of relationship between the heat and water balances. It is apparent from Fig. 94 that the dependence that lies at the base of this equation is in general determined by two limiting conditions, one of which is based on the idea of the valve mechanism of the turbulent exchange of sensible heat in the surface layer of air, and the other on the obvious fact of the smallness of the run-off coefficient in conditions of an arid climate. The choice of one or another interpolation function for the transition from the first of these conditions to the second is not very important, since, over most of the range of variation in the parameters of the relationship equation, the appropriate relation deviates little from one or the other boundary condition.

Thus, although the equation of relationship is a semiempirical relation, the role of empirical data in its formulation is small in comparison to the general considerations mentioned above. We note that the equation of relationship is a supplementary relation, independent of the equations of the heat and water balances. For this reason, there appears a possibility of joint utilization of the equations in geographic investigations.

Equations (6.9) and (6.10), establishing the relationship between the components of the heat and water balances, have been tested in a number of investigations. Among them, we will mention calculations of the run-off coefficient for European rivers (Budyko, 1951a). For 29 rivers with drainage areas exceeding 10,000 km², the mean error in determining the run-off coefficient amounted to 0.04, this coefficient varying from 0.13 to 0.64. The size of the relative error in calculation of the run-off coefficient for rivers with moderate run-off coefficients (more than 0.30) equaled 7%, which was close to the accuracy of measurements of precipitation and run-off. It follows that in large basins with moderate run-off coefficients, the deviation between "climatic" and actual run-off is insignificant, and in several cases could not be found, considering the accuracy in determining precipitation and run-off.

A more complete test of the equation of relationship between the heat and water balances on land was performed on the basis of data for 1200 regions for which evaporation was determined from the water balance as the difference between precipitation and run-off (Budyko and Zubenok, 1961). It was established that the mean discrepancy between the ratio of evaporation to precipitation calculated from the equation of relationship and that derived by the water balance amounted to 10%.

In this paper, it was pointed out that in certain cases, systematic deviations from the mean dependence presented by the equation of relationship are observed. The character of these deviations depends on features of the annual march of potential evaporation [potential evapotranspiration] and precipitation. With a parallel change in the monthly values of potential evaporation and precipitation, the mean annual values of the ratio of evaporation to precipitation increase slightly. With inverse changes of potential evaporation and precipitation (when the increase of potential evaporation during its annual march coincides with a decline of precipitation), mean values of the ratio of evaporation to precipitation decrease. In most cases, these deviations

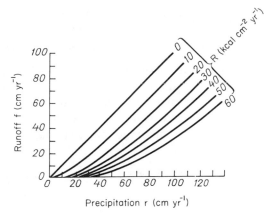

Fig. 95 Dependence of run-off on precipitation and the radiation balance.

are within the range of the accuracy of evaporation calculated by the equation of relationship.

In papers of Bagrov (1953, 1954), Mezentsev (1955), Mezentsev and Karnatsevich (1969), and other authors, different ways are proposed to develop the equation of relationship to take account of the effect of additional factors on the components of the water balance.

The equation of relationship permits us to get a general idea of the form of the dependence of run-off and evaporation on the annual sums of precipitation and radiation balance. The appropriate relations are presented in graphical form in Figs. 95 and 96. These regularities explain a number of empirical relations of run-off to precipitation that were established in earlier studies.

On the basis of the equation of relationship, the dependence of run-off on precipitation for radiation-balance values corresponding to the conditions

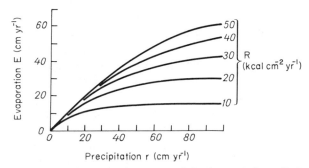

Fig. 96 Dependence of evaporation on precipitation and the radiation balance.

of a given locality can be constructed. This dependence, calculated for the mean conditions of the European plain, is presented in Fig. 97 as curve *A*. For comparison, the following are also presented in this figure:

1. The empirical relationship of Keller (1906), which associates the run-off norm with precipitation according to observational material obtained from rivers of Western Europe (line *B*);
2. The empirical curve of Sokolovskii (1936), which relates run-off with precipitation according to observational material obtained from rivers of Eastern Europe (curve *C*).

The good agreement of the relationship equation with these associations confirms once more its universal character.

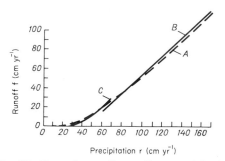

Fig. 97 Dependence of run-off on precipitation.

On the basis of the equation of relationship, one can also explain a considerable dispersion in the relations of run-off to precipitation in data for different regions, which can be found in deriving the mean empirical relations (Poliakov, 1946). A considerable variability of the radiation balance in middle latitudes is the reason for the fact that run-off from basins with a large radiation balance (that is, in more southern regions) turns out much less than from basins with a smaller radiation balance (that is, in more northern regions) with the same precipitation.

The variation in run-off with an increase of precipitation (df/dr) changes in the same way. According to the equation of relationship, it must be greater in northern basins than in southern. This regularity agrees well with the factual data.

Among other possible applications of the equation of relationship to the study of regularities in the run-off regime, we point out the question of change of run-off in mountain regions. It is well known that up to great altitudes in mountains, an increase of run-off with altitude accompanying the increase in precipitation is usually observed.

In Fig. 98 are presented data on the change in run-off and precipitation with altitude for the Aar River, up to an altitude of 2 km (L'vovich, 1945), and data on run-off and precipitation for the five classes of mountain character of the basin of the Tissa River (Poliakov, 1946).

Assuming that for not too great altitudes the value of the radiation balance changes little with altitude (in such conditions, slight increases of incoming radiation and of net long-wave radiation take place, which approximately compensate each other), and taking into account the given data of precipitation, one can calculate the appropriate values of run-off with the use of the relationship equation. The results of this calculation are shown in Fig. 98 as broken lines, which agree closely with the given data on measurements of run-off.

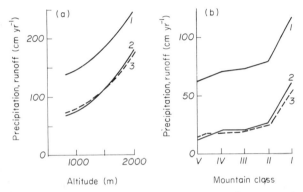

Fig. 98 Change in run-off with altitude. a—Aar River, b—Tissa River; 1—precipitation, 2—measured run-off, 3—calculated run-off.

Thus, it can be concluded that for the mountain basins of the Aar River (up to an altitude of 2 km) and the Tissa River, the observed changes in total run-off and the run-off coefficient are fully explained by the increase of precipitation, that is, by climatic factors. A direct influence of orography on run-off can hardly be seen in these cases.

This conclusion, presumably correct for many mountain basins, has by no means a universal character. It does not extend to high-mountain basins nor to basins with a sharp change in the character of the underlying surface with increase of altitude. The direct influence of orography on run-off can be established, for example, from data for the rivers of the northern Caucasus, presented by Davydov (1947) and elsewhere.

Good agreement of the results of run-off calculated by the equation of relationship of the heat and water balances with factual data confirms the determining influence of climatic factors (and, particularly, energetic factors) on formation of the annual sums of run-off. It must be stressed that this conclusion relates to river basins of considerable size, comparable with the scale of geographical zones. For small areas, river run-off may vary appreciably under the influence of local conditions of a nonclimatic character.

In the next section, we will use the equation of relationship to clarify causal regularities that lie at the base of geographical zonality.

3. The Heat Balance and Geographical Zonality

Climatic indices characterizing geographical zones

One of the main problems of physical geography is explanation of the law of geographical zonality that was found at the beginning of this century by the distinguished soil scientist Dokuchaev (1900, and elsewhere).

Dokuchaev pointed out that within the limits of extensive areas (zones), natural conditions are characterized by many features in common, which change markedly in passing from one zone to another. He established the principal types of geographic zones, which, in the territory of our country, include tundra, forest, forest–steppe, steppe, and desert. Subsequently, in papers by soil scientists, geobotanists, and geographers, the system of geographic zones was worked out in more detail.

In the studies of Dokuchaev, it was established that the boundaries of geographic zones are determined to a considerable extent by climatic factors, and in particular depend on the climatic conditions of moisture. In his papers, he evaluated the relationships between precipitation and potential evaporation for the principal geographic zones. The investigations of Dokuchaev opened a long succession of works aimed at a study of the relations of the distributions of soil and vegetation to the ratio of precipitation to potential evaporation (or its characteristic features).

Among the investigations along this line, we must mention the paper of Vysotskii (1905), in which, for a number of natural zones, the magnitudes of the ratio of annual precipitation to potential evaporation (assumed equal to evaporation from evaporation pans) were calculated. Vysotskii used these values in analyzing the conditions of the formation of soil types and vegetation cover of the different natural zones.

Transeau (1905), in a study of the climatic factors of forest location, constructed a map of the ratio of precipitation to pan evaporation for the eastern part of North America.

A little later, Penck (1910) offered a climatic classification in which climates were divided into three groups: those with precipitation exceeding evaporation; those with precipitation equal to evaporation; and those with precipitation less than evaporation.

In subsequent papers, most of the authors studying climatic moisture conditions on the basis of calculations of the ratio of precipitation to potential
evaporation gave up using data on evaporation from evaporation pans for
determination of potential evaporation.

The reason for this was, on the one hand, an insufficient amount of such
data for many regions, and on the other, the difficulty of physical interpretation of the readings of evaporation pans used in mass meteorological
observations. (Later, as is well known, the utilization of evaporation pans at
meteorological stations for determination of potential evaporation has been
found unsuitable; in particular, in the network of Soviet stations, the Wild
evaporator has been withdrawn from use.)

The great majority of subsequent investigations of the moisture conditions
on land can be divided into three directions, in which the following data
have been used to characterize potential evaporation:

1. the deficit of atmospheric humidity,
2. air temperature,
3. the radiation balance.

Data on the humidity deficit were first used for study of moisture conditions
in the aforementioned paper of Ol'dekop (1911). For determination of evaporation from the surface of river basins, Ol'dekop offered the formula presented in the previous section, which included the ratio r/E_0, representing the
ratio between precipitation and potential evaporation as the characteristic
of climatic moisture conditions. To determine the value of potential evaporation, Ol'dekop used the formula $E = \Omega d$, where d is the humidity deficit,
and Ω is a coefficient of proportionality. According to Ol'dekop, the value
of the coefficient Ω, for the summer half-year, equals 22.7 (if the humidity
deficit is measured in millimeters of mercury and the potential evaporation
in millimeters per month), and for the winter half-year, 16. The annual mean
of the coefficient is consequently 19.3.

Thus, according to Ol'dekop, the annual value of the ratio r/E_0 equals
$r/232d$, where d is the mean annual humidity deficit.

In the paper of Meyer (1926), the ratio of annual precipitation to the mean
annual humidity deficit was used to characterize moisture conditions. This
value, called the NS coefficient, has been rather widely used in the investigation of relationships between the distribution of types of soil and vegetation
and climatic conditions. It is apparent that the NS coefficient is proportional
to the index offered by Ol'dekop and exceeds its value by a factor of 232.

In the paper of Prescott (1931), it was noted that Meyer's index divided by
230 is approximately equal to the value of the ratio of precipitation to evaporation from a water surface.

Later, Ivanov (1941, 1948) offered a formula for the determination of potential evaporation, $E_0 = 0.0018(T + 25)^2(1 - h)$ mm month^{-1}, where T is the mean monthly air temperature, and h is the mean monthly relative humidity of the air. Since the value $(T + 25)^2$, in the range of temperatures at which under natural conditions considerable evaporation occurs, is approximately proportional to the pressure of water vapor at saturation, it is evident that this formula coincides in fact with the formula $E_0 = \Omega d$. In this case, the coefficient Ω turns out equal to 18.4, close to the mean obtained by Ol'dekop. The annual value of the moisture index of Ivanov is consequently equal to $r/221d$.

In these papers, Ivanov made calculations of the ratio of precipitation to potential evaporation for a great number of stations.

Without mentioning numerous other papers, in which the conditions of moisture were characterized by the ratio of precipitation to humidity deficit (or to a value proportional to humidity deficit), we will note one important circumstance.

The only foundation for an assumption that potential evaporation is proportional to the humidity deficit was a notion that the evaporation from a water surface is proportional to the deficit. This notion was widespread in hydrology several decades ago, but in later studies has been considered wrong. Without mentioning current theoretical works on this question, we will note that numerous experimental investigations have established that evaporation from restricted bodies of water is determined by formula $E_0 = \Omega d^n$, where n is a value less than 1. In various hydrologic studies, n has proved to be equal to the following: Poznyshev (1937), 0.5; Mokliak (Ogievskii, 1937), 0.7; Davydov (1944), 0.8; Zaikov (1949), 0.78; and so on. The reason that evaporation from water bodies is actually not proportional to the humidity deficit is explained to some extent in the papers mentioned. We will return to this question later.

The accordance of isolines of the ratio of precipitation to the humidity deficit with the boundaries of vegetation or soil zones has been analyzed in detail for the NS coefficient. In most papers on this question [see Jenny (1941), Volobuev (1953), and others], the following conclusion was drawn: the distribution of the NS coefficient only roughly corresponds with the limits of natural zones; in many cases, this accordance is markedly broken.

Thus, the possibility of using the ratios of precipitation to humidity deficit in order to characterize moisture conditions seems limited, in the light of material from available investigations.

The second group of studies on climatic moisture conditions is based on application of data on air temperature to characterize potential evaporation. Among these studies, we will mention those of Lang (1920) and de Martonne (1926), who suggested the indices r/T and $r/(T + 10)$, respectively, as moisture indices, where T is mean annual temperature. The unsatisfactory character of these indices from the climatological point of view does not require any special proof. It is known that mean annual temperature often depends considerably on thermal conditions of the cold season, which affect the formation of geographic zones comparatively little.

We will give here some examples explaining this circumstance further. It should be considered that rational moisture indices ought to maintain more or less constant values at the borders of specific geographical zones.

According to calculations of Zhegnevskaia (1954), at the border of forest–steppe and steppe, Lang's index varies from 50 to 100 in the European part of the USSR up to infinitely great and then negative values in Siberia. In North America, the magnitude of Lang's index at the same boundary decreases appreciably from north to south, from 100 to 40.

De Martonne's index varies slightly less, but still within a wide range, from 25 to 30 at the border of forest–steppe with steppe in the European part of the USSR up to 40 and more at the same border in Siberia. These variations of Lang's and de Martonne's indices point to insufficient agreement with the real conditions of moisture. We note that similar considerations might be also expressed concerning the method of accounting for moisture conditions in the well-known climatological classification of Köppen (1918). Utilization of mean annual temperature as a characteristic of potential evaporation forms a substantial drawback of this classification.

In comparison with the indices of Lang and de Martonne, greater interest attaches to indices in which temperature characteristics of the growing season are used. Such indices have been worked out in a number of studies, among which might be mentioned those of Selianinov (1930, 1937, and elsewhere).

Selianinov suggested that the sum of temperatures, that is, the product of mean air temperature for a period when it exceeds a specified value (often 10°C) times the duration of this period, be used as a characteristic of potential evaporation. An index proportional to the ratio of precipitation to the sum of temperatures was called the hydrothermal coefficient by Selianinov. The hydrothermal coefficient has been used in many agroclimatic studies, but it has not been tested empirically on the basis of extensive geographic material. We will therefore consider below the question of the relationship between the sum of temperatures and evaporation.

In investigations of the last decades for determining potential evaporation, the formula of Thornthwaite (1948), which associates monthly values of potential evaporation with the mean monthly temperature of the air, has often been used.

In the third group of studies on climatic moisture conditions, data on the balance of radiative energy have been used for evaluating potential evaporation.

The idea of using data on the radiation regime when studying climatic moisture conditions in connection with physico-geographical processes was suggested by Grigor'ev. It was pointed out in his papers (1946, 1954, and elsewhere) that the relationship between radiation balance and precipitation is a determinant of the level of development and intensity of the basic geographical processes.

In the author's work (Budyko, 1948), the following circumstance was noted. The equations of the heat and water balances of land for annual conditions can be written in the following form:

$$\frac{R}{Lr} = \frac{E}{r} + \frac{P}{Lr},$$ (6.11)

$$1 = \frac{E}{r} + \frac{f}{r},$$ (6.12)

(the components of the heat-balance equation are divided by Lr, and those of the water balance by r).

To these ratios we can add the equation of relationship between the heat and water balances, introduced in the previous section:

$$\frac{E}{r} = \Phi\left(\frac{R}{Lr}\right).$$

These three equations connect the four relative values of the components of the heat and water balances. Consequently, for the determination of all these components, it is sufficient to set only one of the equations.

Taking into account the special character of the form of the relationship equation, we can conclude that as a parameter determining all the relative values of the components of the heat and water balances, we can choose the ratio R/Lr or P/Lr. (The ratio E/r or f/r is not a determinant for the first two values under conditions of a dry climate, for which great changes of E/r and f/r correspond to small changes of the ratios R/Lr or P/Lr.)

Since the value of the sensible-heat flux is usually determined less accurately than the radiation balance, it is evident that it is more suitable to take the quantity R/Lr as the principal parameter determining the relative values of components of heat and water balances.

In this case, the given parameter can be considered as the ratio of potential evaporation R/L to precipitation r, or as the ratio of the radiation balance of a moist surface to the heat expenditure for evaporating annual total precipitation.

Thus, when using this parameter, the idea of the moisture index of Dokuchaev–Vysotskii and the idea of Grigor'ev of the importance of the relationship between radiation balance and precipitation to characterize moisture conditions are simultaneously taken into account.

Since the relative values of components of the heat and water balances are determined by only the one parameter R/Lr, the absolute values of these components are then determined by two parameters, for example, R/Lr and R.

This conclusion deserves additional discussion for conditions of a climate with harshly insufficient moisture. In this case, the value of the radiation balance included in the equation of relationship and relating to conditions of a moist surface may differ from the value of the radiation balance for the actual state of the earth's surface.

Observational and calculation data show that this difference increases with growth of the index R/Lr, and becomes substantial at a significant value of this index.

For this reason, under conditions of a climate with markedly insufficient moisture, we can add to the equations presented above a supplementary dependence of the ratio of the radiation balance at the actual state of the earth's surface to its value for a moist surface on the radiative index of dryness. The utilization of this dependence keeps in force the aforementioned conclusion about the parameters determining the components of the heat and water balances, even for conditions of an arid climate. It should be mentioned, however, that in this situation, a consideration of this effect is not very important, because according to the structure of the equation of relationship, the influence of changes in the index R/Lr on values of E/r becomes small in arid conditions.

We can therefore use the values of the radiation balance both for the actual state of the surface and for a moist surface as the characteristic of the radiation balance that determines other components of heat balance.

Methods for determining potential evaporation

To clarify the physical meaning of the radiative index of dryness, we must thoroughly consider the relationships between potential evaporation and the radiation balance at the earth's surface. At the same time, we will be able to draw some conclusions about the relationship between potential evaporation and other characteristics mentioned at the beginning of this chapter.

From a general point of view, it is evident that potential evaporation from the land surface depends on a number of meteorological factors, the most important of which are the surplus of solar energy, humidity, and air temperature. It follows that any method for determining potential evaporation by only one of these elements will inevitably be approximate and will contain more or less error. To evaluate the accuracy of approximate methods, it is necessary to compare them with a method based on consideration of all fundamental factors affecting potential evaporation.

Let us examine the three principal approximate modes of characterizing potential evaporation that have been mentioned above: Humidity deficit, temperature sums, and radiation balance.

To assess the accuracy of these methods, we will compare them to the combination method for calculation of potential evaporation, in which all the principal factors affecting potential evaporation are taken into account, namely, the radiation balance, temperature, and humidity of the air (Budyko, 1951b). We will set forth this method here in a slightly simplified form.

The value of potential evaporation from a land surface, provided that it is sufficiently moist, can be determined by methods similar to those for the determination of evaporation from a water surface. At present, it is established that evaporation from a water or a moist surface is proportional to the deficit of humidity, calculated from the temperature of the evaporating surface (see Chapter II of this book).

We write this dependence in the form

$$E_0 = \rho D(q_s - q), \tag{6.13}$$

where ρ is the air density, D is the integral coefficient of diffusion, q_s is the saturation specific humidity at the temperature of the evaporating surface, and q is the atmospheric specific humidity at the level of measurements in mass observations.

It follows from Eq. (6.13) that to calculate potential evaporation, one needs to know the atmospheric humidity, the integral coefficient of diffusion, and the temperature of the evaporating surface determining the value q_s.

The first two values can usually be found from the results of appropriate observations and calculations. Much more difficult is the determination of the third value—the temperature of the evaporating surface.

It is known that the direct measurement of the temperature of a land surface generally involves considerable difficulty. In this case, the problem is further complicated by the question about the temperature of the surface that is evaporating under conditions of sufficient moisture, that is, under conditions that may differ considerably from the real conditions of terrain in a dry climate.

We note that for determining the temperature of the evaporating surface, it is possible to use the heat-balance equation

$$R = LE + P + A, \tag{6.14}$$

where P is the turbulent flux of sensible heat from the underlying surface to the atmosphere, and A is the heat inflow into the soil.

The value of the radiation balance can be presented in the form $R = R_0 - 4\delta\sigma T^3(T_w - T)$, where δ is the coefficient characterizing the properties of the radiating surface, σ is the Stefan–Boltzmann constant, T is the air temperature, T_w is the temperature of the active surface, and R_0 is the radiation balance for a moist surface calculated when determining net long-wave radiation form the air temperature. (We should indicate that, although in other sections of this book a special designator for this characteristic of the radiation balance is not used, the introduction of such a designator for the formulas comprised in this section turns out to be necessary.)

For the sensible-heat flux, in analogy to Eq. (6.13), we can write the formula $P = \rho c_p D(T_w - T)$, where c_p is the specific heat of the air at constant pressure (see Chapter II of this book).

Taking these expressions into account, we obtain from Eq. (6.14)

$$R_0 - A = L\rho D(q_s - q) + (\rho c_p D + 4\delta\sigma T^3)(T_w - T). \qquad (6.15)$$

From Eq. (6.15), provided we possess data on humidity q and temperature T, and know the values D and $R_0 - A$, we can calculate the values T_w and q_s interrelated by a known physical dependence (the vapor-pressure relation). This calculation will permit us then to calculate potential evaporation E_0 from Eq. (6.13).

A similar method has been offered in the papers of Penman (1948, and elsewhere), who used it for determination of evaporation from a water surface. Penman suggested that potential evaporation from a land surface is proportional to that from a water body under the same external conditions.

Equations (6.13) and (6.15) permit us to investigate the dependence of potential evaporation on the basic meteorological factors (Budyko, 1951b). Not dwelling on this question, we will pass on to an evaluation of the aforementioned simplified methods for determining potential evaporation.

In using the method of the radiation balance for a limited period of time, potential evaporation is determined from the formula $E_0 = (R_0 - A)/L$. Since, for the annual period, A is close to zero, then for these conditions (and also for a number of other cases), we can assume that $E_0 = R_0/L$.

It follows from Eq. (6.15) that the determination of potential evaporation by the radiation balance can yield accurate results when the value $(\rho c_p D + 4\delta\sigma T^3)(T_w - T)$ is much less than the heat expenditure for potential evaporation $L\rho D(q_s - q)$.

Consequently, the absolute error in determination of potential evaporation by the radiation balance ($\Delta E_0'$) equals

$$(1/L)(\rho c_p D + 4\delta\sigma T^3)(T_w - T),$$

and the relative error is determined by the formula

$$\frac{\Delta E_0'}{E_0} = \left(\frac{c_p}{L} + \frac{4\delta\sigma T^3}{L\rho D}\right)\left(\frac{T_w - T}{q_s - q}\right). \qquad (6.16)$$

Equation (6.16) permits the calculation of both the relative errors in determining potential evaporation and the errors in calculating evaporation from a water surface, provided we take its value as equal to $(R_0 - A)/L$. This formula is used below for an evaluation of errors in calculation of potential evaporation. Here, to illustrate it better, we will present data on the error in calculation of potential evaporation by the radiation balance, obtained by comparing the values of potential evaporation calculated by Eqs. (6.13) and (6.15) for the annual period (summing up the monthly values) with the corresponding values of R_0/L.

For this purpose, the values of E_0 and R_0/L have been calculated for 44 points situated in a variety of climatic conditions, from the tundra zone to the equatorial forests and tropical deserts, on all the continents (except the Antarctic).

The results of this comparison, presented in Fig. 99, show that the calculation of potential evaporation by the mean annual values of the radiation balance provides values close to calculations of potential evaporation by Eqs. (6.13) and (6.15). The coefficient of correlation between the values compared equals 0.98.

This conclusion means that the effect of such factors as temperature and humidity of the air on the annual values of potential evaporation turns out to be less important than that of the radiation balance. On the basis of the data from Fig. 99, we can also infer that in most cases, for a sufficiently moist

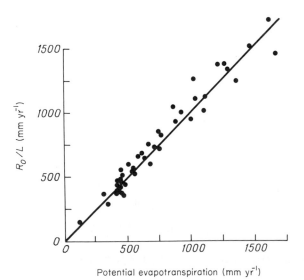

Fig. 99 Comparison of values of potential evaporation determined by the combination method and from the radiation balance.

land surface, the sensible-heat flux P is small in absolute value, compared to the principal components of the heat balance—the radiation balance and the latent-heat flux. (An exception to this rule is observed mainly in comparatively poorly moistened areas under the conditions of a dry climate.)

To clarify the physical meaning of the method for calculating potential evaporation by the humidity deficit, we will consider the relationship between humidity deficit and radiation balance for various climatic conditions.

Figure 100 shows a comparison of the annual means of atmospheric humidity deficit adopted from the paper of Sokolova (1937), with the corre-

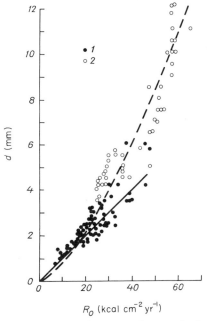

Fig. 100 Comparison of the annual means of atmospheric humidity deficit (*d*) with values of the radiation balance (*R*₀). 1—tundra, forest, forest–steppe, steppe; 2—semidesert, desert.

sponding values of radiation balance R_0. The data on the humidity deficit and radiation balance have been taken from the maps, for 187 points evenly located over the whole area of the USSR except eastern Siberia (where the data are less reliable), mountain regions, and coastal belts.

Data for regions of arid climate (deserts and semideserts) are shown by circles, and the rest of the data, relating to conditions of steppe, forest–steppe, forest, and tundra, by points.

It is apparent from Fig. 100 that for conditions of humid climates, a close relation, near to direct proportionality, exists between the values of the radiation balance and the humidity deficit. The dependence presented in Fig. 99 enables us to think that for the conditions under consideration, the humidity deficit is also connected with potential evaporation by direct proportionality.

Thus, for humid regions, the calculations of potential evaporation by radiation balance and humidity deficit yield close results (provided the coefficient of proportionality Ω in the formula $E_0 = \Omega d$ has been correctly chosen).

Let us now compare the principal errors in calculating potential evaporation by the humidity deficit and by the radiation balance for conditions of a humid climate.

Potential evaporation from a moist surface, equal to $E_0 = \rho D(q_s - q)$ can be presented as the sum of two terms: $E_0 = \rho D(q_s' - q) + \rho D(q_s - q_s')$, where q_s' is the saturation concentration of water vapor at air temperature. Since the value $q_s' - q$ equals the atmospheric humidity deficit, then the last formula can be presented in the following form: $E_0 = E_0'' + \rho D(q_s - q_s')$, where E_0'' is the potential evaporation determined from the deficit of atmospheric humidity, and $\rho D(q_s - q_s') = \Delta E_0''$ is the value characterizing the principal error in calculation of potential evaporation by the atmospheric humidity deficit. This error appears as a consequence of the inequality between temperatures of the air and the active surface.

The relative error in calculation of potential evaporation by the humidity deficit is plainly equal to

$$\frac{\Delta E''}{E_0} = \frac{(q_s - q_s')}{q_s - q}. \tag{6.17}$$

If we compare the relative errors in calculations by the radiation balance and by the humidity deficit, by means of dividing the appropriate values from Eqs. (6.16) and (6.17), we then obtain

$$\frac{\Delta E_0'}{\Delta E_0''} = \left(\frac{c_p}{L} + \frac{4\delta\sigma T^3}{L\rho D}\right)\frac{T_w - T}{q_s - q_s'}. \tag{6.18}$$

It is interesting to note that because of the approximate proportionality of the differences $T_w - T$ and $q_s - q_s'$, within the range of the changes actually possible, the ratio $\Delta E_0'/\Delta E_0''$ for each value of air temperature is approximately constant. Thus, in particular, with the use of Eq. (6.18) we find that for an air temperature of 25°, the value $\Delta E_0'/\Delta E_0''$ is approximately equal to $\frac{1}{2}$. This means that the principal error in calculation of potential evaporation by the radiation balance is less than that in calculation of potential evaporation by the humidity deficit by approximately a factor of 2. This conclusion must be considered in the calculation of potential evaporation, but it does not exclude the possibility of an approximate determination of potential evaporation by the atmospheric humidity deficit under conditions of a comparatively humid climate.

It is much more difficult to use the humidity deficit for calculation of potential evaporation in arid climates, especially under desert conditions.

It is seen from Fig. 100 that for arid conditions, the direct proportionality between the radiation balance and the humidity deficit in the air is broken, and the scatter of points in the graph increases. If we compare Figs. 100 and 99, it is clear that in this case, the direct proportionality between humidity deficit and potential evaporation, found by the combination method, also breaks down.

Can it be considered that a rapid growth of atmospheric humidity deficit accompanying a transition to desert climatic conditions corresponds to a similar rapid growth of potential evaporation? A negative answer to this question is not to be doubted.

If we compare the mean humidity deficits in a desert and in a well-irrigated oasis in the same region, these values, as the observational data show, differ by a factor of several times. At the same time, the values of potential evaporation in both cases are presumably the same, since the actual value of evaporation in the well-irrigated oasis is also the value of potential evaporation, in which we are interested, for the given region of desert. Thus, the humidity deficit in the air under real conditions of the arid climate cannot be considered proportional to the value of potential evaporation.

Actually, most of the meteorological stations in deserts, whose data have become the basis for construction of the map of the humidity deficit that we have used in our work, are under the influence of the proximity of irrigated areas. Therefore, the data of station observations provide values of humidity deficit that are only partially conditioned by the influence of the desert or semidesert climate. Nevertheless, as Fig. 100 and also materials from special observations show, the values of humidity deficit obtained from station observations in deserts turn out appreciably "overestimated" in comparison to those that ought to correspond to conditions of abundant irrigation of a given region.

It is interesting to note that the question of the necessity of accounting for the effect of moistening on the desert climate when determining potential evaporation was long ago considered by Voeikov.

Thus, in particular, in "Климаты земного шара (The Climates of the Earth") (1884), Voeikov examined the interesting example of an error made by the engineers who designed a storage lake of the Suez Canal. According to data of measurements of evaporation by means of small evaporators, they considered that evaporation from the storage lake would be about 7 m per year. The actual evaporation proved to be several times smaller.

This difference can be explained by the fact that for comparatively large evaporating surfaces under desert conditions, water outgo in evaporation from a unit area of surface is much less than that from small surfaces, as a consequence of the effect of evaporation on the climate of the air layer near the surface.

Besides the considerations presented here, there exists a second cause determining a growth of evaporation that is slower than the increase in humidity deficit, with an intensification of climatic dryness. Observational data show that the mean water temperatures of restricted bodies of water in arid regions are usually much lower than the air temperature. This leads to a decrease in the values of humidity deficit calculated from the temperature of the evaporating surface, compared to the humidity deficit of the air. As a result, there is a relative decline of evaporation, which is noticeable for different evaporating surfaces.

Let us turn now to the question of utilization of temperature sums in calculation of potential evaporation. It is well known that, although the temperature sum is a familiar agrometeorological index, widely used in agricultural climatology, the question of its physical interpretation remains obscure. In this connection, it is of interest to compare temperature sums with the energetic characteristic of potential evaporation, the radiation balance. The results of such a comparison are presented in Fig. 101.

Values of R are plotted along one axis of this graph, and along the other

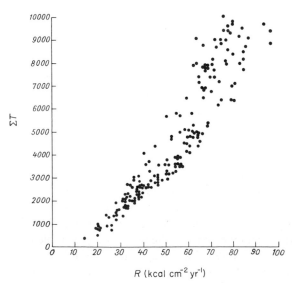

Fig. 101 Comparison of temperature sums (10°C base) with values of the radiation balance.

are plotted the sums of temperatures above 10°C ($\sum T$) taken from the
"Мировой агроклиматический справочник (World Agroclimatic
Handbook") (1937) for 300 stations located in different climatic conditions
and in all the continents (except the Antarctic) from 71° N latitude to 46° S.
All the data contained in the reference book (except the materials for coastal,
island, and mountain stations) have been used.

It is seen from Fig. 101 that there is a close relationship between temperature sums and the radiation balance, which, on the average, is maintained
in all latitudes and on all continents. A distinct dependence of temperature
sums upon radiative energy factors clarifies to some extent the physical
meaning of this characteristic, which sometimes has been considered a
rather conventional index. At the same time, the relationship established
between temperature sums and radiation balance points to the possibility
of using temperature sums for an indirect evaluation of potential evaporation
under various climatic conditions.

It must be indicated, however, that with the scattering of points in Fig. 101,
the relationship between temperature sums and radiation balance cannot be
considered single-valued. Analysis of the original material shows that in
individual regions, a certain discrepancy between radiation regime and
temperature sums is observed.

Thus, for example, in some monsoon regions, the temperature sums turn
out to be reduced in comparison with the values of radiation balance. A still
greater discrepancy between these values is observed in mountain regions,
where the temperature sums usually decrease with altitude appreciably more
rapidly than the radiation balance does.

In such cases, the conditions for an increase in the mean differences between
temperatures of the air and the earth's surface appear, which may lead to
definite errors in evaluating the thermal factors of geographic processes by
the summed air temperatures.

The advantage of temperature sums as a characteristic of potential evaporation consists in the fact that they vary comparatively little with a change
in climatic dryness; less, in particular, than the atmospheric humidity deficit.
This circumstance permits using temperature sums also for the determination
of potential evaporation under conditions of arid climates, deserts included.

Of interest are comparisons of different methods for determining potential
evaporation with data of measurements of evaporation from the earth's
surface under conditions of sufficient moisture.

Among the studies of this kind, that by McIlroy and Angus (1964) (carried
out in Australia), the results of which have been considered in Seller's book
"Physical Climatology" (1965), are worthy of attention.

The authors of this study measured evaporation from irrigated grass
during the yearly march. The data of their measurements were compared

with the results of calculations of potential evaporation made by several methods, their data being in close agreement with the values derived by means of the combination method. Methods for determining potential evaporation based on consideration of individual meteorological elements yielded much poorer results.

Summing up our examination of the question about methods for calculating potential evaporation, we can point out the following.

The best-founded method for determination of potential evaporation is the above-stated combination method, taking into account the effect of radiation balance, temperature, and humidity on potential evaporation.

When determining annual values of potential evaporation, one can use the method of calculation by radiation balance, which, for diverse climatic conditions yields results close to those of calculation carried out by the combination method.

Among empirical methods, the calculation of annual values of potential evaporation by summed temperatures deserves attention. For this purpose, it is possible to employ the mean relation between temperature sums and the radiation balance according to data in Fig. 101.

Calculations of potential evaporation from the atmospheric humidity deficit may yield satisfactory results mainly for a comparatively humid climate. For conditions of an arid climate (especially deserts), this calculation method is less suitable and may lead to noticeable errors.

Let us pause now on the question of the period for which one must take data on the radiation balance for the determination of potential evaporation.

It should be noted that under different climatic conditions in the middle latitudes, radiation-balance values for the year and for the growing season turn out to be close in magnitude (Budyko, 1949). This fact, which at first sight seems paradoxical, is explained in the following way. During the cold season in middle latitudes, the radiation balance is negative, its absolute values being relatively small. In spring, the radiation balance becomes positive, and toward the beginning of the growing period (which is usually characterized by the rise of air temperature to $10°$), it reaches comparatively large positive values in most situations. This leads to the fact that the negative and positive values of the radiation balance for the period of the "nongrowing" season compensate each other to a considerable extent.

Available data on the radiation balance permit us to carry out a comparison of values for the year and for the growing season. The results of this comparison are presented in Fig. 102, where the radiation balance R for the year is plotted along one axis [the abscissa] and the balance R' for the period with temperature exceeding $10°$ along the other axis [the ordinate]. The data from the graph relate to stations situated in the zone from 40 to $70°$ N latitude.

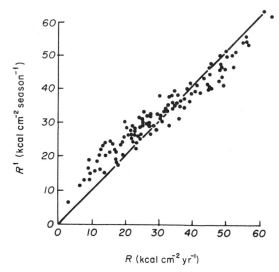

Fig. 102   Comparison of radiation-balance totals for the year and for the growing period.

It is apparent from the graph that for comparatively large values of radiation balance, that is, in lower latitudes, the values of R and R' are always close to each other. For the higher latitudes, where the balance values are smaller, a difference appears between R and R', the latter value being noticeably larger than the former. It can be noted that the greatest discrepancy between these values is seen mainly in conditions of an extremely continental climate (central portions of Eurasia).

In these regions, a rapid rise of temperature in spring leads to the fact that the compensation between the negative and positive values of the radiation balance in the "nongrowing" season turns out to be incomplete. As a result, the radiation balance in the growing season becomes greater than the balance over the year.

This conclusion, however, does not imply the necessity of using radiation-balance values for the growing season for calculation of the annual values of potential evaporation in conditions of an extreme continental climate. It is easy to understand that the values of the radiation balance for the year period in middle latitudes under conditions of sufficient moisture cannot be totally converted into evaporation. In the presence of a pronounced annual march of temperature, a certain part of the heat of the radiation balance in the warm season is spent for heating (and thawing) the soil; this heat returns in the cold season, when the soil is being cooled (and frozen).

In using the available calculation data on heat exchange in the soil, we can infer that under conditions of the continental climate in middle latitudes, the amount of heat that is likely to be converted in evaporation in the warm season is noticeably less than the value of the radiation balance over the growing season, and closer to the annual value of the balance.

These conclusions confirm the fact that to determine potential evaporation for the year under various climatic conditions, it is suitable to use the radiation-balance values that also relate to the annual period.

The relationship between geographic zonality and climatic conditions

For study of the influence of climatic factors on geographic zonality, there has been constructed a world map of the radiative index of dryness (Budyko, 1955), presented in Fig. 103.

In the construction of this map, we used the world map of radiation balance, related to conditions of a moist surface. It follows from this map that the location of isolines of values of the radiation balance at a moist surface has, in general, a latitudinal character. In desert regions, this value is usually slightly larger in comparison to surrounding areas of a more humid climate, although this difference is relatively small.

To construct the maps of the dryness index, we carried out calculations of the index R/Lr for 1600 points, evenly located over the surface of the continents.

On the map of the radiational index of dryness, isolines of values equal to $\frac{1}{3}$, $\frac{2}{3}$, 1, 2, and 3 are seen. The isolines are drawn for the entire surface of the continents, with the exception of mountain regions, which are hatched.

It is seen from this map that the distribution of isolines of the radiative dryness index on the continents is characterized by a great variation of index values on each continent. The most humid conditions, corresponding to the smallest values of the dryness index, are observed mainly in high latitudes, where potential evaporation is very small. The greatest values of the dryness index relate to the conditions of deserts and semideserts.

In comparing the map of the radiative index of dryness (Fig. 103) with the available geobotanic and soil maps, it is easy to see that the location of isolines of the dryness index agrees well with the location of the principal physical–geographic zones. The smallest values of the dryness index (up to $\frac{1}{3}$) correspond to tundra, index values ranging from $\frac{1}{3}$ to 1 to the forest zone, from 1 to 2 to steppe, more than 2 to semidesert, and more than 3 to the desert zone.

Omitting a number of specific conclusions that can be seen from a comparison of the map of the dryness index with the geobotanic and soil maps, we will stress only the point that the radiative index of dryness, characterizing the relative values of components of the heat and water balances, agrees

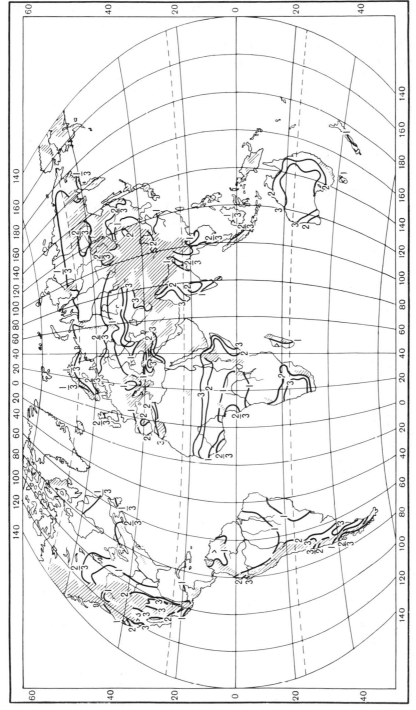

Fig. 103 Radiative index of dryness.

347

well with the locations of the boundaries of the principal natural zones. It is evident that in different latitudes lying within the limits of the same zone, substantially different levels of development of natural processes are observed. These differences are associated with the fact that the energetic basis of natural processes, which can be described by the value of radiation balance R, is different in different latitudes.

Thus, in order to characterize the general zonal conditions of natural processes, it is sufficient to use the one parameter R/Lr (defining the relative values of the components of the heat and water balances). However, in order to characterize the absolute values of the intensity of natural processes, it is necessary to use the two parameters R/Lr and R, which determine the absolute values of the components of the heat and water balances.

The relationship between geobotanic conditions and the parameters R/Lr and R can be shown as a graph, along the axes of which are located the values of R and R/Lr, and on which the principal geobotanic zones are separated by straight lines (Budyko, 1950). A schematic form of such a graph is presented in Fig. 104.

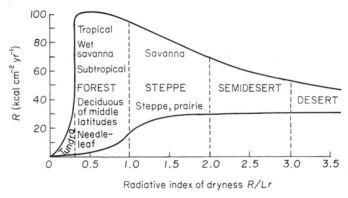

Fig. 104   Diagram of geobotanic zonality.

We note that in constructing this graph, values of the radiation balance for the actual state of the earth's surface, which differ from those for a moist surface, were plotted along the ordinate. The continuous line in the graph bounds the domain of actually existing values of R and R/Lr (except in mountain regions). Within its limits, definite values of the parameter R/Lr shown by the vertical lines distinguish the principal geobotanic zones: tundra, forest, steppe, semidesert, and desert. The great differences in the values of the radiation balance in the forest zone and the slightly lesser differences in the steppe zone correspond to marked geobotanic changes within the area of each zone, the general character of the vegetation cover remaining unchanged.

Since soil zonality is closely connected with the zonality of vegetation cover, the conclusions obtained concerning the relationship between the vegetation zones and definite values of the parameters R and R/Lr can also be carried over completely to the soil zones.

In this respect, it can be established that with an increase of the parameter R/Lr, soil types change in the following sequence: (a) tundra soils; (b) podzols, brown forest soils, yellow earths, red earths [krasnozems], and lateritic soils (the variety of soil types in this group corresponds to the changes in parameter R within its broad limits); (c) black earths [chernozems] and black savanna soils; (d) chestnut soils; (e) grey earths [sierozems]. The relationship between soil zonality and the climatic indices R/Lr and R can be in general depicted in a graph similar to that of the vegetation zones presented in Fig. 104.

The relationship between the hydrologic regime and the parameters R and R/Lr can be established not only in a qualitative but also in a quantitative form.

It follows from the relationship equation that to each level of values of the parameter R/Lr there corresponds a definite level of values of the run-off coefficient. Consequently, for tundra conditions, where $R/Lr < \frac{1}{3}$, the run-off coefficient must be greater than 0.7; in the forest zone at $\frac{1}{3} < R/Lr < 1$, the run-off coefficient must possess a value from 0.3 to 0.7; in the steppe zone (where $1 < R/Lr < 2$), from 0.1 to 0.3; in the semidesert and desert zones, less than 0.1. Factual data confirm this regularity well.

Thus, consideration of the effect of energy factors permits explanation in quantitative form of zonal changes in the run-off coefficient.

The absolute values of run-off are determined by two parameters, R and R/Lr. Therefore, in a graph similar to Fig. 104, we can show the distribution of annual run-off values (Fig. 105). This graph defines the absolute values of run-off in different geographic zones.

It must be indicated that the data on precipitation totals in the calculations presented here do not include the corrections that have been proposed in

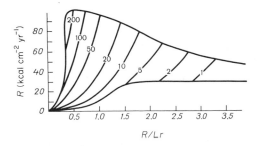

Fig. 105 Run-off (cm yr^{-1}) in different geographical zones.

recent years for improving the accuracy of norms of precipitation determined by means of available instruments. Taking these corrections into account leads to an increase in precipitation totals, especially marked in regions with a large amount of solid precipitation.

Investigations show that, although utilization of the improved precipitation norms changes the typical values of the moisture indices slightly, it does not as a rule change the general regularities connecting the moisture indices with the geographic zonality. In a number of cases, correction of the precipitation sums permits better agreement between the moisture indices and the boundaries of the geographic zones.

4. The Table of Geographic Zonality

The law of geographic zonality

The material set forth in the preceding section makes possible a better conception of the physical meaning of the law of geographical zonality discovered by Dokuchaev. It follows from this material that a close relationship exists between the geographic zones and the two climatic parameters— the radiation balance at the earth's surface and the radiative index of dryness.

This relationship was studied in the papers of Grigor'ev and Budyko (1956, 1962), in which it was referred to as the periodic law of geographic zonality. We note that an idea of the periodicity of changes in some properties of natural zones had been suggested even earlier, in a study of the distribution of soil cover (Zakharov, 1931; Vilenskii, 1945). In all these papers, the concept of periodicity had a definite meaning, which we take up below.

In accordance with the concept set forth in the previous section, Grigor'ev and the author pointed out that within each latitudinal belt, there exists a definite correspondence of the boundaries of natural zones to the isolines of one or another value of the radiative index of dryness. In different latitudinal belts, the same values of the radiative index of dryness correspond to natural zones that are similar in terms of several substantive indicators. Thus, with transition from one latitudinal belt to another (which leads to changes in the values of the radiation balance), the indicators of similarity are repeated in a set of natural zones corresponding to changes in moisture conditions, together with differences caused by changes in conditions of thermal energy.

The general scheme of this regularity is given in Table 31, which represents a further development of the model shown in Fig. 104. It should be noted that in constructing the table of geographic zonality, radiation-balance values relating to moist conditions of the underlying surface were used. This is one of the reasons for differences in the data between the table under consideration and Fig. 104. Other differences are associated with the utilization of more detailed data on precipitation and vegetation cover in different regions in construction of the table of geographic zonality.

The table under consideration permits forming the following conclusions about the regularities of geographic zonality relating to plains areas. Each column in the table defines a gradation of moisture conditions and corresponds to definite values of the run-off coefficient. In each column, the annual norm of run-off increases with the increase in the radiation balance, that is, with decreasing latitude. (This does not extend to conditions of deserts, where run-off in low latitudes is close to zero.)

Each column of the table corresponds to a similar type of vegetation cover. Under conditions of surplus moisture (column 3), forest vegetation prevails in all latitudes, except in conditions of extreme moisture surplus (dryness index less than $\frac{2}{5}$). In this case, forest vegetation is replaced by tundra in the high latitudes and by marsh in the low. (Since a dryness index less than $\frac{2}{5}$ over more or less extensive areas is observed only in comparatively high latitudes, the swamped areas in low latitudes cannot be considered independent geographical zones.)

Not only the type but also the productivity of the vegetation cover are characteristic of each gradation of moisture. In the aforementioned paper of Grigor'ev and the author, it was suggested that the productivity of natural vegetation cover increases the more closely the moisture conditions approach the optimum (at the same radiation balance); and under fixed conditions of moisture, productivity increases with an increase in the radiation balance.

The problem of productivity of the vegetation cover in different geographic zones is discussed in detail in Chapter VIII.

Each column of the table corresponds to a definite sequence of change in soil types, which, within the limits of the same column, possess substantially similar indications. Thus, in particular, the third column contains the following sequence of soil types: tundra, podzolic and brown forest soils, subtropical red earths and yellow earths, tropical podzol-like red earths, and laterites; the fourth column contains black earths and dark chestnut-colored soils, black soils and poorly leached brown soils of the subtropics, red-brown tropical soils, and so on.

Certain quantitative characteristics of the soil-formation process are characteristic of each sequence mentioned.

A special place in the table belongs to the area of eternal snow, which possesses no analogies and is characterized by a negative value of the radiation balance, a negative index of dryness, and practical absence of vegetation and soil cover, and also the subzone of the Arctic deserts, with a negligible value of the annual radiation balance and excessive moisture.

The regularities of geographic zonality presented in the table can be explained by the following simple considerations.

Because of the spherical shape of the earth, its surface is divided into several latitudinal zones, which differ in the values of inflow of radiant energy to the earth's surface. Within the limits of each of these zones (except the zone of eternal snow), different moisture conditions ranging from surplus to extreme insufficiency can be observed. It is easy to understand that the nature of zones with similar conditions of moisture in different latitudes possesses features of a definite similarity (which are joined with the differences caused by the difference in the inflow of radiation energy). If we successively compare regions in two latitudinal belts with increasing moisture (or with increasing dryness), the features of similarity repeat themselves periodically. Thus, a periodic change in the characteristics of geographic processes is

TABLE
Geographical

Thermal energetic basis—the radiation balance	Less than 0 (extremely large surplus of water)	Moisture conditions—		
				From 0
				Surplus
		$0-\frac{1}{5}$	$\frac{1}{5}-\frac{2}{5}$	$\frac{2}{5}-\frac{3}{5}$
1	2			3
Less than 0 (high latitudes)	I Eternal snow	—	—	—
From 0 to 50 kcal cm^{-2} yr^{-1} (Southern Arctic, Subarctic, and middle latitudes)	—	II, a Arctic desert	II, b Tundra (with small islands of sparse forest in the south)	II, c Northern and middle taiga
From 50 to 75 kcal cm^{-2} yr^{-1} (subtropical latitudes)	—	—	VI, a Regions of subtropical forest with a great amount of marshland	Pluvial
More than 75 kcal cm^{-2} yr^{-1} (tropical latitudes)	—	—	X, a Regions of predominance of equatorial forest swamps	X, b Strongly super humid (heavily swamped equatorial forest)

revealed in successively passing round the globe by different parallels of latitude, when, during the circuit on a given parallel, the direction of the monotonically changing index of moisture is followed. It is easy to understand that such a periodicity cannot be compared to that of the properties of the chemical elements, with which it has nothing in common.

Seasonal change in the climatic factors of geographic zonality

The table of geographic zonality establishes a relationship between natural zones and the mean annual values of the elements of the climatic regime. It must be borne in mind that as a rule, these values are the result of averaging variable values of the elements of climate, characteristic of individual seasons of the year.

31
ZONALITY

the radiative index of dryness

to 1 moisture $\frac{3}{5}-\frac{4}{5}$	Optimal moisture $\frac{4}{5}$–1	From 1 to 2 (moderately insufficient moisture)		From 2 to 3 (insufficient moisture)	More than 3 (extremely insufficient moisture)
		4		5	6
—	—	—		—	—
II, d Southern taiga and mixed forest	II, e Deciduous forest and forest–steppe	III Steppe		IV Semidesert of middle latitudes	V Desert of middle latitudes
VI, b subtropical forest		VII, a Sclerophyll subtropical forest and shrub	VII, b Subtropical steppe	VIII Subtropical semidesert	IX Subtropical desert
X, c Moderately super-humid (swamped) equatorial forest	X, d Equatorial forest, becoming forest savanna	XI Dry savanna		XII Desert-like savanna (tropical semi-desert)	XIII Tropical desert

Taking into account the special features of the climatic regime in different seasons, we can more distinctly realize the effect of climatic factors on geographic zonality (Grigor'ev and Budyko, 1962).

To characterize the climatic conditions of the seasons, we will single out the following basic types of climatic regime.

1. The Arctic climatic regime, characterized by the presence of snow cover, negative air temperatures, and a negative or near-zero radiation balance.
2. The tundra climatic regime, with mean monthly temperatures from zero to 10° and a small positive radiation balance.
3. The climatic regime of the forest zones, with mean monthly temperatures exceeding 10°, a positive radiation balance, and sufficient moisture, when evaporation amounts to not less than half of the value of potential evaporation.
4. The climatic regime of the dry zones (steppe and dry savanna), where with a positive radiation balance evaporation ranges from one tenth to one half of the value of potential evaporation.
5. The climatic regime of deserts, where with a positive radiation balance evaporation is less than one tenth of potential evaporation.

If any of the above-listed types of climatic regime were observed throughout the whole year, then the climatic conditions relating to each month would correspond with the natural zonality. But in most geographic regions, a change among several types of climatic regime is observed throughout the year. Thus, for example, in the steppe zone of the European part of the USSR, four types of climatic regime are observed during the year: in the winter period, the Arctic regime; at the beginning of spring, the tundra regime, which gives way to the forest-zone regime, after which, in summertime, conditions of the climatic regime typical of the steppe zone are observed. In this case, only the last of the seasonal types of climatic regime corresponds to the type of geographic zone.

General characteristic changes in climatic conditions during the annual march at different latitudes of the Northern Hemisphere are presented in Fig. 106. Fig. 106a characterizes plains regions in the zone of 20–40° E, situated in Europe and Africa. Figure 106b shows the changes in climatic conditions for the eastern periphery of Asia, Fig. 106c for the eastern areas of North America and for South America.

The models shown in these figures reveal substantial differences in the seasonal changes of climatic regime in different longitudes. These differences are especially noticeable in middle and low latitudes, where the type of regime depends on moisture conditions.

In Europe and Africa, a regime with reduced moisture is observed in a wide latitudinal zone, which shifts north during the summer and south in winter. This shift corresponds with the most favorable conditions of moisture in the subtropics in winter and spring, and in the tropical latitudes in summer.

In eastern Asia and in North America, the structure of the moisture regime differs sharply from the first diagram. This corresponds to substantial differences in circulation processes.

It is apparent from Fig. 106 that in most regions in all longitudes, conditions of either insufficient moisture (regimes 4, 5) or insufficient heat (regimes 1, 2) are observed during a significant part of the year. Only in a

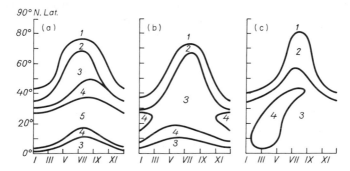

Fig. 106   Seasonal changes in the climatic factors of geographic zonality. 1–5—climatic regimes. (See p. 354.)

narrow belt near the Equator are conditions corresponding to regime 3 observed all through the year.

It is evident that with regimes 2 and 4, and especially with regimes 1 and 5, the productivity of natural vegetation is reduced, which causes a corresponding reduction in the intensity of other biogeographical processes (zoogeographic and soil). In this case, the following regularity is observed. Under conditions of insufficient heat, the type of geographical zone is determined by the climatic regime of that period when the productivity of natural vegetation is the greatest, even if this period is relatively short. Thus, for example, the zonal landscape of tundra is determined by conditions of the warm season, which may not exceed one fifth to one fourth of the duration of the year. In this situation, the climatic regime of the cold season, embracing the greater part of the year, does not determine the zonal character of the landscape.

A similar regularity is usually noted also under conditions of insufficient moisture, when the more humid period turns out to be determinant for the type of zone, though it might be shorter than the period with insufficient moisture.

It should be noted, however, that under conditions of natural zones with insufficient moisture, short periods with sufficient or surplus moisture may be observed, which do not ensure the development of typical forest vegetation requiring a more or less long moistening of the soil.

The indicated regularities that associate the type of geographic zone with seasonal change in climatic factors of zonality contribute to the concept stated above of the influence of climatic factors on geographic zonality.

A formulation of the periodic law of geographic zonality set forth in 1956 is used generally in contemporary studies. In a number of papers, the possibility of using this law for a clarification of regularities of the distribution of vegetation cover is discussed (Armand, 1967; Bazilevich et al., 1970; and others). Recently, the possibility of using the law for study of the zonality of geomorphologic processes has been clarified (Budyko et al., 1970).

Climatic classification

Among various supplements to the table of geographical zonality given above, we will discuss in more detail the classification of the climates of the Soviet Union worked out on the basis of it (Grigor'ev and Budyko, 1959). In working out this classification, data on the sums of temperatures at the level of the earth's surface, which are closely connected with values of the radiation balance, were employed to characterize thermal conditions. In calculation of the dryness index, potential evaporation was determined by the combination method (refer to Section 2 of this chapter).

A comparison has shown that the boundaries of geobotanic zones agree well with the distribution of climatic characteristics used in this classification. The area where the mean daily air temperature remains lower than 10°C proved to correspond to the zone of Arctic deserts. The isoline of the sum of temperatures at the earth's surface equal to 1000° is close to the southern border of the tundra zone (forest–tundra included). The same natural border proved to be close to the isoline of the dryness index equal to 0.45. The area with dryness index slightly lower than 0.45 but with greater values of temperature sums accords with the location of the high-mountain zone of alpine meadows. Isolines of the dryness index equal to 1 closely coincide with the border between the forest and steppe zones. And within the limits of the forest zone, the area with temperature sums less than 2200° coincides with needleleaf forest (taiga); from 2200 to 4400°, the mixed and broadleaf forest of middle latitudes; more than 4400°, forest with elements of subtropical vegetation.

Values of the dryness index ranging from 1 to 3 agree with the location of the vegetation zones of insufficient moisture, mainly steppe and forest–steppe. Under such conditions, with summed temperature less than 2200°, conditions of mountain steppe and forest–steppe (and also Siberian steppe and forest–steppe, being to a considerable extent of a mountain character) are observed. At temperature sums exceeding 4400°, the steppe of middle latitudes changes into a steppe with elements of subtropical vegetation or with xerophytic woody vegetation having some subtropical features.

Dryness index values exceeding 3 correspond to conditions of the desert zone, where, at comparatively low temperature sums (less than 2200°), mountain deserts are observed. In the zone of lowland deserts in the north at lower temperature sums (approximately up to 4400°), conditions of Artemisia and saltbush deserts prevail; at greater sums, conditions of saxaul, shrub, and ephemeral deserts prevail.

In accordance with the regularities indicated here, the gradations of the basic climatic indices given in Tables 32 and 33 have been used for designing a system of climatic regionalization.

TABLE 32
MOISTURE CONDITIONS

Moisture conditions	Index of dryness $\left(\dfrac{\text{potential evaporation}}{\text{precipitation}}\right)$	Geographical conditions
I Too moist	Less than 0.45	Arctic desert, tundra, forest–tundra, alpine meadows
II Moist	0.45–1.00	Forest
III Insufficiently moist	1.00–3.00	Forest–steppe, steppe, xerophytic subtropical vegetation
IV Dry	More than 3.0	Desert

Along with the basic climatic indices given, which define the conditions of geographical zonality, characteristics of the climatic conditions of winter have been used in addition for constructing a detailed map of climatic regions.

Although the differences in meteorological regime of the cold season in our latitudes affect geographical processes much less than do the differences in climatic conditions of the warm season, the severity of winter and the character of winter precipitation are important for the regime of rivers, soil formation, vegetation, and so on. In this regard, six principal types of meteorological regime in wintertime, presented in Table 34, have been distinguished in the area of the Soviet Union.

It must be noted that certain relationships exist between the meteorological conditions of winter and the natural vegetation cover. The area of severe

TABLE 33
THERMAL CONDITIONS OF THE WARM PERIOD

Thermal conditions	Sum of temperature at the surface of the earth for the period with the air temperature exceeding 10°C	Geographical conditions
1. Very cold	Air temperature does not exceed 10°C throughout the year	Arctic desert
2. Cold	0–1000°	Tundra and forest–tundra
3. Moderately warm	1000–2200°	Needleleaf forest, alpine meadows, mountain steppe, and Siberian steppe
4. Warm	2200–4400°	Mixed and broadleaf forest, forest–steppe, steppe, northern desert
5. Very warm	More than 4400°	Subtropical vegetation, desert

climate in the forest zone corresponds to a considerable degree to the territory of the Dahurian larch—one of the trees most capable of enduring low temperatures.

The border between the zones of moderately severe and moderately mild winters in the forest zone of the European USSR corresponds approximately to that between the east European and west European taiga. Farther south, in the steppe zone, this border coincides with a change in type of vegetation from the Black-Sea steppe to the Kazakhstan steppe.

In using the criteria of climatic classification and the numerical and letter designations corresponding to the criteria mentioned, we can characterize

TABLE 34
WINTER CONDITIONS

Characteristics of the winter	January temperature (°C)	Greatest mean decadal depth of snow cover (cm)
A. Severe winter with little snow	< −32	< 50
B. Severe snowy winter	< −32	> 50
C. Moderately severe winter with little snow	−13 to −32	< 50
D. Moderately severe snowy winter	−13 to −32	> 50
E. Moderately mild winter	0 to −13	—
F. Mild winter	> 0	—

the climatic conditions of each area by a three-symbol combination, for example, II, 4, D (climatic conditions humid, with a warm summer, and a moderately severe, snowy winter).

A general scheme of classification of the climates of the USSR is presented in Table 35, analogous to a certain part of the table of geographical zonality. It should be noted that the quantitative definitions of climatic conditions in these tables are slightly different. Such differences are associated first with the fact that the climatic indices used in Tables 31–33 do not coincide, though they are analogous. Besides, it should be borne in mind that in designing a climatic classification for the USSR, precipitation values in regions with a great quantity of solid precipitation have been determined by an indirect method. This permitted us to avoid the large errors in precipitation sums that are found in observational data.

Other differences are of a terminological character (for example, the term "too moist" in Table 32 possesses a narrower meaning than in Table 31), or are a consequence of more detailed analysis of schemes of climatic classification for the area of the USSR.

All these differences, however, are of a specific character and do not disrupt the connection in principle of the model for classification of climate with the table of geographical zonality.

It is seen from Table 35 that in the territory of the USSR, twelve types of basic climatic regions, corresponding to the different geographical zones, are delineated. The basic climatic regions are divided into 32 types of interzonal climatic regions on the basis of winter conditions.

The spatial location of climatic zones and regions is shown on the map of the climatic regionalization of the USSR (Fig. 107).

It is apparent from this map that the zone of excessively moist climate with a very cold summer (I, 1) corresponds with the area of Arctic desert situated on islands of the Arctic Ocean and in the northern mountain part of Taimyr Peninsula. A considerable portion of the zone's territory is occupied by glaciers. The glacier-free area is covered for most of the year by snow and possesses a weakly developed soil mantle (the Arctic soils). A very meager vegetation (lichen, moss, and so on) does not form a closed cover and usually occupies less than half the total soil surface. Because of low temperatures and high humidity in this zone, evaporation is rather small and in some periods may be replaced by condensation. Thus, precipitation is mainly disposed of as run-off.

The zone of excessively moist climate with a cold summer (I, 2) coincides in general with the tundra and forest–tundra zones, embracing the northern and northeastern coasts of the USSR and also some interior continental regions of the northeast (mountain tundra). The tundra soils typical of this zone usually contain comparatively little organic matter and are character-

TABLE 35

CLASSIFICATION OF THE CLIMATES OF THE USSR

Thermal conditions of the warm period—the sum of temperatures at the surface of the earth	Moisture conditions (index of dryness)			
	I Too moist (<0.45)	II Moist (0.45–1.00)	III Insufficiently moist (1.00–3.00)	IV Dry (>3.00)
1. Very cold. Air temperature <10°C all year	I, 1, C Arctic desert	—	—	—
2. Cold, 0–1000°	I, 2, A–E Tundra and forest–tundra	—	—	—
3. Moderately warm, 1000–2200°	I, 3, E Alpine meadows	II, 3, A–E Needleleaf forest	III, 3, A–E Mountain steppe and Siberian steppe	IV, 3, C–D Mountain desert
4. Warm, 2200–4400°	—	II, 4, C–E Mixed and broad-leaved forest	III, 4, C–E Steppe and forest–steppe	IV, 4, C–E Northern desert
5. Very warm, >4400°	—	II, 5, F Subtropical forest	III, 5, E–F Xerophytic subtropical vegetation	IV, 5, E–F Desert

360

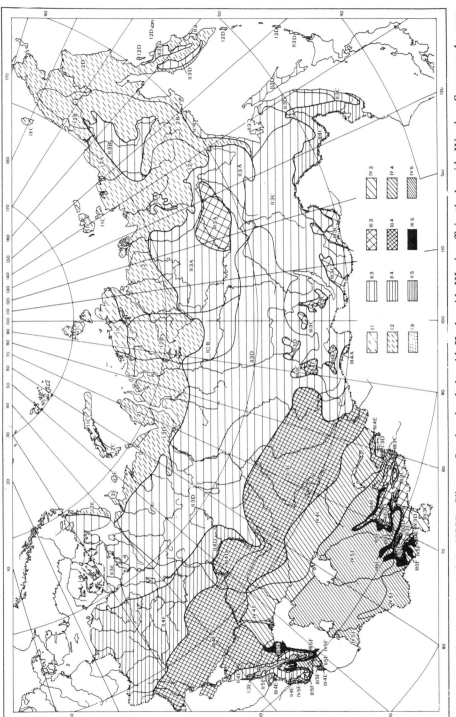

Fig. 107 Climatic regions of the USSR. Climate: I—abundantly humid, II—humid, III—insufficiently humid, IV—dry. Summer: 1—very cold, 2—cold, 3—moderately warm, 4—warm, 5—very warm. Winter: A—severe with little snow, B—severe and snowy, C—moderately severe with little snow, D—moderately severe and snowy, E—moderately mild, F—mild.

ized by low activity of biological processes. The tundra vegetation developing during the relatively short period of absence of snow cover is characterized by a predominance of moss, lichen, and also (in the southern part of the zone) shrubs and dwarf trees. Although the magnitudes of annual evaporation for the tundra zone are only approximately known, it is evident, however, that this process disburses a minor fraction of the precipitation received, probably no more than 30% on the average. Comparatively high values of the run-off coefficient are therefore noted in this zone.

The third climatic zone of surplus moisture, the zone with a moderately warm summer (I, 3), corresponds to the regions of alpine meadows. Such conditions are observed in a number of mountain regions of the USSR, but only on the ridge of the Great Caucasus do they embrace an extensive area that can be shown in the accompanying map. In this area, a vegetation of subalpine and alpine meadows that is rather rich in terms of type composition is developed on mountain-meadow soils. The precipitation ensures abundant run-off at a high value of the run-off coefficient.

Absence of forest vegetation is typical of the landscapes of climatic zones with surplus moisture. It must be indicated that the absence of forest in these zones is associated, not only with a deficiency in heat, but also with a moisture regime unfavorable to forest vegetation. In these zones, a significant predominance of precipitation over evaporation maintains a high water content in the soil throughout the year. Development of the root system of trees is therefore complicated by a deficiency of oxygen in the soil.

The effect of moisture conditions on the distribution of forest vegetation is distinctly expressed in the location of the southern border of the tundra, which shifts toward higher latitudes in regions with a less moist climate. This regularity also is of great importance for an explanation of the absence of forest in those regions of the alpine meadows where temperature sums are quite sufficient for development of forest vegetation.

The following group of climatic zones with a moist climate (II) includes, like the previous group, three zones.

Conditions of a moist climate with a moderately warm summer (II, 3) are characteristic of an extensive area of needleleaf forest, embracing the northern part of the European USSR (except the northern coastal regions) and the greater part of the Asian area of the USSR.

In the zone in question, podzolic soils are characteristic where forest vegetation consisting of evergreen and deciduous needleleaf species is developed. The deciduous needleleaf (larch) forest is situated mainly in regions with the most severe winter conditions. Although mean precipitation totals over the area of needleleaf forest vary over a wide range, significant water content in the soil and sufficiently high values of the run-off coefficient are nevertheless observed in all parts of this zone. For this reason, flow in many large rivers is reliably formed in the needleleaf forest zone.

The climatic zone of moist climate with a warm summer (II, 4) is situated in the middle part of the European USSR and in the southern part of the Priamur'ia and Primor'ia territories. In this district, mixed and broadleafed forests of diverse species compositions develop on turf-podzol and gray-forest soils.

A comparatively small part of the territory of the USSR is occupied by the zone of moist climate with a very warm summer (II, 5), which covers the western Transcaucasus and the southern region of the eastern Transcaucasus. Yellow and red earths, that is, soils of a subtropical type, are characteristic. In this area, the broadleafed forests to a great extent also have a subtropical character. Abundant precipitation, much exceeding potential evaporation, maintains a comparatively high soil moisture and ensures high run-off.

The climatic zones with a moist climate are characterized by development of forest vegetation. The principal factor favoring predominance of forest landscapes in these zones is the high soil moisture during the warm season, which, however, does not exceed those limits beyond which insufficient soil air prevents the development of the root system of trees.

It should be noted that forest vegetation can exist only with significant transpiration, because the intensity of turbulent diffusion at the level of tree crowns far exceeds that near the earth's surface. The increased turbulent exchange and the large total area of leaves make possible a relatively high level of assimilation, assuring the development of a considerable mass of nonproducing plant organs (trunks and branches).

With insufficient soil moisture, restricting the transpiration necessary for trees, forest vegetation is replaced by steppe vegetation, which is better accommodated to conditions of soil-moisture deficiency.

The zone of insufficient moisture with a moderately warm summer [III, 3] corresponds to the climatic conditions of a number of mountain regions of Central Asia and south-central Siberia. This zone also includes an extensive area in the middle reaches of the Lena River and the lower reaches of the Viliui River. In the mountains of Central Asia in this zone, mountain steppe and sparse high-mountain vegetation develops. In the south of Siberia, turfy–grassy and tansy steppes are widely distributed. In southern Siberia, a part of this climatic zone is occupied by pine forest, known to be of an intrazonal character. Vegetation cover of the territory situated along the middle reaches of the Lena River, referred to above, is rather complicated and is characterized by a mixture of needleleaf forest with lacustrine meadows (forest–steppe).

The basic part of the zone of insufficient moisture and warm summer (III, 4) is situated in the south of the European USSR and western Siberia. Analogous climatic conditions are also observed in some mountain regions of the Caucasus and Central Asia. Black earth [chernozem] and chestnut soils, on which various kinds of steppe and forest–steppe vegetation are developed, are characteristic of this zone.

The zone of insufficient moistening with a very warm summer (III, 5) is present on comparatively small areas of the southern shore of the Crimea, the central Transcaucasus, a part of the east coast of the Caucasus, and in some piedmont regions of Central Asia. In this zone, subtropical steppe, thin xerophytic forest, and other types of xerophytic vegetation cover are widely distributed. A part of the territory is occupied by intrazonal vegetation (floodplains of the Terek River, and so on).

All the zones of climate with insufficient moisture are characterized by relatively small run-off coefficients, which usually do not exceed 0.10–0.20. Because annual precipitation is less than potential evaporation, most of the precipitation goes for evaporation.

Climatic zones with an arid climate occupy the greater part of the areas of Central Asia and the eastern Transcaucasus.

The zone of arid climate with a moderately warm summer (IV, 3), situated in the Pamirs, corresponds to the conditions of high-mountain deserts.

The zone of arid climate with a warm summer (IV, 4) embraces semi-deserts and deserts with Artemisia and solonchak vegetation. Conditions of arid climate with a very warm summer (IV, 5) correspond in the main to the regions of deserts with saxaul, shrub, and ephemeral vegetation. In all zones of arid climate, the light-chestnut, brown-desert-steppe, gray-brown desert soils, gray earths, takyr, and other types of soils typical of arid conditions are widely distributed. Meager precipitation in these areas is almost entirely spent for evaporation; run-off is usually close to zero.

In climatic zones with insufficient precipitation and in zones with an arid climate, the development of vegetation is determined to a considerable extent by the regime of soil moisture. In proportion to the reduction of soil moisture with an increase in climatic aridity, the possible value of transpiration from a unit area of a given region diminishes. For this reason, the character of the vegetation cover changes, its composition begins to include different xerophytes, and it ceases to be continuous. Thus, all the principal climatic zones are in a certain accordance with general geographical zonality and, in particular, with geobotanic zonality. Areas in which this accordance is noticeably disturbed are comparatively few.

They include, for example, the area situated in the region of the middle Lena River and lower Viliui River, where conditions of insufficient moisture occur that usually correspond to forest–steppe vegetation. However, it follows from the "Геоботаническая карта СССР (Geobotanical Map of the USSR") by Lavrenko and Sochava (1954) that in this region, a needle-leaf forest prevails, for which conditions of a moist climate are typical.

In this connection, we should note that in this area regions with lake–meadow (*alas*) vegetation (that is, forest–steppe) and also regions with solonchaks, which usually develop under conditions of insufficient moisture, are comparatively widely distributed. Presumably, this was the basis for plotting the forest–steppe zone over a considerable part of this area in earlier geobotanic maps. It might be considered that the vegetation cover in this region is of a complicated character that depends not only on climatic conditions but also on the peculiarities of relief and on the effect of permafrost, which here extends down to great depths.

Some discrepancies between types of vegetation and climatic conditions are also observed in individual regions with pronounced effect of edaphic factors, in particular, in regions with sandy soils (where intrazonal pine forests are widely distributed), in the floodplains of rivers, and so on.

It should be borne in mind that the effect of many nonclimatic factors on vegetation cover shows up, not immediately, but through local changes of the meteorologic and hydrologic regimes. These changes correspond to peculiarities of the local climate and microclimate that cannot be reflected in climatic maps of limited scale. Therefore, it can be considered that in reality, there exist still closer relations between climate and vegetation, as compared to the regularities that can be established through comparison of schematic maps of climatic regions and vegetation cover.

REFERENCES

Арманд Д. Л. 1967. Некоторые задачи и методы физикн ландшафта. Сб. «Геофизика ландшафта». Изд. «Наука», М.

Armand, D. L. (1967). Some questions and methods in physics of the landscape. *In* "Geofizika Landshafta," (D. L. Armand, ed.) pp. 7–24. Izdat. Nauka, Moscow. MGA 19.12-16.

Багров Н. А. (1953). О среднем многолетнем испарении с поверхности суши. Метеорология и гидрология, № 10.

Bagrov, N. A. (1953). Mean long-term evaporation from the land surface. *Meteorol. Gidrol.* No. 10.

Багров Н. А. (1954). О расчете испарения с поверхности суши. Метеорология и гидрология, № 2.

Bagrov, N. A. (1954). Calculation of evaporation from the land surface. *Meteorol. Gidrol.* No. 2.

Базилевич Н. И., Родин Л. Е., Розов Н. Н. (1970). Географические аспекты изучения биологической продуктивности. Изд. Геогр. о-ва СССР, Л.

Bazilevich, N. I., Rodin, L. E., and Rozov, N. N. (1970). "Geograficheskie Aspekty Izucheniia Biologicheskoi Produktivnosti (Geographical Aspects of the Study of Biological Productivity)." Izdat. Geograf. Obshchestva SSSR, Leningrad.

Будыко М. И. (1948). Испарение в естественных условиях. Гидрометеоиздат, Л.

Budyko, M. I. (1948). "Isparenie v Estestvennykh Usloviiakh." Gidrometeoizdat, Leningrad. MGA 3.7-153; "Evaporation under Natural Conditions" (OTS 63-11061). Isr. Program Sci. Transl., Jerusalem, 1963. MGA 16.2-17.

Будыко М. И. (1949). Тепловой баланс северного полушария. Труды ГГО, вып. 18.

Budyko, M. I. (1949). The heat balance of the Northern Hemisphere. *Tr. Gl. Geofiz. Observ.* **18.**

Будыко М. И. (1950). Климатические факторы внешнего физико-географического процесса. Труды ГГО, вып. 19.

Budyko, M. I. (1950). Climatic factors of the external physical-geographical processes. *Tr. Gl. Geofiz. Observ.* **19**, 25–40. MGA 2.8-130.

Будыко М. И. (1951a). О климатических факторах стока. Проблемы физической географии, вып. 16.

Budyko, M. I. (1951a). On climatic factors of runoff. *Probl. Fiz. Geogr.* **16**.

Будыко М. И. (1951б). О влиянии мелиоративных мероприятий на испаряемость. Изв. АН СССР, сер. геогр., № 1.

Budyko, M. I. (1951b). On the influence of reclamation measures upon potential evapotranspiration. *Izv. Akad. Nauk. SSSR Ser. Geogr.* No. 1, 16–35. MGA 3.6-130.

Будыко М. И. (1955). Климатические условия увлажнения на материках. Изв. АН СССР, сер. геогр., № 2, 4.

Budyko, M. I. (1955). Climatic conditions of moisture on the continents, Pt. 2. *Izv. Akad. Nauk SSSR Ser. Geogr.* No. 2, 4. MGA 6: 1642.

Будыко М. И. (1956). Тепловой баланс земной поверхности. Гидрометеоиздат, Л.

Budyko, M. I. (1956). "Teplovoi Balans Zemnoi Poverkhnosti." Gidrometeoizdat, Leningrad; "Heat Balance of the Earth's Surface," translated by N. A. Stepanova. U.S. Weather Bur., Washington, D.C., 1958. MGA 13E-286.

Будыко М. И., Зубенок Л. И. (1961). Определение испарения с поверхности суши. Изв. АН СССР, сер. геогр., № 6.

Budyko, M. I., and Zubenok, L. I. (1961). The determination of evaporation from the land surface. *Izv. Akad. Nauk SSSR Ser. Geogr.* No. 6, 3–17.

Будыко М. И., Котляков В. М., Мещеряков Ю. А. (1970). О применении количественных методов в физико-географических исследованиях. Изд. Геогр. о-ва СССР, Л.

Budyko, M. I., Kotliakov, V. M., and Meshcheriakov, Iu. A. (1970). "O Primenenii Kolichestvennykh Metodov v Fiziko-geograficheskikh Issledovaniiakh (On the Application of Quantitative Methods to Physical-Geographical Investigations)." Izdat. Geogr. Obshch. SSSR, Mater. V S''ezda, Leningrad, *Sov. Geogr. Rev. Transl.* **12** (No. 5), 266–277 (1971).

Виленский Д. Г. (1945). Русская почвенно-картографическая школа и ее влияние на развитие мировой картографии почв. Изд. АН СССР, М.—Л.

Vilenskii, D. G. (1945). "Russkaia Pochvenno-kartograficheskaia Shkola i ee Vliianie na Razvitie Mirovoi Kartografii Pochv (The Russian Soil-Mapping School and its Influence on the Development of World Soil Mapping)." Izdat. Akad. Nauk SSSR, Moscow and Leningrad.

Воейков А. И. (1884). Климаты земного шара, в особенности России. СПб.

Voeikov, A. I. (1884). "Klimaty Zemnogo Shara, v Osobennosti Rossii (The Climates of the Earth, Especially Russia)." Izdat. Kartograf. Zavedeniia, S.-Peterburg. MGA 3.4-4, 11A-97. Ch. 8 publ. as: Flüsse und Landseen als Produkte des Klima's. *Z. Ges. Erdk. Berlin* 1885, No. 2, 92–110. See also A. Woeikof, "Die Klimate der Erde," 2 vols., Jena, H. Costenoble, 1887.

Волобуев В. Р. (1953). Почвы и климат. Изд. АН АзССР. Баку.

Volobuev, V. R. (1953). "Pochvy i Klimat (Soils and Climate)." Izdat. Akad. Nauk Azerb. SSR, Baku.

Высоцкий Г. Н. (1905). Степи Европейской России. Полная энциклопедия русского сельского хозяйства, т. 9.

Vysotskii, G. N. (1905). The steppes of European Russia. *In* "Polnaia Entsiklapediia Russkogo Sel'skogo Khoziaistva," vol. 9 (A. F. Rudskiy, ed.), Izdanie A. F. Devriena, S.-Peterburg.

Геоботаническая карта СССР. (1954). Под ред. Е. М. Лавренко, В. Б. Сочавы. Изд. Ботанического ин-та АН СССР, М.

"Geobotanicheskaia Karta SSSR (Geobotanical Map of the USSR)" (E. M. Lavrenko, and V. B. Sochava, eds.). Izdat. Botan. Inst. Akad. Nauk SSSR, Moscow, 1954.

Герасимов И. П. (1945). Мировая почвенная карта и общие законы географии почв. Почвоведение, № 3, 4.

Gerasimov, I. P. (1945). A world soil map and general laws of the geography of soils. *Pochvovedenie* No. 3, 4.

Герасимов И. П. (1960). Гидрометеорологические факторы почвообразования. Сб. Тепловой и водный режим земной поверхности. Гидрометеоиздат, Л.

Gerasimov, I. P. (1960). "Hydrometeorological factors in soil formation. *In* "Teplovoi i Vodnyi Rezhim Zemnoi Poverkhnosti (Heat and Water Regime of the Earth's Surface)." Gidrometeoizdat, Leningrad. [Cf. Moisture and heat factors of soil formation. *Sov. Geogr. Rev. Transl.* **2**, No. 5, 3–12 (1961).] MGA 13.5-593.

Григорьев А. А. (1946). Некоторые итоги разработки новых идей в физической географии. Изв. АН СССР, сер. геогр. и геофиз., №2.

Grigor'ev, A. A. (1946). Some results of analysis of new ideas in physical geography. *Izv. Akad. Nauk SSSR Ser. Geogr. Geofiz* No. 2.

Григорьев А. А. (1954). Географическая зональность и некоторые ее закономерности. Изв. АН СССР, сер. геогр., № 5, 6.

Grigor'ev, A. A. (1954). Geographical zonality and some of its characteristics. *Izv. Akad. Nauk SSSR Ser. Geogr.* No. 5, 17–39; No. 6, 41–50.

Григорьев А. А., Будыко М. И. (1956). О периодическом законе географической зональности. ДАН СССР, т. 110, № 1.

Grigor'ev, A. A., and Budyko, M. I. (1956). On the periodic law of geographic zonality. *Dokl. Akad. Nauk SSSR*, **110**, No. 1.

Григорьев А. А., Будыко М. И. (1959). Классификация климатов СССР. Изв. АН СССР, сер. геогр., № 3.

Grigor'ev, A. A., and Budyko, M. I. (1959). Classification of the climates of the USSR. *Izv. Akad. Nauk SSSR Ser. Geogr.* No. 3, 3–19; *Sov. Georgr. Rev. Transl.* **1**, No. 5, 3–24 (1960). MGA 12:2117, 14.7-739.

Григорьев А. А., Будыко М. И. (1962). О сезонных изменениях климатических факторов географической зональности. ДАН СССР, т. 143, № 2.

Grigor'ev, A. A., and Budyko, M. I. (1962). Seasonal variations in the climatic factors of geographic zonality. *Dokl. Akad. Nauk SSSR* **143**, No. 2, 391–393 (1962). MGA 14.5-80.

Давыдов В. К. (1944). Испарение с водной поверхности в Европейской части СССР. Труды НИУ ГУГМС, сер. IV, вып. 12.

Davydov, V. K. (1944). Evaporation from water surfaces in the European part of the USSR. *Tr. Gl. Upr. Gidrometeorol. Sluzhby Nauch. Issl. Uchrezhdenii* [4], **12**.

Давыдов Л. К. (1947). Водоносность рек СССР, ее колебания и влияние на нее физико-географических факторов. Гидрометеоиздат, Л.

Davydov, L. K. (1947). "Vodonosnost' Rek SSSR, ee Kolebaniia i Vliianie na nee Fiziko-geograficheskikh Factorov (The Water Supply of the Rivers of the USSR, Its Variations, and the Influence of Physical-geographical Factors on It)." Gidrometeoizdat, Leningrad.

Докучаев В. В. (1900). Zones naturelles des sols. (Перевод в кн. В. В. Докучаев. Учение о зонах природы. Изд. АН СССР, М., 1948.)

Dokuchaev, V. V. (1900). Zones naturelles des sols. Transl. in "Uchenie o Zonakh Prirody." Izdat. Akad. Nauk SSSR, Moscow, 1948.

Жегневская Г. С. (1954). К вопросу о климатических факторах увлажнения юга Европейской части СССР. Изв. ВГО, т. 86, вып. 6.

Zhegnevskaia, G. S. (1954). The problem of climatic factors of the moisture conditions of the southern part of the European USSR. *Izv. Vses. Geogr. Obschestva.* **86** (No. 6) 537–542. MGA 8.4-253

Зайков Б. Д. (1949). Испарение с водной поверхности прудов и малых водохранилищ на территории СССР. Труды ГГИ, вып. 21.

Zaikov, B. D. (1949). Evaporation from the surface of ponds and small water bodies in the USSR. *Tr. Gos. Gidrol. Inst.* **21.**

Захаров С. А. (1931). Курс почвоведения. Сельхозгиз, М.

Zakharov, S. A. (1931). "Kurs Pochvovedeniia (Soil Science)." Sel'khozgiz, Moscow.

Иванов Н. Н. (1941). Зоны увлажнения земного шара. Изв. АН СССР, сер. геогр. и геофиз., № 3.

Ivanov, N. N. (1941). Moisture zones of the earth. *Izv. Akad. Nauk SSSR. Ser. Geogr. Geofiz.* No. 3.

Иванов Н. Н. (1948). Ландшафтно-климатические зоны земного шара. Зап. ВГО, нов. сер., т. I.

Ivanov, N. N. (1948). Landscape-climatic zones of the earth. *Zap. Vses. Geograf. Obshchest.* [N.S.], **1.**

Калесник С. В. (1947). Основы общего землеведения. Учпедгиз, М.—Л.

Kalesnik, S. V. (1947). "Osnovy Obshchego Zemlevedeniia (Foundations of General Geography)." Uchpedgiz, Moscow and Leningrad.

Калесник С. В. (1970). Общие географические закономерности Земли. Изд. «Мысль», М.

Kalesnik, S. V. (1970). "Obshchie Geograficheskie Zakonomernosti Zemli (The General Geographic Regularities of the Earth)." Izdat. Mysl', Moscow.

Львович М. И. (1945). Элементы водного режима рек земного шара. Труды НИУ ГУГМС, сер. IV, вып. 18.

L'vovich, M. I. (1945). Elements of the water regime of the rivers of the earth. *Tr. Gl. Upr. Gidrometeorol. Sluzhby Nauch. Issled. Uchrezhdenii* [4], **18.**

Мезенцев В. С. (1955). Еще раз о расчете среднего суммарного испарения. Метео-рология и гидрология, № 5.

Mezentsev, V. S. (1955). More on the calculation of average total evaporation. *Meteorol. Gidrol.* No. 5, 24–26. MGA 8.5-133.

Мезенцев В. С., Карнацевич И. В. (1969). Увлажненность Западно-Сибирской равнины. Гидрометеоиздат, Л.

Mezentsev, V. S., and Karnatsevich, I. V. (1969). "Uvlazhnennost' Zapado-Sibirskoi Ravniny (Moisture Conditions of the West Siberian Plain)." Gidrometeoizdat, Leningrad.

Мировой агроклиматический справочник. (1937). Под ред. Г. Т. Селянинова. Гидро-метеоиздат, Л.—М.

"Mirovoi Agroklimaticheskii Spravochnik (World Agroclimatic Handbook)" (G. T. Selianinov, ed.). Gidrometeoizdat, Leningrad, 1937. MGA 4C-203.

Огиевский А. В. (1937). Гидрология суши. Гидрометеоиздат. Л.—М.

Ogievskii, A. V. (1937). "Gidrologiia Sushi (Hydrology)." Gidrometeoizdat, Leningrad and Moscow.

Ольдекоп Э. М. (1911). Об испарении с поверхности речных бассейнов. Труды Юрьевской обсерватории.

Ol'dekop, E. M. (1911). Ob Isparenii s Poverkhnosti Rechnykh Basseinov (On Evaporation from the Surface of River Basins). *Tr. Meteorol. Observ. Iur'evskogo Univ. Tartu,* **4.**

Познышев О. С. (1937). Испарение и его связь с метеорологическими факторами. Труды комиссии по ирригации, № 10.

Poznyshev, O. S. (1937). Evaporation and its relation with meteorological factors. *Trudy Kom. Irrigatsii* No. 10, 1937.

Поляков Б. В. (1946). Гидрологический анализ и расчеты. Гидрометеоиздат, Л.

Poliakov, B. V. (1946). "Gidrologicheskii Analiz i Raschety (Hydrologic Analysis and Calculations)." Gidrometeoizdat, Leningrad.

Селянинов Г. Т. (1930). К методике сельскохозяйственной климатологии. Труды по с.-х. метеорол., вып. 22, № 2.

Selianinov, G. T. (1930). On the methodology of agricultural climatology. *Tr. Sel'skokhoz. Meteorol.* **22**, No. 2.

Селянинов Г. Т. (1937). Методика сельскохозяйственной характеристики климата. Мировой агроклиматический справочник. Гидрометеоиздат, Л.—М.

Selianinov, G. T. (1937). Methods of agricultural characterization of climate. *In* "Mirovoi Agroklimaticheskii Spravochnik (World Agroclimatic Handbook)" (G. T. Selianinov, ed.), pp. 5–49. Gidrometeoizdat, Leningrad and Moscow. MGA 4C-203.

Соколова Е. М. (1937). Недостаток насыщения влагой воздуха на территории СССР. Труды ГГИ, вып. 3.

Sokolova, E. M. (1937). Saturation deficit of the air over the USSR. *Tr. Gos. Gidrol. Inst.* **3**.

Соколовский Д. Л. (1936). Связь стока с осадками в различных географических условиях. Метеорология и гидрология, № 6.

Sokolovskii, D. L. (1936). The relation of runoff with precipitation in different geographic conditions. *Meteorol. Gidrol.*, No. 6.

Сочава В. Б. (1948). Географические связи растительного покрова на территории СССР. Уч. зап. ЛГПИ, т. 73.

Sochava, V. B. (1948). Geograficheskie Sviazi Rastitel'nogo Pokrova na Territorii SSSR (Geographic relations of the plant cover of the USSR). *Uch. Zap. Leningrad. Gos. Univ. Pedagog. Inst. im. A. I. Gertsena* **73**.

Сочава В. Б. [и др.] (1970). Топологические особенности тепла и влаги в таежных геосистемах. Доклады Ин-та географии Сибири и Дальнего Востока, вып. 26.

Sochava, V. B., *et al.* (1970). Topologic features of heat and moisture in taiga geosystems. *Dokl. Akad. Nauk SSSR Inst. Geogr. Sibiri Dal'nego Vostoka* **26**.

Шулейкин В. В. (1941). Физика моря. Изд. АН СССР, М.—Л.

Shuleikin, V. V. (1941). "Fizika Moria (Physics of the Sea)." Izdat. Akad. Nauk SSSR, Leningrad and Moscow. MGA 13E-289.

de Martonne, E., (1926). Aréisme et indice d'aridité. *C. R. Acad. Sci.* **182**.

Jenny, H. (1941). "Factors of Soil Formation" McGraw-Hill, New York and London. (Русский перевод: Иенни. Факторы почвообразования. ИЛ, М., (1948.)

Keller, H. (1906). Niederschlag, Abfluss und Verdunstung in Mitteleuropa. *Besondere Mitteil. Jahrb. Gewässerkunde Norddeuts.* **1**, Pt. 4.

Köppen, W. (1918). Klassifikation der Klima nach Temperatur, Niederschlag und Jahreslauf. *Petermanns Mitt.* **64**, 193–203, 243–248.

Lang, R. (1920). "Verwitterung und Bodenbildung als Einführung in die Bodenkunde." Stuttgart, E. Schweizerbart.

McIlroy, J. C., and Angus, D. E. (1964). Grass, water and soil evaporation at Aspendale. *Agric. Meteorol.* **1**, 201–224.

Meyer, A. (1926). Über einige Zusammenhänge zwischen Klima und Böden in Europa. *Chem. Erde* No. 2.

Penck, A. (1910). Versuch einer Klimaklassifikation auf physiogeographischer Grundlage. *Sitzungsber. Preuss. Akad. Wiss. Phys. Math. Kl.* No. 12.

Penman, H. L. (1948). Natural evaporation from open water, bare soil and grass. *Proc. Roy. Soc. Ser. A*, **193**, 120–145.

Prescott, J. (1931). The soils of Australia in relation to vegetation and climate. *Bull. Council Sci. Ind. Res., Austr.* **52**.

Schreiber, P. (1904). Über die Beziehungen zwischen dem Niederschlag und der Wasser-führung der Flüsse in Mitteleuropa. *Z. Meteorol.* **21**, Pt. 10.

Sellers, W. D. (1965). "Physical Climatology." Univ. Chicago Press, Chicago, Illinois.

Thornthwaite, C. W. (1948). An approach toward a rational classification of climate. *Geogr. Rev.*, **38**, No. 1.

Transeau, E. N. (1905). Forest centers of eastern America. *Amer. Natur.* **39**, No. 468.

VII

The Thermal Regime of Living Organisms

1. The Influence of Thermal Factors on Plants and Animals

The thermal conditions of life are restricted within comparatively narrow limits. Most reactions in biological systems occur at temperatures no lower than 0°C and no higher than 50°C. Although many organisms can exist at temperatures of an external medium that go beyond these limits, their activity usually ceases. This interval is expanded for organisms that can control their temperature; but even for them, the thermal zone of life is narrower than the range of temperatures observed on the globe. In the regions with the highest and lowest temperatures, biological processes are therefore either inhibited or absent.

Within the range of temperatures permitting development of biological reactions, the rate of these reactions, as a rule, depends essentially on the temperature. For quantitative evaluation of these dependences, so-called temperature coefficients are often used, which indicate by what factor the reaction rate increases when the temperature rises by 10°.

The value of temperature coefficients for various biological processes varies within wide limits, from 1.2–1.4 to several units, in many cases being close to 2. Usually, the increase of reaction rate with temperature rise is restricted to a certain limit, beyond which the growth of the reaction rate stops and changes into a decrease.

Temperature greatly affects almost all the biological processes in plants. This influence is associated with a number of different mechanisms. Thus, for example, the solubility in the cell solution of the principal components of

371

mass exchange or metabolism in plants—carbon dioxide and oxygen—decreases appreciably with a rise in temperature. When carbon-dioxide content in the cell solution changes, acidity changes accordingly, which affects several biochemical processes in plants.

The fundamental process of the life activity of autotrophic plants, photosynthesis, which determines their productivity, depends essentially on thermal conditions.

According to experimental data, the dependence of photosynthesis on temperature is most important at low temperatures, slightly above the freezing point. Under such conditions, photosynthesis is mainly limited by enzyme reactions, the temperature coefficients of which usually exceed 2. As a result, photosynthesis rapidly increases with a temperature rise. At higher temperatures, the increase in photosynthesis with a temperature becomes slower, and at a temperature around 20–25°, photosynthesis reaches its maximum. Deceleration of the increase in photosynthesis at higher temperatures can be explained by the limiting effect of light reactions, which depend little on thermal conditions. A further rise of temperature leads to a decline of photosynthesis, which presumably is explicable by thermal inactivation of enzymes.

It should be noted that in some plants, photosynthesis can also occur at negative temperatures, though under such conditions its value is very small.

More simple is the dependence of plant respiration on temperature. The value of respiration increases regularly as temperature rises, with comparatively large values of the temperature coefficient.

Temperature greatly influences the growth and development of plants. The effect of thermal conditions on the growth of plants is similar to that of temperature on the activity of enzymes.

At temperatures from 0 to 15°C, the rate of growth rapidly increases with a rise in temperature; at temperatures from 15 to 30°C, the increase of the growth rate becomes slower; and at temperatures above 30° the rate of growth starts decreasing. Lowering of temperature at night produces a favorable effect on the growth of plants. The mechanism of this effect is still insufficiently studied. The only thing clear is that it is not limited to the action of lowered temperature on the decrease of plant respiration in the period of absence of photosynthesis.

The dependence of plant growth on temperature has long been taken into account in agriculture when estimating the heat resources of different regions. In the middle of the 19th century, de Candolle (1874) suggested that the temperatures of single days be summed up for this purpose. The method of "temperature sums" in its various forms has been used in agrometeorology up to the present time.

The effect of temperature on the development of plants is rather complicated. The character of this effect changes substantially in different phases of a plant's life. Thus, for example, for normal development of many plants, periods of an appreciable lowering of temperature are necessary; otherwise the ability to flower is lost or other functions of the plants arc disturbed.

For all plants, there are temperature limits that determine their existence.

At low temperatures, plants are damaged as a result of formation of ice crystals in their tissues. The crystals destroy the cell walls both directly and as a result of water transfer in the tissues during the freezing process.

The size of the temperature drop that can be endured by plants varies within wide limits for different plants. It also depends on the rate of lowering of temperature (plants more easily endure a slow cooling than a fast one) and on the degree of chilling of the plant, that is, on the cooling that it has experienced earlier.

Temperature rises exceeding definite limits also do harm to plants, including the destruction of chlorophyll, leaf burn, and other damage that with a further rise of temperature lead to the destruction of the plant.

Stability under the action of high temperatures is different for different plants. Succulent plants of the desert can endure the highest temperatures without damage.

Thermal factors thus exert a deep and determining influence on the vital activity of plants. The geographical distribution of plants, their seasonal changes, and the species composition and productivity of vegetation cover therefore all depend on thermal conditions.

The effect of temperature on the life activity of animals is no less important than its influence on plants. All animals are divided into two groups with reference to heat regime: poikilothermal animals, whose body temperature varies over a wide range, and homoiothermal animals, who maintain their body temperature at an approximately stable level. Sometimes an intermediate group of heterothermal animals, who can control their body temperature to a limited extent, is added to the groups mentioned.

The body temperature of poikilothermal animals usually does not coincide with the temperature of the external medium, because of the effect of metabolic processes, which are associated with the secretion of heat. However, the heat production of such animals is as a rule insignificant, so that the difference is usually small. This rule has some exceptions, at moments of high activity of animals. Thus, for example, the body temperature of many insects sharply increases during flight.

There also exist other factors whose effect may contribute to a change in the temperature of poikilothermic animals in comparison to the external medium. Thus, for example, body temperature can fall as a result of heat loss caused by evaporation from the animal's body surface, and with the outgo of long-wave radiation to space. Absorption of solar radiation can lead to a rise of the body temperature.

Fluctuations of the body temperature of large poikilothermal animals (such as some reptiles) may noticeably lag behind changes in the temperature of the external medium because of the effect of thermal inertia of the animal's body.

The homoiothermal animals include the two highest classes, birds and mammals, which, during the course of evolution, have worked out an effective mechanism to maintain a stable body temperature independent of external conditions. This mechanism is based on the activity of the heat regulation center, located in one of the sections of the brain, the hypothalamus. When the external factors of the thermal regime change, this center ensures an appropriate change in the systems of physical and chemical heat regulation, which enables the animal to maintain a constant body temperature. The basic means of heat regulation is the wide variability of metabolism, which sharply increases with falling temperature. Along with the means of heat regulation mentioned, many animals possess other means, changing evaporation from the body surface, state of the coat of hair, and so on. Different homoiothermal animals have different body temperatures. For birds, it is commonly equal to 40–42°, and for mammals it more often ranges from 36 to 39°. The stability of body temperature is relative for homoiothermal animals. It often varies during the diurnal march, when muscular activity changes, in the regime of nutrition, and with other factors. Under external environmental conditions anomalous for the homoiothermal animal, its body temperature can fluctuate markedly.

Vital activity of both poikilothermal and homoiothermal animals is possible within the limits of a certain range of body temperature, bounded by the so-called lethal temperatures.

These temperatures for one and the same species of animal can differ significantly, depending on the acclimatization of the animal, that is, on its earlier existence at higher or lower temperatures.

The lethal temperatures of poikilothermal animals are diverse. Some animals die at comparatively small changes in their body temperature, and others bear temperature changes amounting to tens of degrees without harm.

For homoiothermal animals, the difference between the upper and lower lethal temperatures lies most often within the limits of 15–25 C°. For man, with a normal body temperature of about 37°, the lower lethal temperature is 24–25° and the upper is 43–44°.

The biological functions of both poikilothermal and homoiothermal animals change considerably with fluctuations in body temperature.

The temperature effect is very great on the vital activity of poikilothermal animals, whose activity is possible only within a definite and sometimes rather narrow range of temperature. For this reason, the behavior of poikilothermal animals is often determined by the necessity of maintaining the optimal body temperature. Thus, for example, with a shortage of heat, many insects, reptiles, and other animals move into sites in the sun and take a position that ensures the greatest radiative heating of their bodies. When the earth's surface is overheated by the sun, these animals abandon it. They either go to their holes or move to the branches of plants where the temperature of the air is lower than the temperature of the earth's surface. We should especially point out the great influence of thermal conditions on the reproduction processes of poikilothermal animals, which in many respects determines their ecology in a particular period.

Although the ecology of homoiothermal animals depends to a lesser extent on thermal regime, under unfavorable conditions these animals also use microclimatic features of the landscape to approximate their body temperature to the optimum.

The necessity of such actions is especially great for small animals, whose body thermal inertia is insignificant. They accordingly become cooled more easily at low temperatures of the environment, because of the large value of the ratio between the body surface, through which the outflow of heat takes place and the body mass, which determines the heat production from metabolism (Rubner's law).

The substantial influence of thermal factors on the vital activity of animals determines the importance of thermal conditions of the external environment to the geographic distribution of animals and their ecology.

2. The Thermal Regime of Plants

In investigations of the effect of thermal factors on the vital activity of plants, data on the air temperature observed at a certain height in an instrument shelter are most often used.

At the same time, it was noted long ago that air temperature only approximately defines those thermal conditions that take form immediately on the surface of plants as a result of the complex interrelation of the heat exchange processes.

For example, this viewpoint was expressed in the outstanding work by Veselovskii, "О климате России (On the Climate of Russia)" (1857), published more than a hundred years ago. He wrote: "Since the vegetative processes and the phenomena of organic life in general occur more or less under the influence of the direct action of the sun's rays, the study of climate in terms of thermal conditions would be incomplete if we restricted ourselves

to air temperature alone. Therefore, in the chapter about heat we will first
speak about the heat of the air and then about the heating power of the
sun's rays, or the temperature received from the sun by bodies on the earth's
surface." In developing this idea, Veselovskii pointed out that "even on
the basis of differences between the causes acting on the heating of the air
and the conditions determining the heating of the earth's surface, it must be
supposed that . . . the lines of a specific annual air temperature and the lines
of the same temperature of the upper layer of the earth will not be parallel."
To illustrate this statement, Veselovskii gave some examples indicating sharp
differences between the states of vegetation cover at the same air temperature
but different incomes of solar radiation.

It should be recognized that these considerations of Veselovskii were far
ahead of contemporary science, and that the task he set to determine the
characteristics of the thermal regime that immediately affect the life of plants
was not solved for a long time.

Experimental data characterizing the actual temperature of plants can be
obtained by application of special instruments, such as thermoelectric
thermometers, probes of which look like thin nets or "spiders," or radiation
thermometers, measuring temperature by the flux of long-wave radiation.

Some results of observations conducted with such instruments are presented in Figs. 108–110 (Budyko, 1958).

Figure 108 shows the mean diurnal march of the difference between the
temperatures at the earth's surface and in the air in the period May 21–26,

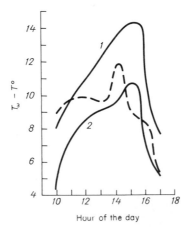

Fig. 108 Diurnal march of the difference between temperatures of the earth's surface
and the air at Koltushi. Solid lines show measured values, broken line indicates calculated
values (see text).

1956, according to observations over a plot with grass cover at Koltushi (Leningrad region). The solid curves define the observational results (1— measuring plant-surface temperature with the radiation thermometer; 2— with the thermo-spider).

The data from Fig. 108 show what values may be reached by the differences between the earth's surface temperature and the air temperature in regions of abundant precipitation. It is apparent from the graph that under moist climatic conditions, the mean differences between these temperatures in the daytime hours may exceed 10°. A certain difference between the readings of the radiation and the thermoelectric thermometers shown in the figure is worthy of attention. This difference is likely not only to be associated with errors in observations of each of the methods, but also to reflect (to some extent) the difference between the physical meanings of temperature determined by the different methods.

It follows from the data presented in Fig. 108 that even under conditions of abundant moisture, the temperature of plants may differ from that of the air by a figure comparable with the geographic variation of temperature over distances of thousands of kilometers. The cause of the difference obviously lies in the heating of the plant surface by the sun's rays.

Figure 109 shows data on observations of the mean difference between temperatures of the earth's surface and the air in a desert region, and Fig. 110, in an oasis in Central Asia, according to the data from the expedition of the Main Geophysical Observatory in July, 1952.

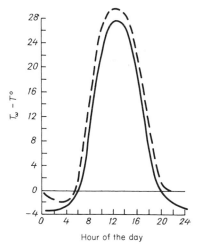

Hour of the day

Fig. 109 Diurnal march of the difference between temperatures of the earth's surface and the air in the desert. Solid line shows measured values, broken line indicates calculated values (see text).

The data of Fig. 109 relate to a dry surface of the desert. They are interesting as defining the limit reached by the difference between air and plant
temperatures under desert conditions, if the plants are adjacent to the earth's
surface and lose little heat in evaporation. Figure 110 demonstrates the
difference between the temperatures of cotton leaves and the air under
conditions of abundant moisture with irrigation. It is apparent from Figs.
109 and 110 that the thermal regime of plants in the desert varies greatly,
depending on moisture conditions. Without irrigation, the temperature of a
plant in the daytime may be much higher than air temperature; with irrigation, which ensures a greater heat conversion in evaporation, plant temperature turns out to be noticeably lower than air temperature.

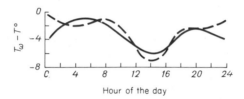

Fig. 110 Diurnal march of the difference between the temperatures of the earth's
surface and the air in an oasis. Solid line shows measured values, broken line indicates
calculated values (see text).

Thus, it becomes clear that the actual temperature of plants often does not
coincide with the temperature of the air. This conclusion is confirmed by
observations conducted by many investigators under different climatic
conditions.

Since we do not possess mass observational material on plant temperatures
obtained with the aid of special instruments, which might be used instead of
data on the air temperature in studying the effect of climatic factors on plants,
there arises a question about the possibility of obtaining such material by
calculation, on the basis of data from standard observations conducted in
the network of meteorological stations. One may solve this problem by calculating the heat balance of vegetation cover (Budyko, 1958).

The determination of plant temperature by the heat-balance method is
based on the following considerations.

The equation of the heat balance of the land surface has the form

$$R = LE + P + A, \qquad (7.1)$$

where R is the radiation balance, L is the latent heat of vaporization, E is the
evaporation, P is the turbulent sensible-heat flux, and A is the inflow of heat
to the soil.

After transforming the components characterizing radiation balance and sensible-heat exchange, this equation can be presented in the form

$$R_0 - 4\delta\sigma T^3(T_w - T) = LE + \rho c_p D(T_w - T) + A, \qquad (7.2)$$

where R_0 is the radiation balance at the earth's surface calculated by determining net long-wave radiation from air temperature, δ is the coefficient characterizing the difference between the properties of the radiating surface and a black body, σ is the Stefan–Boltzmann constant, T is the air temperature, T_w is the temperature of the earth's surface, ρ is the air density, c_p is the heat capacity of the air, and D is the integral coefficient of diffusion. It follows that

$$T_w - T = \frac{R_0 - LE - A}{\rho c_p D + 4\delta\sigma T^3}. \qquad (7.3)$$

This formula can be applied to calculate the temperature of the earth's surface in the cases when the air temperature, the heat-balance components R_0, LE, and A, and the integral coefficient of diffusion D are known.

The methods for calculating the above-mentioned components of the heat balance from the data of standard meteorological observations are set forth in Chapter II of this book. The value of the coefficient D can often be considered constant. Its mean for daytime conditions in summer approaches 1 cm sec^{-1}, and for mean 24-hour conditions in summer, about 0.6 cm sec^{-1} (see Chapter II).

In some cases, especially under conditions of abundant moisture in the terrain, the temperature of the active surface can be calculated from Eq. (7.2) on the assumption that

$$E = \rho D(q_s - q) \qquad (7.4)$$

(where q_s is the saturation specific humidity at the temperature of the active surface, and q is the specific humidity), taking into account the dependence of q_s on T_w.

In a closed vegetation cover, the leaves of plants usually constitute a basic part of the "active surface," where heat and water exchanges with the atmosphere occur. In this case, it can be considered that the mean temperature of the plant leaves is approximately equal to the temperature of the earth's surface determined from Eq. (7.3).

The results of applying the heat-balance method to calculate the temperature of the earth's surface are presented in Figs. 108–110, where they are shown by a broken line. It is apparent from the figures that the calculated material agrees well with the observational data. This clarifies the possibility of using the heat-balance method for determination of the temperature of the vegetation cover.

In this connection, the problem of obtaining mass material on the active-surface temperature and constructing a map of its distribution has been raised. For this purpose, Efimova calculated the monthly means of the difference between temperatures of the active surface and the air in the European USSR, and constructed a series of maps of this difference and of the active-surface temperature in each month of the warm season. In her calculation, she used a mean of the coefficient D equal to 0.63 cm sec^{-1}.

One of these maps, showing the monthly means of the difference $T_w - T$ in July, is presented in Fig. 111. The regularities of the geographical distribution of the difference $T_w - T$ shown in this map are also typical of other months of the warm season.

It is apparent from the map that the difference $T_w - T$ increases from the central and western regions of the European USSR toward the south and southeast. Such changes are probably to be explained by a decline of heat converted in evaporation, owing to a reduction of soil moisture in these directions. At first glance, the increase of temperature difference in the

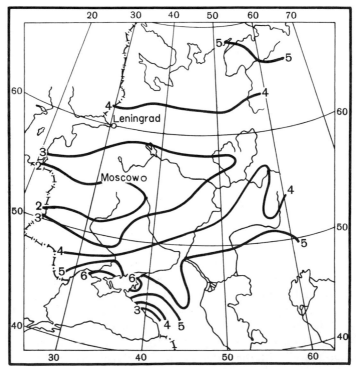

Fig. 111 Difference between the temperatures of the earth's surface and the air in July.

northern regions of the European USSR is somewhat unexpected. This regularity is presumably connected with conditions of the transformation of [marine] air masses with comparatively low temperatures that come into the continent in summer and are gradually heated as they move into the interior.

The heat-balance method can be also used for working out another problem in the investigation of the temperature of vegetation cover. It is known that the conditions of the thermal regime on the more or less steep south and north slopes lead to development of different kinds of vegetation on them, whereas observations of air temperature conducted at the level of the meteorological shelter do not indicate any substantial difference between the temperature regimes of north and south slopes in conditions of hilly relief. It is apparent from general considerations that the difference between the conditions of heating on the hillsides is associated with the differences in the radiation regime and therefore ought to be manifested in the greatest degree at the level of the earth's surface. At higher levels, the turbulent mixing of the atmosphere smoothes out temperature differences arising at individual elements of the earth's surface. Thus, for a quantitative evaluation of the effect of the thermal regime of slopes on the development of vegetation, one must have data on the surface temperature of slopes of different steepness and orientation.

To obtain such data, a series of calculations based on utilization of the aforementioned equations of the heat balance was carried out. In these, the changes in the radiation-balance values on hillsides, associated with the change in direct-beam solar radiation and in net long-wave radiation, were considered.

Some results of these calculations are given in Table 36, where the differences are presented between monthly mean temperatures at the earth's

TABLE 36

DIFFERENCES BETWEEN TEMPERATURES AT THE EARTH'S SURFACE ON
SLOPES FROM THOSE ON LEVEL GROUND

Region	Month	North slopes		South slopes	
		20°	10°	10°	20°
Volgograd	May	−1.3	−0.7	0.3	0.8
	July	−1.3	−0.8	0.1	0.5
	Sept.	−3.3	−1.7	1.7	2.9
Tashkent	March	−2.3	−1.2	0.9	1.8
	May	−1.8	−1.0	0.5	1.2
	July	−1.9	−0.7	0.4	0.8
	Sept.	−4.1	−1.8	2.0	3.6

surface of north and south slopes with a steepness of 10 and 20° and in a flat place. The data relate to several months of the warm season in the regions of Volgograd and Tashkent.

It is seen from this table that the temperature differences between the hill-sides increase with a decline in mean sun altitudes, and reach rather large values in spring and autumn.

It is evident that such data can be useful for an explanation of the effect of microclimate on vegetation cover under conditions of rugged relief.

It has already been mentioned that agrometeorologists use the values of air-temperature sums as the principal indicator of the thermal regime. Using the material on the temperature at the earth's surface obtained by the heat-balance method, we compare the sums of air temperatures exceeding 10° ($\sum T$) and the sums of active-surface temperatures (exceeding 10°) ($\sum T_w$) for the same period and at a number of points. The results of the comparison are given in Table 37.

TABLE 37

SUMS OF AIR TEMPERATURES ABOVE 10°C ($\sum T$) AND SUMS OF ACTIVE-SURFACE TEMPERATURES [ABOVE 10°C] ($\sum T_w$) IN THE SAME PERIOD

Region	$\sum T$	$\sum T_w$	Region	$\sum T$	$\sum T_w$
Murmansk	780	1090	Kiev	2600	2790
Arkhangel'sk	1250	1570	Voronezh	2630	3020
Leningrad	1820	2140	Poltava	2730	3060
Moscow	1990	2250	Emba	2980	3700
Gor'ky	2030	2300	Volgograd	3300	4060

The data show that the sums of temperatures at the earth's surface, which in all cases are greater than the sums of air temperatures, do not change in proportion to the latter.

The greatest relative discrepancy between the temperature sums at the earth's surface and in the air is observed in the extreme north (Murmansk). In eastern regions, the relative difference between the temperature sums increases slightly in comparison to western regions.

The great absolute differences between the temperatures of the earth's surface and the air and the great relative differences between the corresponding temperature sums in the Far North presumably indicate an important influence of the landscapes of these regions. It is well known that the characteristic feature of tundra vegetation is its dwarfed nature, which may be associated with a tendency to improve a thermal regime that is unfavorable for plant development.

It has frequently been pointed out in agrometeorological investigations (Davitaia, 1948; Selianinov, 1930) that the same temperature sum often turns out more effective for the development of vegetation in northern regions compared to southern ones, and in eastern regions of the USSR compared to western.

Such a regularity has been explained by the greater length of day in the north in summer, and by a more favorable diurnal temperature march in the east owing to the more continental character of its climate. Although we do not reject these fully trustworthy explanations, we believe that they only partially define the indicated differences in the effectiveness of the temperature sums. It is highly probable that a considerable part of the differences can be explained by the different relationships between the temperature sums of the earth's surface and the air in these regions. Thus, using material on the temperature of the earth's surface may prove to be important for specification of agrometeorological calculations. Such data may prove especially useful for an evaluation of peculiarities of the thermal conditions associated with the development of vegetation on hillsides.

In accordance with the data of this calculation, Table 38 shows the differences between the sums of the temperatures at the earth's surface on slopes and in a flat place for the period when air temperature was above 10° in the regions of Volgograd and Tashkent.

TABLE 38

DIFFERENCES BETWEEN THE SUMS OF THE EARTH'S SURFACE TEMPERATURES
ON SLOPES FROM THOSE ON LEVEL GROUND

Region	North slopes		South slopes	
	20°	10°	10°	20°
Volgograd	− 300	− 170	110	250
Tashkent	− 570	− 260	220	430

This table shows that comparatively steep north and south slopes are characterized by substantial differences between the temperature sums and, consequently, by substantial differences in the conditions of growth of agricultural and natural vegetation.

The above procedure for determining temperature at the earth's surface for evaluation of the thermal regime of plants has been used in a number of studies (Zubenok, et al., 1958; Mishchenko, 1962, 1965, 1966; "Микро-климат СССР (Microclimate of the USSR)," 1967; and others).

These studies have confirmed the good agreement between vegetation temperature measured by direct methods and temperature calculated from the heat balance at the earth's surface. Data in these investigations confirm the existence of great differences between the temperatures of plants and the air in many geographical regions in different weather conditions. Maps of the differences between the temperatures of the earth's surface and the air in the area of the USSR were drawn in the studies mentioned.

The paper of Davitaia and Mel'nik (1962), in which the question of the effect of radiative heating of the earth's surface on the location of the forest boundary was considered, is worthy of attention. The authors of this paper established the fact that the northern boundary of lowland forest corresponds to a summed air temperature above 10° approximately equal to 600–700°. At the same time, in mountain conditions, forest reaches altitudes with much lower air temperatures, whose sum for the vegetation period equals 200–300°.

Davitaia and Mel'nik suggested that this difference was determined by different conditions of radiative heating of plants in lowlands and mountains. To test this hypothesis, they carried out observations of plant-surface temperature in the region of the northern boundary of forest on the Kola Peninsula and in the zone of the upper boundary of forest in the mountains of the Caucasus. The observational data confirmed their hypothesis and showed that in both cases the boundary of forest corresponds to practically the same sum of temperatures of the vegetation surface.

Although in most bioclimatic investigations one may confine oneself to an evaluation of the mean temperature of the vegetation cover, in some cases there is interest in a more detailed study of the temperature distribution within the plant space. This question has been considered in some papers, in which the heat exchange in the layer of vegetation has been calculated for this purpose.

We will set forth the basic idea of the calculation according to material of an investigation along this line (Budyko and Gandin, 1968). If we average the meteorological parameters in the vegetation cover along the horizontal, then we can consider that the temperature T and the specific humidity q inside the vegetation depend only on the vertical coordinate z. In this situation, we can set the heat-balance equation for a thin layer dz within the vegetation cover in the form

$$dQ - dI = L\, dE + dP, \qquad (7.5)$$

(where Q is the total short-wave radiation, and I is the net long-wave radiation), wherefrom it follows that

$$\frac{dQ}{dz} - \frac{dI}{dz} = L\frac{dE}{dz} + \frac{dP}{dz}. \qquad (7.6)$$

In addition to this equation, the relations of the components of the heat balance to their determinant factors should be taken into account. These relations include these formulas:

1. for the turbulent flux of sensible heat,

$$P = -\rho c_p k \frac{dT}{dz};$$ (7.7)

2. for the turbulent flux of water vapor,

$$E = -\rho k \frac{dq}{dz}$$ (7.8)

(where k is the coefficient of turbulent exchange inside the foliage space);

3. for short-wave radiation,

$$\frac{dQ}{dz} = \gamma s Q$$ (7.9)

(where s is the specific surface of the leaves, that is, the leaf surface in a unit volume [leaf-area density], and γ is a coefficient of proportionality);

4. for the flux of long-wave radiation,

$$\frac{dI}{dz} = 4\delta\sigma T^3 \frac{dT_w}{dz}$$ (7.10)

(where T_w is plant temperature).

We must add to these equations the relations that connect the heat exchange and water exchange between the vegetation cover and the air in the foliage space with the differences of temperature and specific humidity at the leaf surfaces and in the air.

Simultaneous solution of the listed equations under the given boundary conditions permit us to obtain a nonlinear integral equation, which can be solved numerically. As a result, we obtain the values of plant temperature at different levels in the vegetation, as a function of a number of meteorological and biological parameters. The practical importance of such an investigation is limited by insufficient knowledge of some parameters that affect the results of calculation.

3. The Heat Regime of Animals and Man

The heat regime of animals, like that of plants, is closely connected with their heat balance. Contrary to plants, the heat regime of the animal's body may depend substantially on the level of metabolism, especially for homo-iothermal animals possessing heat regulation (Slonim, 1952, and elsewhere).

Since the principal physical regularities in the heat regime of animals and man coincide, we will first consider the problem of the heat regime of the human body.

In experimental investigations (Buettner, 1952; Burton and Edholm, 1955), it has been established that the mean temperature of the surface of the human body varies within rather wide limits (more than 20°), depending on the relationship between the components of the heat balance. Usually, this temperature differs noticeably from that of the internal organs (or from the temperature of the body as a whole), which is more stable than the tem-perature of the body surface. Different values of mean surface temperature correspond to different conditions of heat perception, that is, to a warm, a cold, or an intermediate state that is often called the zone of comfort. The most favorable state of heat sensation is usually observed at a mean tem-perature of the body surface near 33°. At a surface temperature below 29°, conditions of cold are felt, and at temperatures above 34–35°, excessive heat.

It should be noted that notwithstanding the existence of numerous investi-gations in this field, the methods that have been applied have not permitted us to answer the question about what heat sensation a person experiences in one or another region under the influence of the whole complex of meteoro-logical conditions, physiological factors, and given type of clothing.

To solve this problem, a method for calculating the heat balance of the human body (Budyko, 1958; Budyko and Tsitsenko, 1960; and others) has been applied in recent years.

Under conditions of a stationary regime, when the temperature of the human body changes little in time, the equation of heat balance of the human body has the form

$$R + M = LE + P, \tag{7.11}$$

where R is the radiation balance at the surface of the body, LE is the con-version of heat for evaporation, P is the turbulent sensible-heat flux from the body surface to the atmosphere, and M is the heat production, which is determined on the average by the quantity and calorific value of food assimilated during a given period of time. Equation (7.11) does not include components that are small compared to the values of the principal components of the balance. Among these we should mention the heat loss owing to res-piration, which can amount to noticeable values at low air temperatures.

In order to consider the thermally insulating effect of clothing on the heat balance, we must make up a balance equation for the outer body surface of a clothed man and an equation for the outer surface of his clothing. The first of the equations can be presented in the form

$$M = LE' + P', \tag{7.12}$$

in which we assume the evaporation E' and the turbulent sensible-heat flux P' equal to

$$E' = \rho D'(q_s - q_x)a \tag{7.13}$$

and

$$P' = \rho c_p D'(T_s - T_x), \tag{7.14}$$

where D' is the coefficient characterizing the heat conductivity of the clothing, q_s is the saturation specific humidity at the temperature of the body surface, q_x and T_x are the mean specific humidity and temperature of the air at the level of the outer surface of the clothing, T_s is the mean temperature of the body surface, and a is a coefficient equal to the ratio of the rate of evaporation from the body surface to the rate of evaporation from a wet surface under the same conditions.

Let us express the heat-balance equation at the outer surface of the clothing as follows:

$$R_0 + \rho c_p D'(T_s - T_x) = (\rho c_p D + 4\delta\sigma T^3)(T_x - T). \tag{7.15}$$

In this equation R_0 designates the radiation balance at the clothing surface, calculated on the assumption that its temperature is equal to that of the environment. This value is added to the heat flux received at the outer surface of the clothing from the body, equal to $\rho c_p D'(T_s - T_x)$. The right-hand part of the equation expresses the heat loss from the clothing surface, which represents the sum of the sensible-heat flux $\rho c_p D(T_x - T)$ and the radiative flux $4\delta\sigma T^3(T_x - T)$, D designating the integral coefficient of turbulent diffusion. Equation (7.15) does not include the value of evaporation, since water vapor is not generated on the clothing surface.

We must add to Eqs. (7.12–7.15) a formula that expresses the fact that the flux of water vapor passing through the clothing surface does not change in value. We present this regularity in the form

$$\rho D'(q_s - q_x)a = \rho D(q_x - q)a, \tag{7.16}$$

where q is the specific humidity of the surrounding air. From Eqs. (7.12–7.16), we obtain the relationship

$$R_0 + M\left[1 + \frac{\rho c_p D + 4\delta\sigma T^3}{\rho c_p D'}\right] = L\rho D(q_s - q)a\left[1 + \frac{4\delta\sigma T^3}{\rho c_p(D + D')}\right]$$
$$+ (\rho c_p D + 4\delta\sigma T^3)(T_s - T). \tag{7.17}$$

Equation (7.17) permits us to calculate the value of T_s, that is, the mean temperature of the surface of the body, in relation to the meteorological parameters R_0, T, q, and D; the physiological characteristics M and a; and the parameter D', characterizing properties of the clothing. In this calculation, we take account of the known dependence of q_s on T_s expressed by the vapor-pressure formula or the psychrometric table.

Having made such a calculation, we can evaluate the heat sensation of a clothed man under various climatic conditions and also determine the comparative effect of different factors on heat sensation.

Equation (7.17) is simplified if it is applied to calculate the heat regime of a man whose clothing does not have a heat-insulating effect. In such a case, one assumes that $1/D' = 0$, which corresponds to an infinitely great heat conductivity of the clothing. We obtain the formula

$$R_0 + M = L\rho D(q_s - q)a + (\rho c_p D + 4\delta\sigma T^3)(T_s - T). \qquad (7.18)$$

An equation similar to Eq. (7.18) was found in the work of Büttner (1938), who used it for evaluation of the effect of individual factors on the heat perception of man.

Application of Eqs. (7.17) and (7.18) to calculate the thermal regime of the human body under different natural conditions involves some difficulties, among which the determination of the radiation balance R_0 must be especially noted. Now, thanks to the availability of mass data on the radiation regime, this task becomes simplified and can be approximately solved as follows.

If we assume that the human body in a vertical position has a form approximately corresponding to that of a relatively thin vertical cylinder, the calculation of the value R_0 in this case becomes much simplified.

From simple geometrical considerations, we obtain the relation that on a unit area of the lateral surface of the vertical cylinder falls a quantity of direct solar radiation equal to $S \cot h/\pi$, where S is the sum of direct radiation incident on a unit area of a horizontal surface, and h is the angular altitude of the sun. The amount of scattered radiation from the sky incident on a unit area of the cylinder's surface is approximately equal to half the scattered radiation Q' incident on a horizontal element of the surface. The income of radiation reflected from the earth's surface and approximately equal to $\frac{1}{2}(S + Q')\alpha$, where α is the albedo of the earth's surface, is added to this value.

Net long-wave radiation at the unit area of the cylinder's surface is equal to half of the net long-wave radiation at a horizontal surface I_0. To this is added the algebraic sum of two terms expressing the effect on net long-wave radiation of the difference between the temperatures of the cylinder surface and the air, and the difference between the temperatures of the cylinder surface and the earth's surface.

The first of these equals $\frac{1}{2}\delta\sigma(T_s^4 - T^4)$, and the second, $\frac{1}{2}\delta\sigma(T_s^4 - T_w^4)$, where T_w is the temperature of the earth's surface. Their sum is approximately equal to $4\delta\sigma T^3(T_s - T) - 2\delta\sigma T^3(T_w - T)$. The first of these components has been already included in the heat-balance equation.

Taking this into account, we obtain the following formula:

$$R_0 = \left[S\frac{\cot h}{\pi} + \frac{1}{2}Q' + \frac{1}{2}(S + Q')\alpha \right](1 - \alpha_0) - \frac{1}{2}I_0 + 2\delta\sigma T^3(T_w - T),$$

$$(7.19)$$

where α_0 is the reflectivity (albedo) of the surface of the human body.

In deriving Eq. (7.19), among other simplifying assumptions, we adopted a hypothesis on the isotropy of the fluxes of scattered radiation and long-wave emission incident on the cylinder surface. Evaluations that have been made show that considerations of anisotropy of these fluxes affect the results of calculating the thermal regime of the human body very little.

To determine the values of S, Q', and I_0 in Eq. (7.19), one can use observational material and calculation methods. The value of $T_w - T$ can be calculated by the method set forth in the previous section.

If we substitute the value R_0 into Eqs. (7.17) and (7.18), we will obtain the following:

$$\left[S\frac{\cot h}{\pi} + \frac{1}{2}Q' + \frac{1}{2}(S + Q')\alpha \right](1 - \alpha_0) - \frac{I_0}{2} + 2\delta\sigma T^3(T_w - T) + M$$

$$= L\rho D(q_s - q)a + (\rho c_p D + 4\delta\sigma T^3)(T_s - T). \qquad (7.20)$$

$$\left[S\frac{\cot h}{\pi} + \frac{1}{2}Q' + \frac{1}{2}(S + Q')\alpha \right](1 - \alpha_0) - \frac{I_0}{2}$$

$$+ 2\delta\sigma T^3(T_w - T) + M\left[1 + \frac{\rho c_p D + 4\delta\sigma T^3}{\rho c_p D'} \right]$$

$$= L\rho D(q_s - q)a\left[1 + \frac{4\delta\sigma T^3}{\rho c_p(D + D')} \right] + (\rho c_p D + 4\delta\sigma T^3)(T_s - T). \quad (7.21)$$

To solve Eq. (7.20) or (7.21), it is necessary to determine the physiological parameters they contain, namely, heat production M and the characteristic of the evaporation condition a.

According to data of a series of investigations, the heat production of a person in a state of rest and in conditions of thermal comfort is more or less stable and approximately equal to 40–50 kcal m^{-2} hr^{-1} (that is, 1.1×10^{-3} to 1.4×10^{-3} cal cm^{-2} sec^{-1}).

The data of the work of Winslow et al. (1937a) permit us to clarify the relationship between heat production and the mean temperature of the body surface.

Figure 112 demonstrates the dependence of heat production M on mean temperature of the body surface T_s, constructed on the basis of experimental data contained in the paper mentioned. It is seen from the graph that

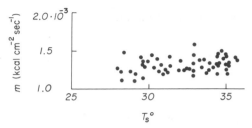

Fig. 112   Dependence of heat production on the temperature of the body surface.

heat production of a man not engaged in physical work depends relatively little on the temperature of the body surface in the interval corresponding to the zone of comfort. The mean value of heat production turns out approximately equal to 1.3×10^{-3} cal cm^{-2} sec^{-1}, which corresponds to the evaluations noted earlier.

The question about determination of the conditions of evaporation from the body surface can be solved with the use of the material from another paper by Winslow *et al.* (1937b). On the basis of experimental data from this research, a graph, presented in Fig. 113, has been constructed. It shows the dependence of the coefficient *a* on the temperature of the body surface. It should be noted that, unlike heat production, the parameter *a* changes rather markedly, even in a comparatively narrow range of body-surface temperature. Such a change corresponds to differences in the activity of the sweat secretion system, which is an important regulator of man's thermal regime. At a body temperature above 35°, the dependence of *a* on T_s becomes nonsingular, which is presumably associated with disruption of the stationary thermal state of the human body under conditions of overheating.

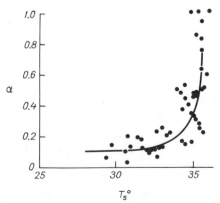

Fig. 113   Dependence of evaporation conditions on the temperature of the body surface.

A comparison of Figs. 112 and 113 shows that within the range of temperatures of the body surface from 29 to 35°, a change in the rate of evaporation from the surface proves to be a more substantial factor in human heat regulation than the change in heat production.

It is evident that in solving Eqs. (7.20) and (7.21), one must consider the dependence of the coefficient a on the temperature of the surface of the body. This can be done by the use of Table 39, comprising data from Fig. 113.

TABLE 39

DEPENDENCE OF THE COEFFICIENT a ON THE
TEMPERATURE OF THE BODY SURFACE T_s

T_s	29°	30°	31°	32°	33°	34°	35°
a	0.10	0.11	0.11	0.12	0.13	0.18	0.31

With the use of Eqs. (7.20) and (7.21), one can calculate the mean temperature of the surface of the human body, which defines its thermal condition. In some investigations, the results of such calculations have been compared to data from direct measurements of body temperature (Efimova and Tsitsenko, 1963; Kandror et al., 1966; and elsewhere).

Experimental investigations carried out in different climatic zones of the USSR have shown that at positive air temperatures, there usually exists good agreement between the measured and calculated values of the mean temperature of the body surface. At negative air temperatures, the correlation between the measured and calculated values decreases, which is presumably associated with the difficulty of achieving a stationary state of the human body under such conditions.

The latter conclusion does not interfere with the possibility of using calculated temperatures of the human body at low temperatures as a general characteristic of the degree of severity of a climate.

Equations (7.20) and (7.21) can be used to calculate the thermal state of the human body under specific climatic conditions. As an example, we present here the results of such calculations for the territory of the European USSR for mean conditions of July at 1300 hours [1:00 p.m.] (Budyko and Tsitsenko, 1960). The values of meteorological parameters necessary for the calculation were determined in the following way.

Total short-wave radiation incident on a unit-area horizontal surface at different hours of the day was calculated by the model developed by Biriukova (1956). To determine the values of direct and scattered radiation, data of total solar radiation were used, along with the latitudinal relation of the ratio of direct to total radiation given in Fig. 114. This relation was constructed

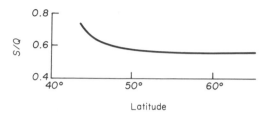

Latitude

Fig. 114 Latitudinal dependence of the ratio of direct radiation to total solar radiation.

from data of actinometric observations at 1300 hours in the summer months (May to August) at a number of stations in the European USSR.

The albedo of the surface of the human body, in accordance with available evaluations, was assumed equal to 0.30 (Büttner, 1938). The albedo of the surface of clothing can vary within wide limits, depending on its color. For the given calculation, an albedo value equal to 0.30 was used. Net long-wave radiation I_0 and the value $T_w - T$ were determined by the methods set forth in previous sections of this book.

To calculate the integral coefficient of diffusion D, we used the formula

$$D = m\sqrt{u}, \qquad (7.22)$$

(where u is wind speed in meters per second and m is a coefficient approximately equal to 0.7 if D is expressed in centimeters per second). This formula was obtained as a result of experimental investigations (Buettner, 1952) of the heat exchange between a standing man and the surrounding air. (It should be noted that later investigations provide slightly greater values of the coefficient m, close to 1.0).

Climatic data show that in the European USSR during daytime in summer, the mean wind speed changes comparatively little, and at anemometer height it usually equals 4–5 m sec^{-1}. With the use of a logarithmic formula for the change of wind speed with height, we can establish that under these conditions, the mean wind speed at a height of 1 m is approximately equal to 2 m sec^{-1}.

The coefficient D in this calculation can thus be considered approximately equal to 1 cm sec^{-1}. It is interesting to note that this value is close to the mean values of this coefficient for the earth's surface under similar conditions,

The coefficient D', characterizing the heat-insulation properties of clothing. should obviously change within wide limits depending on the type of clothing.

Using Eq. (7.21), we can calculate what values of coefficient D' correspond to clothing that ensures thermal comfort under common room conditions or under mean conditions of a summer day in a continental climate of the middle latitudes. Such a calculation shows that the appropriate values of the coefficient D' are of the order of several tenths of one centimeter per second. In this calculation, its mean value was considered equal to 0.4 cm sec^{-1}. To determine the coefficient a, the table given above was used, and the value of heat production M was taken as equal to 1.3×10^{-3} cal cm^{-2} sec^{-1}.

The solutions of Eqs. (7.20) and (7.21) were found graphically, since the relations $a(T_s)$ and $q_s(T_s)$ considered in them are given by tabular aids.

As a result of calculation, maps of the mean temperature of the surface of the human body protected and unprotected by clothing at 1300 hours in different months of the warm season were drawn. Figures 115 and 116 show

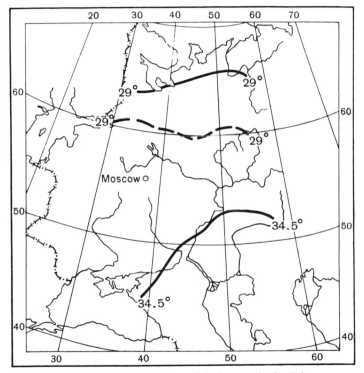

Fig. 115   Thermal state of the human body. July.

the pertinent maps for July and May. They present isolines of the mean temperature of the body surface for 29 and 34.5°.

It has already been pointed out that it can be assumed that at temperatures below 29°, conditions of heat deficiency are observed, and at temperatures above 34.5°, those of heat excess.

The data relating to a man in light clothing are shown by solid lines, those relating to a man without clothing by a broken line.

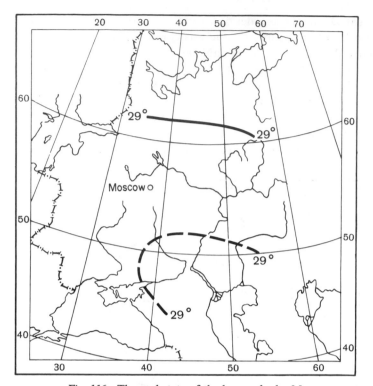

Fig. 116 Thermal state of the human body. May.

It is apparent from the first map that in July, the zone of a favorable thermal regime for a man in light clothes extends over the greater part of the European USSR. Only in the extreme north are conditions of heat deficiency observed, and in the northern Caucasus and in lower Povol'zh'ie an area with excessively warm conditions is marked out. In the absence of the heat-insulating effect of clothing, the heat-perception regime changes. North of 60°, insufficiently warm conditions occur, while no area of excess heat is observed in the territory under consideration.

A slightly different picture is observed in May (Fig. 116). In this case, conditions of heat excess are not observed at all. Heat conditions favorable for a man in light clothes are outlined in the central and southern regions, while for a man unprotected by clothing, favorable conditions are found only in the extreme southeast.

Such calculations can be used for determining the thermal efficiency of different kinds of clothing under one or another climatic condition and also for evaluating the possibility of using such practices as sunbathing, air-bathing, and so on.

Calculations by Eqs. (7.20) and (7.21) also permit evaluating the comparative effect of different factors on the thermal state of man under actual climatic conditions.

Thus, in particular, it can be established that on a summer day, the chief heat source for man is not his own heat production but the income of short-wave radiation. For mean conditions of the European USSR in this situation, heat production makes up 25–30% and the income of radiative heat 70–75% of the total income of energy.

The relative value of different forms of heat outgo changes considerably, depending on external conditions. At high temperatures, heat conversion for evaporation becomes a principal form of heat outgo, which is obviously associated with the activity of the sweat-secretion system. In the far southeast of the European USSR, the values of heat outgo for evaporation amount to 75–80% of the total heat outgo. At lower temperatures, the relative role of heat conversion in evaporation decreases sharply, reaching 20–25%, and even smaller values. In this case, the turbulent flux of sensible heat, amounting to 50–60%, becomes the principal form of heat outgo. Heat loss in the form of net long-wave radiation has a smaller value in all cases, varying within limits of 5–20% of the total heat outgo.

If we evaluate the effect of different meteorological factors on the heat state of man with use of Eqs. (7.20) and (7.21), it becomes clear that under the climatic conditions of the European USSR in summer considered above, changes in air temperature, solar radiation, and wind speed have considerable importance. Fluctuations in humidity affect the heat regime of the human body relatively little.

The above procedure for calculating the characteristics of the thermal state of the human body has been used in various bioclimatic investigations, among which we should mention the papers of Liopo (1966, 1968, and elsewhere). In these papers, a nomogram was constructed that permitted the calculation of the characteristics of the human thermal regime as a function of meteorological conditions and physiological factors. Along with this, Liopo used computers for calculating the characteristics of the thermal regime, which enabled her to study the variability of man's thermal state under various weather–climatic conditions.

In the papers of Liopo, Tsitsenko (1963, and others), Aizenschtat (1965, and others), and other authors, data were obtained characterizing both the mean conditions of the thermal state of man in different regions of the USSR and the temporal variability of these conditions.

We note that the procedure under consideration can be applied with some modifications to study the heat regime of both poikilothermal and homoiothermal animals. In such studies, one should first carry out a calculation of the radiation regime of the body of the animal with consideration of its form.

It is evident that, as for the human body, this form can be presented in an approximation as a simple geometrical model. An albedo value relating to the surface of the animal's body, necessary for determining absorbed radiation, should be found experimentally.

Conditions of evaporation from the surface of the animal's body must then be taken into account. For many animals (for example, reptiles), evaporation is insignificant, which permits considering the coefficient a in the above formulas as equal to zero. In cases when heat outgo for evaporation from the animal's body is comparable in size with the other heat-balance components, the value of coefficient a should be determined from empirical data.

If the animal under consideration has a coat of hair, then its effect on the thermal regime can be evaluated similarly to the consideration of the effect of clothing on the human thermal regime. For this purpose, employing experimental data, one must evaluate the magnitude of the coefficient D', which in such conditions characterizes the heat conductivity of a coat of hair. Without any hair, the value $1/D'$ equals zero.

The appropriate value of heat production for poikilothermal organisms can be often considered close to zero, and for homoiothermal animals should be determined from experimental data depending on the level of the animal's activity.

It is apparent from the considerations presented here that a calculation of the heat balance and an evaluation of the thermal state of the body of an animal is, in the main, no more complicated than a similar calculation for man. However, it must be noted that such calculations are sometimes impeded by the absence of the necessary experimental data.

It follows from calculated material on the thermal regime of poikilothermal animals (Budyko, 1959) that the temperature of their bodies can exceed air temperature by 10–20 C° and more, if they are heated by the sun's rays, especially when evaporation from their bodies is small. At night, the temperature of poikilothermal animals can be less than air temperature by approximately 5–7 C°.

The body-surface temperature of homoiothermal animals that depend substantially on heat regulation is less variable. Nevertheless, the influence of meteorological conditions on their thermal regime is very important. An approximate idea of the quantitative regularities of this influence can be obtained from the above data on the thermal state of the human body.

Among the studies of the thermal state of homoiothermal animals, the monograph by Iaroshevskii (1968) is worthy of mention. In studying the heat balance of sheep, Iaroshevskii established that the heat conversion for evaporation from the sheep's body increases noticeably with an increase in body surface temperature. An important role in the heat exchange of sheep is played by the outgo of latent heat in respiration, which in young animals can amount to a half of the total heat loss.

The state of the sheep's fleece, namely, its length, thickness and degree of soiling, affects thermal regime greatly. By varying body position, sheep can noticeably change their thermal state. Thus, at low air temperatures, sheep cluster in tight groups or lie down on the ground, which diminishes the heat loss from the animal's body.

Iaroshevskii pointed out that the thermal regime exerts a great influence on the biological activity of sheep and in many cases restricts their productivity considerably. It can be considered that the conclusions resulting from Iaroshevskii's experiments on sheep are in many respects true for other mammals, the regularities of whose thermal regimes have not yet been investigated.

REFERENCES

Айзенштат Б. А. (1965). Метод расчета и результаты определений некоторых биоклиматических характеристик. Труды САНИГМИ, вып. 22 (37).

Aizenshtat, B. A. (1965). Calculation methods and results of determination of certain bioclimatic characteristics. *Tr. Tashkent. Sredneaziatskii Nauch. Issled. Gidrometeorol. Inst.* **22**, 3–41. MGA 17.4-74.

Бирюкова Л. А. (1956). О методике климатического расчета суточного хода суммарной и поглощенной радиации. Труды ГГО, вып. 66.

Biriukova, L. A. (1956). A climatological method of calculating the daily march of incoming and absorbed solar radiation. *Tr. Gl. Geofiz. Observ.* **66**, 33–36. MGA 10:1619.

Будыко М. И. (1956). Тепловой баланс земной поверхности. Гидрометеоиздат, Л.

Budyko, M. I. (1956). "Teplovoi Balans Zemnoi Poverkhnosti." Gidrometeoizdat, Leningrad; "Heat Balance of the Earth's Surface," translated by N. A. Stepanova. U.S. Weather Bur., Washington, D.C., 1958. MGA 8.5-20, 13E-286.

Будыко М. И. (1958). Температура деятельной поверхности и ее биоклиматическое значение. Сб. «Современные проблемы метеорологии приземного слоя воздуха». Гидрометеоиздат, Л.

Budyko, M. I. (1958). Temperature of the active surface and its bioclimatic significance. *In* "Sovremennye Problemy Meteorologii Prizemnogo Sloia vozdukha (Contemporary Problems of the Meteorology of the Layer of Air Near the Ground)," pp. 201–211. Gidrometeoizdat, Leningrad; U.S. Weather Bur., WB/T No. 19. U.S. Weather Bur., Washington, D.C., 1960. MGA 14.5-100.

Будыко М. И. (1959). О тепловом балансе живых организмов. Изв. АН СССР, сер. геогр., № 1.

Budyko, M. I. (1959). The heat balance of living organisms. *Izv. Akad. Nauk SSSR Ser. Geogr.*, No. 1, 29–35. MGA 14.5-712.

Будыко М. И., Гандин Л. С. (1968). К теории теплового режима растительного покрова. Труды ГГО, вып. 229.

Budyko, M. I., and Gandin, L. S. (1968). Theory of the thermal regime of plant cover. *Tr. Gl. Geofiz. Observ.* **229**, 4–6. MGA 20.5-490.

Будыко М. И., Циценко Г. В. (1960). Климатические факторы теплоощущения человека. Изв. АН СССР, сер. геогр., № 3.

Budyko, M. I., and Tsitsenko, G. V. (1960). Climatic factors of the thermal sensitivity of man. *Izv. Akad. Nauk SSSR Ser. Geogr.* No. 3, 3–11; U.S. Weather Bur., WB/T No. 92. U.S. Weather Bur., Washington, D.C., 1962. MGA 14.5-711.

Веселовский К. С. (1857). О климате России. Изд. АН, СПб.

Veselovskii, K. S. (1857). "O Klimate Rossii (On the Climate of Russia)." Izdat. Akad. Nauk, St. Peterburg.

Давитая Ф. Ф. (1948). Климатические зоны винограда в СССР. Пищепромиздат, М.

Davitaia, F. F. (1948). "Klimaticheskie Zony Vinograda v SSSR (Climatic Zones of Grapes in the USSR)." Pishchepromizdat, Moscow.

Давитая Ф. Ф., Мельник Ю. С. (1962). Радиационный нагрев деятельной поверхности и границы леса. Метеорология и гидрология, № 1.

Davitaia, F. F., and Mel'nik, IU. S. (1962). Radiative heating of the active surface and the timberline. *Meteorol. Gidrol.* No. 1, 3–9. MGA 13.9-94.

Ефимова Н. А., Циценко Г. В. (1963). Сравнение экспериментального и расчетного методов определения температуры поверхности тела. Труды ГГО, вып. 139.

Efimova, N. A., and Tsitsenko, G. V. (1963). Comparison of experimental and computational methods for determining the temperature of the surface of the body. *Tr. Gl. Geofiz. Observ.* **139**, 115–121.

Зубенок Л. И., Ефимова Н. А., Мухенберг В. В. (1958). Материалы к климатическому районированию СССР. Труды ГГО, вып. 76.

Zubenok, L. I., Efimova, N. A., and Mukhenberg, V. V. (1958). Data for climatic regionalization of the USSR. *Tr. Gl. Geofiz. Observ.* **76**, 98–112. MGA 10:807; *In* "Problems of Dynamic Meteorology and Climatic Theory" (Trans. of vyp. 76), pp. 151–171, Amer. Meteorol. Soc., Boston, Massachusetts, 1961. MGA 13:1447.

Кандрор И. С., Demina D. M., Ratner, E. M., Evlampieva, M. N., and Murav'eva, G. J. (1966). Экспериментальная проверка применимости уравнения теплового баланса М. И. Будыко и Г. В. Циценко для определения теплового состояния человека в натурных условиях. Гигиена и санитария, № 3.

Kandror, I. S., *et al.* (1966). Experimental verification of the applicability of the heat-balance equation of M. I. Budyko and G. V. Tsitsenko for the determination of the thermal state of man in natural conditions. *Gig. Sanit.* **31**, No. 3. Transl. in *Hygiene and Sanitation*, **31**, No. 3, 352–358, 1966.

Лиопо Т. Н. (1966). Статистические вероятностные методы медико-географической оценки климата. Сб. «Итоги и перспективы внедрения новых методов географических исследований». Иркутск.

Liopo, T. N. (1966). Statistical probability methods for medico-geographical evaluation of climate. *In* "Itogi i Perspektivy Vnedreniia Novykh Metodov Geograficheskikh Issledovanii (Tasks and Prospects of Inculcating New Methods of Geographic Investigation)." Irkutsk.

Лиопо Т. Н. (1968). Номограмма для определения характеристик теплозащитных свойств одежды, обеспечивающей тепловой комфорт. Труды ГГО, вып. 233.

Liopo, T. N. (1968). A nomogram for determining characteristics of the thermally protective properties of clothing insuring thermal comfort. *Tr. Gl. Geofiz. Observ.* **233**, 156–160. MGA 20.6-66.

Микроклимат СССР. (1967). Под ред. И. А. Гольцберг. Гидрометеоиздат, Л.

"Mikroklimat SSSR" (I. A. Gol'tsberg, ed.). Gidrometeoizdat, Leningrad, 1967. MGA 19.9-13; "Microclimate of the USSR." Isr. Program Sci. Transl., Jerusalem, 1969. MGA 20.10-1.

Мищенко З. А. (1962). Суточный ход температуры воздуха и его агроклиматическое значение. Гидрометеоиздат, Л.

Mishchenko, Z. A. (1962). "Sutochnyi Khod Temperatury Vozdukha i Ego Agroklimaticheskoe Znachenie (The Daily March of Air Temperature and Its Agroclimatic Significance)." Gidrometeoizdat, Leningrad. MGA 14.12-20.

Мищенко З. А. (1965). О темпсратуре деятельной поверхности в микроклиматических исследованиях. Труды ГГО, вып. 180.

Mishchenko, Z. A. (1965). Temperature of the active surface in microclimatic investigations. *Tr. Gl. Geofiz. Observ.* **180**, 58–76. MGA 17.6-316.

Мищенко З. А. (1966). О тепловом балансе и температуре растений. Труды ГГО, вып. 190.

Mishchenko, Z. A. (1966). The heat balance and temperature of plants. *Tr. Gl. Geofiz. Observ.* **190**, 41–57. MGA 18.1-236; *Can. Meteorol. Branch Meteorol. Transl.* **No. 13**, 53–73 (1968). MGA 20.3-357.

Селянинов Г. Т. (1930). К методике сельскохозяйственной климатологии. Труды по с.-х. метеорол., вып. 22, № 2.

Selianinov, G. T. (1930). On the methodology of agricultural climatology. *Tr. Sel'skokhoz. Meteorol.* **22**, No. 2.

Слоним А. Д. (1952). Животная теплота и ее регуляция в организме млекопитающих. Изд. АН, М.—Л.

Slonim, A. D. (1952). 'Zhivotnaia Teplota i Ee Reguliatsiia v Organisme Mlekopitaiushchikh (The Heat of Life and Its Regulation in Mammals)." Izdat. Akad. Nauk, Moscow and Leningrad.

Циценко Г. В. (1963). Методика расчета температуры поверхности тела человека на основании уравнения теплового баланса. Труды ГГО, вып. 139.

Tsitsenko, G. V. (1963). Methods for calculating the surface temperature of the human body on the basis of the heat-balance equation. *Tr. Gl. Geofiz. Observ.* **139**, 108–114.

Ярошевский В. А. (1968). Погода и тонкорунное овцеводство. Гидрометеоиздат, Л.

Iaroshevskii, V. A. (1968). "Pogoda i Tonkorunnoe Ovtsevodstvo (Weather and Fine-Wool Sheep Breeding)." Gidrometeoizdat, Leningrad.

Burton, A. C., and Edholm, O. G. (1955). "Man in a Cold Environment." Edward Arnold, London. (Русский перевод: Бартон, Эдхолм. Человек в условиях холода. ИЛ, М., 1957.)

Büttner, K. (1938). "Physikalische Bioklimatologie." Akad. Verlagsges., Leipzig.

Buettner, K. (1952). Physical aspects of human bioclimatology. *Compendium Meteorol.* (T. F. Malone, ed.), 2d Printing, Am. Meteorol. Soc., Boston, 1112–1125.

de Candolle, A. (1874). Géographie botanique raisonée. Arch. sci. bibl. univ. de Genève, Geneva.

Winslow, C. E. A., Herrington, L. P., and Gagge, A. (1937a). Physiological reactions of the human body to varying environmental temperatures. *Amer. J. Physiol.* **120**, No. 1.

Winslow, C. E. A., Herrington, L. P., and Gagge, A. (1937b). Physiological reactions of the human body to various atmospheric humidities. *Amer. J. Physiol.* **120**, No. 2.

VIII

Climatic Factors of Photosynthesis

1. The Physical Mechanism of Photosynthesis

In nature, organic matter appears as a result of the activity of autotrophic plants, which are the only group of organisms capable of synthesizing organic matter from mineral. Of the two ways of creating organic matter, based on utilization of radiative energy (photosynthesis) and chemical energy (chemosynthesis), only the first is important for the general level of biomass production, because chemosynthesis, which is very significant for the circulation of nitrogen and other processes, yields a relatively negligible quantity of organic matter. In order to build organic matter, photosynthesizing plants use carbon dioxide from the air,* water, and a small amount (compared to the general mass of synthesizing matter) of the mineral substances of the soil. A certain part of the energy of incoming short-wave solar radiation is converted for photosynthesis in vegetation cover.

The basic content of the total photosynthetic reaction can be expressed in a simplified way in the equation

$$6CO_2 + 6H_2O = C_6H_{12}O_6 + 6O_2$$

In numerous experimental investigations, it has been established that the "coefficient of useful activity" of photosynthesizing vegetation (that is, the ratio of the heat converted in synthesizing biomass to the general amount of incoming solar energy) is very small and usually does not exceed 0.1–1%

---

* Besides the carbon dioxide of the air, plants can also obtain a certain quantity of carbon dioxide from the soil. However, the first source has the fundamental place.

(see Section 3 of this chapter). Under favorable conditions, the coefficient increases up to several per cent (Vinberg, 1948; Nichiporovich, 1963, and elsewhere).

At the same time, it should be indicated that according to the extensive available experimental material, vegetation also expends water resources rather uneconomically. The productivity of transpiration (the ratio of the increase in the weight of the dry mass of the plant to the water expended in transpiration in a given interval of time) usually has a value from $\frac{1}{200}$ to $\frac{1}{1000}$ (most often about $\frac{1}{300}$). For this reason, the opinion exists that such copious transpiration does not correspond to physiological needs of the plant and is, to a considerable extent, a waste of water (Maksimov, 1926, 1944, and elsewhere).

These two fundamental facts indicate that in natural conditions, vegetation assimilates only a small part of the available energy and water resources. It is evident that for investigation of the question of the relation of plant productivity to climatic factors, it is very important to clarify the causes that so greatly restrict the utilization of natural resources in the synthesis of biomass.

For this purpose, we turn to an analysis of the physical mechanism of carbon-dioxide assimilation and transpiration (Budyko, 1949, 1956).

The assimilation organ of a photosynthesizing plant—a leaf—represents a case made of thick cuticular tissue pierced by numerous small openings, stomata, which can open and close. The case encloses a very large surface of chloroplasts containing grains of chlorophyll. The surface of the chloroplasts communicates with the atmospheric air through intercellular spaces and the stomata.

It is essential for the development of photosynthesis that the surface of the chloroplasts should be maintained in a wet state, since carbon dioxide can be assimilated only in dissolved form. For this reason, the relative humidity of the air in the intercellular spaces is high and usually far exceeds the relative humidity in the atmosphere. Diffusion of carbon dioxide into a leaf with open stomata is inevitably accompanied by diffusion in the opposite direction of water vapor, that is, transpiration.

If a vegetation cover is sufficiently closed, then for the layer containing the plants we can set up a heat-balance equation in the form

$$R = LE + P + lA, \tag{8.1}$$

where R is the radiation balance, E is the evaporation (transpiration), L is the latent heat of vaporization, P is the sensible-heat flux from the earth's surface to the atmosphere, A is the assimilation, and l is the heat converted in assimilation of a unit mass of CO_2.

In Eq. (8.1), together with other small components of the heat balance, the heat exchange between the earth's surface and the underlying layers of soil is neglected. In this case such neglect is possible, since the heat inflow into the soil during the warm season is usually considerably less than the basic components of the heat balance.

Considering that for a sufficiently dense vegetation cover, evaporation is essentially determined by the process of transpiration, we will point out the following important fact. The three components comprising the right-hand part of Eq. (8.1), namely, evaporation, sensible-heat flux, and assimilation, depend on diffusion processes having similar mechanisms.

In plant transpiration, water vapor diffuses from the moist walls of the inner leaf surface to its outer surface through the intercellular spaces and stomata, the concentration of water vapor varying from q_s (the mean concentration in the air at the internal surface of the leaf) to q_0 (the mean concentration at the outer leaf surface).

The evaporation rate will be equal to

$$E = \rho D'(q_s - q_0), \tag{8.2}$$

where ρ is the air density, and D' is the integral coefficient of diffusion for water vapor on the path from the inner to the outer leaf surface. It is evident that the value D' depends on the morphology of the leaf (the number and size of stomata, the thickness of the leaf, the density of the cuticle, and so on).

The second stage of water-vapor diffusion is associated with the change in water-vapor concentration from q_0 (on the leaf surface) to q, the concentration outside the vegetation layer. For this stage, we can write the equation

$$E = \rho D''(q_0 - q), \tag{8.3}$$

where D'' is the integral coefficient of external diffusion, depending mainly on the intensity of turbulent exchange.

Excluding q_0 from Eqs. (8.2) and (8.3), we obtain

$$E = \frac{\rho(q_s - q)}{(1/D') + (1/D'')}. \tag{8.4}$$

The diffusion of carbon dioxide from the air outside the vegetation cover to the absorbing surfaces inside the leaf can also be divided into two stages.

On the one hand, the diffusion rate (equal to the rate of assimilation) equals

$$A = \rho D_c'(c_0 - c_1), \tag{8.5}$$

where D_c' is the effective coefficient of diffusion through the intercellular channels and stomata for carbon dioxide on the path from the outer leaf surface to the surface of the parenchyma, c_0 is the mean concentration of carbon dioxide in the air at the outer leaf surface, and c_1 is the mean concentration of carbon dioxide in the air at the surface of the parenchymal cells.

On the other hand, the assimilation rate equals

$$A = \rho D_c''(c - c_0), \tag{8.6}$$

where c is the concentration of carbon dioxide outside the vegetation, and D_c'' is a quantity analogous to D''.

From Eqs. (8.5) and (8.6), it follows that

$$A = \frac{\rho(c - c_1)}{(1/D_c') + (1/D_c'')}. \tag{8.7}$$

The ratio between the rate of assimilation and the rate of evaporation from Eqs. (8.4) and (8.7) equals

$$\frac{A}{E} = a \frac{c - c_1}{q_s - q}, \tag{8.8}$$

in which it should be noted that the coefficient of proportionality a comprised in the formula

$$a = \frac{D_c' D_c''(D' + D'')}{D' D''(D_c' + D_c'')}$$

can change only within very narrow limits. Since the process of diffusion of water vapor and of carbon dioxide between the outer leaf surface and the free-flowing air is determined by turbulent mixing, then it is evident that coefficients D'' and D_c'' possess the same values. It is natural to consider that the diffusion of water vapor and carbon dioxide between the walls of the parenchyma and the outer leaf surface has a molecular character. In this case, the ratio D_c'/D' must be equal to the ratio of the coefficient of molecular diffusion of carbon dioxide in air to the coefficient of molecular diffusion of water vapor in air, that is, approximately 0.64.

Taking this into consideration, we can infer that, depending on the relationship between the values of D' and D'', the coefficient a can vary only from 0.64 to 1, approaching unity when external diffusion has the leading role (a thin leaf with mostly open stomata), and reducing to 0.64 when internal diffusion has the leading role (a thick leaf with poor ventilation). If we assume that under average conditions the rate of evaporation from the leaf amounts to approximately 50% of the rate of evaporation from a smooth wet surface, then it is easy to calculate that under this condition the coefficient a approximately equals 0.8.

Considering that the rate of evaporation from a wet surface equals

$$E_f = \rho D''(q_s - q), \tag{8.9}$$

at $E_f = 2E$ we obtain $a = 0.78$.

Taking into consideration the fact that the turbulent heat flux from the vegetation mantle to the atmosphere equals

$$P = \rho D'' c_{\mathrm{p}}(T_{\mathrm{w}} - T) \tag{8.10}$$

(where c_{p} is the heat capacity of the air, T is the air temperature, and T_{w} is the temperature of the leaf surface), we find from Eqs. (8.1), (8.4), (8.7), and (8.10) a formula for the assimilation rate,

$$A = \frac{R(c - c_1)}{(L/a)(q_{\mathrm{s}} - q) + l(c - c_1) + b(T_{\mathrm{w}} - T)}, \tag{8.11}$$

where

$$b = \frac{c_{\mathrm{p}}}{a}\left(1 + \frac{D''}{D'}\right).$$

It follows from Eq. (8.11) that the assimilation rate depends on the difference between the concentrations of carbon dioxide outside the vegetation cover and on the internal surface of the leaf $(c - c_1)$, increasing with an increase of this difference. Since the concentration of carbon dioxide outside the vegetation cover is relatively stable, it is evident that the assimilation rate will increase with the reduction of c_1, that is, with intensification of CO_2-absorption by protoplasm.

When "physiological absorption" goes on at a significant rate and the general rate of assimilation is limited, not by physiological processes, but by the diffusion flux of carbon dioxide, the value c_1 must be much less than c, and the formula for assimilation takes the form

$$A = \frac{Rc}{(L/a)(q_{\mathrm{s}} - q) + lc + b(T_{\mathrm{w}} - T)}. \tag{8.12}$$

By use of Eq. (8.12), we can determine what quantity of solar energy can be assimilated by a plant at the most effective utilization of carbon dioxide from the air.

Taking into account that c, on the average, is equal to 0.46×10^{-3}, $L = 600$ cal g^{-1}, $a = 0.78$, $l = 2500$ cal g^{-1}, and $b = 0.62$ cal g^{-1} deg^{-1}, we find that

$$lA = \frac{1.2R}{770(q_{\mathrm{s}} - q) + 1.2 + 0.62(T_{\mathrm{w}} - T)}. \tag{8.13}$$

When calculating the energy converted in assimilation by Eq. (8.13), it should be borne in mind that the general heat outgo for evaporation and the turbulent sensible-heat flux in the warm season are determined only by daytime totals, since evaporation and sensible-heat exchange at night are comparatively insignificant because of the activity of the "valve effect."

Therefore, the values of $q_s - q$ and $T_w - T$ in Eq. (8.13) must be taken as means for daytime conditions.

It should be considered that under optimal conditions for photosynthesis, when $c_1 \ll c$, the internal leaf area is sufficiently wet, and as a result, the value q_s should approach the concentration of saturated water vapor at the temperature of the leaf (or, more accurately, the difference between q and the saturation concentration of water vapor should be considerably less than the humidity deficit of the air under summer daytime conditions, calculated according to leaf temperature).

The mean daytime difference between the temperatures of leaves and air under summer conditions of middle latitudes is of the order of several degrees (see Chapter VII). Considering this difference equal to 5°, and assuming the mean daytime relative humidity of the air in summer close to 50% and the mean air temperature equal to 20°, we obtain the values $q_s = 2.0 \times 10^{-2}$ (at a leaf temperature of 25°) and $q = 0.7 \times 10^{-2}$. Substituting these values into Eq. (8.13), we find that $lA = 0.08R$, that is, the energy fixed in assimilation under mean climatic conditions of middle latitudes can reach 8% of the radiation balance.

From available data, we find that for most of the European USSR, the radiation balance in summer amounts to 55–60% of the total incoming short-wave radiation during this season. Using this evaluation, we find that under average summer conditions of middle latitudes, the natural vegetation can assimilate approximately 5% of the incoming solar radiation, provided that carbon dioxide is most effectively absorbed. This evaluation, obtained by theoretical means, agrees well with empirical data on the "coefficient of useful activity" of photosynthesis under the most favorable conditions.

However, the available factual material indicates that such comparatively high coefficients of solar energy utilization are observed only in individual cases, while the mean ratio of heat conversion in photosynthesis by natural vegetation cover to the incoming solar energy is usually of the order of 0.5% (see Section 3 of this chapter).

On this basis, we should infer that under mean conditions, the relationship $c_1 \ll c$ is not fulfilled, and, on the average, the difference $c - c_1$ is about 10% of the value of c.

In other words, a comparison of the theoretical model of diffusion with factual data permits us to determine that plants, as a rule, use only a small part (of the order of 10%) of the possible diffusion income of carbon dioxide.

It can be noted that the conclusion obtained agrees with the results of a number of experiments by Liubimenko and other authors, who, on the basis of physiological investigations, have established that leaves do not fully utilize the possible diffusion of carbon dioxide. As a result of these observations, Liubimenko (1935) concludes that "under natural conditions, production of dry matter is limited not so much by the small content of CO_2 in the atmosphere as it is by an insufficiently fast rate of work of the enzymatic apparatus, which controls the outflow of assimilators and their assimilation".

The model of the physical mechanism of assimilation and transpiration that has been set forth here permits us to explain why plants expend water uneconomically in the process of their development, that is, why the observed values of transpiration productivity are so small.

If we substitute the mean evaluations found for q_s and q under daytime conditions into Eq. (8.8) and assume $c - c_1 = 0.1c$, then the ratio A/E turns out approximately equal to $\frac{1}{360}$. This means that when assimilating 1 g of carbon dioxide, the plant loses through transpiration an average of about 360 g of water.

It should be noted that, although the ratio A/E does not exactly coincide with transpiration productivity,* one can consider its magnitude to be of the same order as this value. Thus, the estimate obtained provides a theoretical explanation of the observed magnitudes of transpiration productivity.

Worthy of attention also is the explanation by Eq. (8.8) of the substantial dependence of transpiration productivity on the humidity deficit. The dependence has been noticed many times by various investigators, who have observed an appreciable decrease in transpiration productivity with a reduction of the humidity deficit, both under greenhouse conditions and with a transition from dry climates to more moist ones (Maksimov, 1926; and others).

The general conclusion from the above can be put into the following words.

Plants usually exploit a very small fraction of the natural energy and water resources. This part is small even in comparison to the small "coefficient of useful activity" that could be reached at the greatest possible diffusion of carbon dioxide from the air. The calculated results given in this section indicate that in the case of complete utilization of atmospheric carbon dioxide, vegetation can assimilate no less than 5% of the incoming solar energy, and that under these conditions, the transpiration productivity must equal, not several thousandths (as it usually does), but several hundredths. Since, under natural conditions, such high indices of photosynthetic efficiency are usually not observed, we must conclude that plant productivity is substantially limited by factors whose nature will be discussed below in detail.

---

* The productivity of transpiration is connected with the growth in dry organic matter, which differs somewhat from the value of assimilation because of the utilization by the plant of water and mineral substances of the soil and because of the loss of a fraction of the dry matter during plant development for respiration and in atrophy of individual plant organs.

2. Photosynthesis in the Layer of Vegetation Cover

The theory of photosynthesis in the layer of vegetation

In the previous section, we examined photosynthesis in a group of leaves existing under uniform external conditions.

To determine total photosynthesis in the layer of vegetation cover, one must take into consideration the difference between the meteorological factors of photosynthesis at different levels in the vegetation.

This task was first proposed in the investigations of Monsi and Saeki (1953) and Davidson and Philip (1958), in which the calculation of total photosynthesis in a vegetation layer was carried out with consideration of the effect of the change in the quantity of radiation along the vertical, but without consideration of the dependence of photosynthesis on the change in the concentration of carbon dioxide. Later, papers of the scientific workers at the Main Geophysical Observatory (Budyko, 1964; Budyko and Gandin, 1964, 1965, 1966; Budyko *et al.*, 1966a, b) offered a more general theory of photosynthesis in vegetation, including consideration of the effect of both the radiative factors and the change in carbon dioxide concentration at different levels in the vegetation. The results of these papers are set forth in this section.

In investigations of photosynthesis at different levels of vegetation, it is necessary to take into consideration the physical regularities of meteorological processes in the layer of the air that the plants occupy, that is, in the vegetation layer [or canopy]. The height of the layer usually varies from several centimeters up to several tens of meters (with arboreal vegetation).

Notwithstanding the great progress being made now in the physics of the boundary layer, the regularities of the meteorological regime in the vegetation layer have not yet been sufficiently studied. From general considerations, it is possible to clarify qualitative features of the regime of the vegetation layer in comparison with the layer lying above it, which is free of vegetation and is usually called the surface layer of air.

When studying the physical processes in the layer of vegetation cover, it is convenient to average the values of meteorological elements at different levels along the horizontal, which permits the exclusion of the effect of individual plants on the meteorological regime.

In applying such an averaging, it is possible to establish that, in contrast with the surface layer of air, the mean vertical fluxes of short-wave and long-wave radiation, sensible heat, water vapor, and momentum in the vegetation cover change substantially with height. The amount of short-wave radiation decreases towards the earth's surface due to absorption and scattering of radiation at the surfaces of the plants. The resultant flux of radiation (radiation balance) also decreases in this direction because of the screening effect of plants.

The fluxes of water vapor and momentum change similarly. The water-vapor flux in vegetation increases with height because of the effect of plant transpiration, and the flux of momentum decreases downward from the upper boundary of vegetation as a consequence of the braking effect of vegetation on air motion. This effect is associated with weakened turbulent exchange in the vegetation layer compared to higher layers of air, the turbulent exchange coefficient in this situation decreasing with approach to the earth's surface.

As an example, Fig. 117 shows data of Efimova (1968) for a field covered by wheat 1.2 m high. The data represent the dependence of the turbulent exchange coefficient k and photosynthetically active radiation Q on height H.

We note that photosynthetically active radiation is the fraction of the total flux of short-wave radiation restricted to wavelengths within whose limits radiation can be used in photosynthesis. Its value is approximately half as large as the values of short-wave radiation. Since the formulas given in this chapter employ only the values of photosynthetically active radiation, we keep for it the designation adopted in the previous chapters for short-wave radiation.

In elaborating a theory of photosynthesis in the layer of vegetation cover, it is necessary to establish a quantitative relation between photosynthesis in a single plant leaf and the external factors affecting it.

It has been established in numerous laboratory investigations [see Rabinowitch (1951), and others] that at small values of photosynthetically active radiation Q, photosynthesis is proportional to radiation and depends little on other external factors, that is, that as $Q \to 0$,

$$A = \beta Q. \tag{8.14}$$

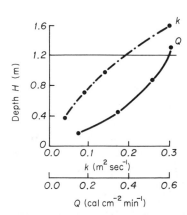

Fig. 117   Coefficient of turbulent exchange k and photosynthetically active radiation Q in a layer of vegetation cover.

Such a condition corresponds to the so-called rising portion of the light curve of photosynthesis.

With large amounts of radiation, photosynthesis depends little on the income of radiation (plateau of the light curve) but substantially on the concentration of carbon dioxide, temperature, and other external factors.

In experimental investigations, it has been established that under conditions of "light saturation," photosynthesis is proportional to the concentration of carbon dioxide for the range of concentrations observed under natural conditions. Taking this conclusion into account, we assume that as $Q \to \infty$,

$$A = \tau c, \tag{8.15}$$

where the coefficient of proportionality τ is a function of temperature and other external factors, but does not depend on radiation or concentration of carbon dioxide.

It is obvious that the values β and τ can be determined from light curves of photosynthesis obtained experimentally, β being the tangent of the slope angle of the initial section of the light curve, and τ corresponding to the height of the light-curve plateau at a given concentration of carbon dioxide.

It must be borne in mind that the coefficient τ characterizes the diffusion conditions of carbon dioxide assimilated by a plant in the course of photosynthesis at light saturation.

The above conditions are satisfied by a formula (Budyko, 1964) describing the light curve of photosynthesis in the form

$$A = \frac{\beta Q}{1 + (\beta Q/\tau c)} \tag{8.16}$$

and representing a generalization of the hyperbolic formula offered by Tamiya in 1951 [see Monsi and Saeki (1953)].

The vertical flux of carbon dioxide in the vegetation layer at level z is equal to

$$A_z = \rho k \frac{dc}{dz}. \tag{8.17}$$

The change of this flux in the layer dz, caused by assimilation of carbon dioxide by leaves, follows from Eq. (8.16), and equals

$$dA_1 = \frac{\beta Q s \, dz}{1 + (\beta Q/\tau c)}, \tag{8.18}$$

where s is the surface of leaves in a unit volume [leaf-area density].

The change in photosynthetically active radiation with height in the vegetation layer is determined by the equation

$$dQ = \phi(Q)\, s\, dz, \tag{8.19}$$

where the function $\phi(Q)$ describes the dependence of the radiation absorption in a layer of thickness dz on the amount of photosynthetically active radiation incident on the upper boundary of this layer. Taking into consideration that on the upper boundary of the vegetation cover at $z = H$ the radiation flux is known ($Q = Q_H$), we obtain from Eq. (8.19)

$$\int_Q^{Q_H} \frac{dQ}{\phi(Q)} = \int_z^H s\, dz. \tag{8.20}$$

In solving Eq. (8.20) for Q, we obtain the relationship

$$Q = \psi\left(Q_H, \int_z^H s\, dz\right), \tag{8.21}$$

describing the dependence of photosynthetically active radiation on height. If we assume that

$$\phi(Q) = \gamma Q, \tag{8.22}$$

then the dependence acquires the form

$$Q = Q_H \exp\left(-\gamma \int_z^H s\, dz\right) \tag{8.23}$$

It was used in this form by Monsi and Saeki (1953). If we set

$$\phi(Q) = \gamma' Q^2, \tag{8.24}$$

then we obtain the expression

$$Q = \frac{Q_H}{1 + \gamma' Q_H \int_z^H s\, dz}. \tag{8.25}$$

Further, for the sake of certainty, we will use the dependence in the form of Eq. (8.23). In this case, from Eq. (8.18), we obtain

$$dA_1 = \frac{\beta Q_H \exp\left(-\gamma \int_z^H s\, dz\right)}{1 + (\beta Q_H/\tau c) \exp\left(-\gamma \int_z^H s\, dz\right)}\, s\, dz. \tag{8.26}$$

The change of flux A_2 caused by plant respiration will be presented in the form

$$dA_2 = -\varepsilon s\, dz, \tag{8.27}$$

where ε is a coefficient of proportionality.

The general change in the vertical flux of carbon dioxide is determined by the relation

$$dA_z = dA_1 + dA_2. \tag{8.28}$$

From the above formulas, we obtain a nonlinear differential equation,

$$\frac{d}{dz}\left(\rho k \frac{dc}{dz}\right) = -\frac{\beta s Q_H \exp\left(-\gamma \int_z^H s\, dz\right)}{1 + (\beta Q_H/\tau c) \exp\left(-\gamma \int_z^H s\, dz\right)} - \varepsilon s. \tag{8.29}$$

To solve Eq. (8.29), we will use the following boundary conditions:

$$\left(\rho k \frac{dc}{dz}\right)\Bigg|_{z=0} = -A_0, \tag{8.30}$$

and

$$\left(\rho k \frac{dc}{dz}\right)\Bigg|_{z=H} = \rho D_H(c_\infty - c_H), \tag{8.31}$$

where A_0 is the flux of carbon dioxide from the soil; c_∞ is the concentration of carbon dioxide in the air at a height z_1 where it depends little on the properties of the vegetation cover; c_H is the concentration of carbon dioxide at level H; and D_H is the integral coefficient of turbulent diffusion in the air layer between levels H and z_1.

The first of these conditions expresses the equality of the income of carbon dioxide from the soil with the value of the turbulent flux of carbon dioxide in the air near the soil surface. The second condition corresponds to the equality of the turbulent flux of carbon dioxide at the upper boundary of the vegetation cover with the turbulent flux coming from the atmosphere into the vegetation layer.

From the condition of balance of carbon dioxide in the spaces between leaves for the whole layer of vegetation, we find that

$$A = A_H + A_0 + \int_0^H \varepsilon s\, dz, \tag{8.32}$$

where A is the total value of assimilation, and A_H is the vertical flux of carbon dioxide at the level H.

From the solution of Eq. (8.29), one can determine the magnitude of A_H, after which the magnitude of total assimilation will be found by Eq. (8.32). In this case, one must take into consideration the dependence of k, s, and ε on height in the vegetation layer, which can be done by the use of available empirical data.

In the general case, Eq. (8.29) can be integrated only numerically. Of interest are the particular cases associated with simplifications of Eq. (8.29), allowing analytic solution.

Such particular cases include the following:

1. A well-ventilated vegetation cover with no flux of carbon dioxide from the soil. In this case, we may assume $k = \infty$, $dc/dz = 0$, $A_0 = 0$.
Then from Eq. (8.29), we derive

$$A_z = \frac{\tau c}{\gamma} \ln \frac{1 + (\beta Q_H/\tau c) \exp\left(-\gamma \int_z^H s\, dz\right)}{1 + (\beta Q_H/\tau c) \exp\left(-\gamma \int_0^H s\, dz\right)} - \int_0^z \varepsilon s\, dz. \qquad (8.33)$$

From Eqs. (8.31) and (8.33), we obtain the equation

$$\rho D_H(c_\infty - c) = \frac{\tau c}{\gamma} \ln \frac{1 + (\beta Q_H/\tau c)}{1 + (\beta Q_H/\tau c) \exp\left(-\gamma \int_0^H s\, dz\right)} - \int_0^H \varepsilon s\, dz. \qquad (8.34)$$

After this, we find c, and then the assimilation by Eq. (8.32). If the turbulent exchange above the vegetation is sufficiently intensive and does not limit photosynthesis, then we can consider $D_H = \infty$ and $c = c_\infty$, as a result of which we find

$$A = \frac{\tau c_\infty}{\gamma} \ln \frac{1 + (\beta Q_H/\tau c_\infty)}{1 + (\beta Q_H/\tau c_\infty) \exp\left(-\gamma \int_0^H s\, dz\right)}. \qquad (8.35)$$

We note that in this case, total assimilation does not depend on respiration.

2. A well-illuminated vegetation cover, in which conditions of light saturation are observed at all levels. In this case, $Q = Q_H$ in the entire layer of vegetation, and Eq. (8.29) acquires the form

$$\frac{d}{dz}\left(k \frac{dc}{dz}\right) - \frac{\tau s}{\rho} c = -\frac{\varepsilon}{\rho} s. \qquad (8.36)$$

Equation (8.36) can be accurately solved only with some assumptions concerning the dependences of $\varepsilon(z)$, $\tau(z)$, $s(z)$, and $k(z)$. In particular, if we consider the first three quantities constant with height and assume that in the vegetation layer

$$k = k_0 + k_1 z \qquad (8.37)$$

(in this case, the coefficients k_0 and k_1 satisfy the relation $k_0/k_1 \ll H$), we obtain from Eq. (8.36) and the boundary conditions the formula

$$A = \frac{B_1 \rho D_H I_1(\eta) [c_\infty - (\varepsilon/\tau)] - A_0}{I_0(\eta) + B_1 I_1(\eta)} + A_0 + \varepsilon s H, \qquad (8.38)$$

where I_0 and I_1 are cylindrical [Bessel] functions of the imaginary argument of the first kind, and

$$\eta = 2\left(\frac{\tau s H}{\rho k_1}\right)^{1/2}, \qquad B_1 = \frac{k_1 \eta}{2 D_H}.$$

Utilization of the above-stated theory permits us to investigate the dependence of photosynthesis in the layer of vegetation cover on the value of the leaf-area index S (the ratio of the area of leaf surface to the area occupied by the vegetation cover), and on various external factors.

We should point out that in recent years, along with the aforementioned theory of photosynthesis in the vegetation cover, some investigators have offered other schemes for numerical modelling of the process under consideration (Ross, 1964; Ross and Bikhele, 1968–1969; Monteith, 1965; DeWit, 1965; Uchijima, 1966; Duncan et al., 1967; and others). All these models are based on the general idea of a transition from photosynthesis in a single leaf to photosynthesis in a layer uniform in the horizontal and with physical conditions changing with height. Differences between these models are associated with the different detailing of the numerical models used, among which some are of a more general and others of a more specific character.

Regularities of photosynthesis in the layer of vegetation cover

Turning to the question of utilization of this theory for studying the regularities of photosynthesis in a vegetation layer, we note that because of the nonlinear character of Eq. (8.29), its solution in the general case cannot be obtained in a closed form. It therefore turned out to be necessary to elaborate an algorithm of the numerical solution of the equation, which was accomplished with the aid of the electronic computer "Ural-4." Below we present some of the results of computations by Gandin et al. (1969). These results relate to the particular case in which the values τ, s, and ε do not depend on height and the vertical profile of the turbulent diffusion coefficient in the plant–air space is linear, that is, $k = k_0 + k_1 z$, where $k_0 \ll k_1 H$. These restrictions are not matters of principle for either the theory or the computation method.

Figure 118 shows the calculated dependence of assimilation A on the flux of photosynthetically active radiation at the upper boundary of the vegetation cover (Q_H), at different values of the leaf-area index $S = \int_0^H s \, dz$ and the ratio τ/ρ.

The dependence is calculated with the following values of other parameters: $A_0 = \varepsilon = 0$; $D_H = 0.6$ cm sec^{-1}; $k_1 = 3$ cm sec^{-1}; $\gamma = 1$; $\beta = 8 \times 10^{-5}$ g cal^{-1}; $k_1 H/k_0 = 200$; $\rho = 1.29 \times 10^{-3}$ g cm^{-3}; and $c_\infty = 0.46 \times 10^{-3}$ (which corresponds to 0.03 of one volume per cent).

It is easy to see that the lines in Fig. 118 are light curves. But, in contrast to the light curves for a single leaf, which have been thoroughly studied in plant physiology (Rabinowitch, 1951), they are light curves obtained by theoretical means for the vegetation cover as a whole. These curves show the

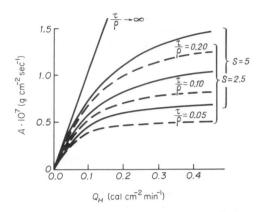

Fig. 118   Dependence of assimilation on radiation.

existence of a strong dependence of total assimilation on the radiation flux at small values, when assimilation depends little on other factors. In contrast, at large values of radiation, the total assimilation hardly depends on it at all and is determined by other factors, in particular temperature, which affects the coefficient τ.

The data presented in Fig. 119 permitted us to evaluate how the vital activity of plants is affected by a factor that is usually not a concern of agrometeorology, namely, the intensity of turbulent exchange in the leaf–air space of a vegetation cover. The coefficient k_1 is a measure of this intensity. The figure shows the effect of k_1 on total assimilation A, and also on the concentration of carbon dioxide at the upper and lower boundaries of the vegetation cover (corresponding to c_H and c_n, respectively). For other parameters of the problem, the values $Q_H = 0.35$ cal cm^{-2} min^{-1}, $\tau/\rho = 0.1$ cm sec^{-1}, and $S = 5$ were adopted.

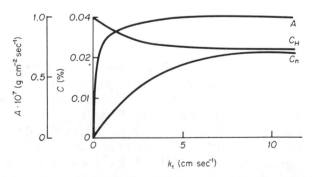

Fig. 119   Dependence of assimilation on turbulent exchange.

It is seen from Fig. 119 that with a poorly ventilated vegetation cover (small k_1), the concentration of carbon dioxide is considerably reduced near the soil surface (without soil "respiration"), and depends strongly on k_1. Total assimilation also depends noticeably on k_1, and is less as turbulent exchange is weaker. With a well-ventilated vegetation cover (large magnitudes of k_1), the concentration of carbon dioxide is practically constant with height and, like total assimilation, ceases to depend on k_1.

Considering that the conditions of ventilation of vegetation depend not only on its structure but also on wind speed and the vertical temperature stratification over the vegetation cover, we should consider the turbulence regime to be one of the factors in plant yield.

The effect of plant respiration on total assimilation at the "standard" magnitudes of the other parameters given above is presented in Fig. 120. It

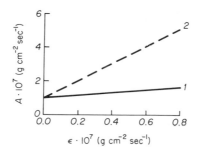

Fig. 120   Influence of plant respiration on assimilation.

presents two lines, line 1 describing the real dependence of A on the coefficient of respiration ε, and line 2 a dependence that corresponds to complete assimilation of all the "secondary" carbon dioxide being released by respiration. It is clear that the actual increase of assimilation is much less than this limiting increase. This means that the effect on photosynthesis of an increase in concentration of CO_2 in the leaf–air space owing to respiration is to a great extent leveled out by a decrease in the diffusion flux of CO_2 from the outside.

Figure 121 demonstrates the effect of the carbon-dioxide flux from the soil A_0 on the total assimilation. Line 1 here also characterizes the actual dependence of A on A_0, and line 2 corresponds to the case of complete assimilation of carbon dioxide coming from the soil. As is seen from a comparison of lines 1 and 2, the increase of A with growth of A_0 is considerably less than the increase that would have occurred if all the additional carbon dioxide coming from the soil were converted in assimilation. This is easy to understand if we take into account that the flux of carbon dioxide from below first meets on its path the shaded leaves, which are incapable of intensive photosynthesis because of a shortage of radiation. Regarding a general increase in concentration due to the flux from below, it is essentially leveled out, as in the case of respiration, by reduction of the carbon dioxide income from above.

As a result, the influence of the carbon dioxide flux from the soil on assimilation is usually small, when compared to the flux of carbon dioxide coming from the atmosphere. This conclusion agrees with one by Monteith *et al.* (1964) from experimental studies on the diffusion of carbon dioxide in vegetation cover.

These results indicate the broad possibilities of applying the theory of photosynthesis to clarify some general regularities of this process.

Let us now turn to an examination of the climatic factors determining the productivity of vegetation cover Π. We assume productivity to be equal to the difference between total assimilation and the loss of organic matter in

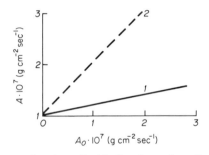

Fig. 121   Influence of carbon-dioxide flux from the soil on assimilation.

respiration, and neglect the losses of matter by atrophy of individual plant organs that occurs in the course of its development.

Since productivity of the vegetation cover depends significantly on the value of the leaf-area index, decreasing at small and large magnitudes of the index (see below), we then calculate the value of productivity at the optimal size of the leaf-area index, corresponding to the greatest values of productivity.

The above equations show that, besides the parameters characterizing the properties of the vegetation cover itself, the value of Π is affected by a great number of meteorological parameters. It therefore seems rational to single out the most important of these. It follows from the analysis carried out that under conditions of sufficient moisture, vegetation productivity is most affected by two factors—photosynthetically active radiation and temperature. The value of the radiation flux Q_H is directly included in the equation of the problem. As far as temperature T is concerned, it influences the parameters τ and ε included in the calculation model.

In accordance with this, we should consider the combination of the two parameters Q_H and T as the principal agroclimatic index under conditions of sufficient moisture. With such an analysis, one should use the means of the other parameters, which have less effect on II.

Unfortunately, notwithstanding many appropriate investigations, we do not have at present sufficient routine and reliable quantitative data on the effect of temperature on the parameters τ and ε for different species of plants. Therefore, we have used the dependences of $\tau(T)$ and $\varepsilon(T)$ in a generalized form that is particularly characteristic of several grain crops. These relations, constructed in accordance with data in the literature, are presented in Fig. 122, which demonstrates the dependence of ratios A_m/A_M and ε/A_M

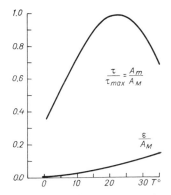

Fig. 122   Influence of temperature on the parameters determining plant productivity.

on temperature T (A_M is the maximum value of assimilation A_m, not limited by the flux of photosynthetically active radiation).

Applying these relations and utilizing the above-mentioned equations, we can calculate the dependence of total productivity II on the flux of photosynthetically active radiation on the upper boundary of the vegetation cover and on temperature. This dependence is presented in Fig. 123, where the relationship between the ratio Π/A_M to the temperature T and photosynthetically active radiation Q_H at the outer boundary of the vegetation cover is shown. It is apparent from this figure that an increase of the flux Q_H leads in all cases to a growth of productivity II. At the same time, with rising temperature T, the productivity II first increases and then, after having reached a certain maximum value depending on Q_H, decreases. This is a consequence both of the similar character of the dependence of τ on T and of the increase in respiration with rising temperature.

It is seen from Fig. 123 that the effect of radiation and temperature on the productivity of vegetation is complex. Radiation under actually existing conditions is always a factor that is in the "minimum." This is associated with the constant shortage of radiation at the lower and partly shaded leaves of vegetation. The temperature influence on productivity has a quite different character: a rise in temperature above a certain limit lowers productivity substantially.

Figure 123 can be used as a nomogram for determination of the value of Π from known values of Q_H, T, and A_M. Thus, sums of Π for the vegetation period were calculated at a number of points in the European USSR. In this calculation, long-term monthly means of Q_H and T in their diurnal march were used, and the value A_M was taken as 0.24 mg CO_2 cm^{-2} hr^{-1}.

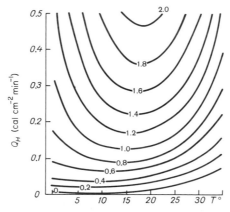

Fig. 123 Dependence of plant productivity upon photosynthetically active radiation and air temperature.

The schematic distribution of the total values of Π (in centner ha^{-1} [1 metric centner = 100 kg]) for the European USSR is presented in Fig. 124.

It should be indicated that in carrying out these calculations, mean values of Q_H and T in a given month for different hours of the 24 were used. Since there is a positive correlation between Q_H and T (the higher temperature values, on the average, correspond to the greater radiation values), the calculation of Π by averaged Q_H and T leads to a certain distortion of the results.

The values presented in Fig. 124 can be considered as the values of possible yield (that is, the yield obtained with the application of optimal agrotechnology), expressed in the mass of carbon dioxide assimilated per unit of area. With the use of the basic photosynthesis equation, one can easily transform them into values of dry mass of vegetable matter. A comparison of these values with the data of record yields shows that only at times do the latter constitute an appreciable fraction of the yields possible under the given climatic conditions. Such a conclusion, confirming the great possibility of increasing yield by improving agrotechnical methods, coincides with the conclusion given in Section 1 of this chapter.

Let us dwell now on the question of the reasons why the productivity of plants is lower than the values obtained in the above calculation. These reasons are associated with the effect of climatic, biological, and soil factors.

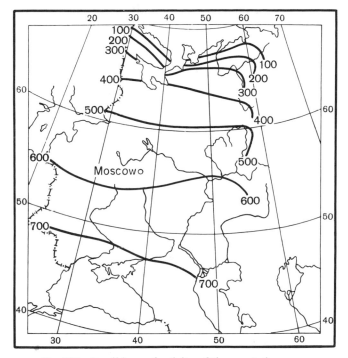

Fig. 124 Possible productivity of the vegetation cover.

The values of productivity found above relate to the optimal conditions of moisture, which are comparatively rarely present over the course of the entire period of plant development, even in the most favorable climatic regions.

The values of possible productivity relate to plants that possess a structure optimal for photosynthesis throughout the vegetation period, and activity of photosynthesizing organs that also remains stable throughout this period. Such conditions are usually not fulfilled for real plants.

In addition, the possible productivity of plants corresponds to conditions of sufficient mineral nutrition, which is rarely completely assured, even under conditions of satisfactory agrotechnics of agricultural fields.

All these reasons account for a considerably lower productivity of both agricultural plants and the natural vegetation cover, compared with the possible productivity calculated by the model given above.

Thus, the potential productivity is a conditional index of productivity, which characterizes the climatic resources of different geographical regions for creation of organic matter by autotrophic plants. For this reason, it seems possible to use data on potential productivity as a composite agro-climatic index defining the effect of radiation and temperature regimes on agricultural plants.

From this viewpoint, it is interesting to compare the values of possible plant production with a common agroclimatic index of thermal regime—the sum of temperatures. The results of such a comparison from calculated material for the European USSR are presented in Fig. 125. It is seen from

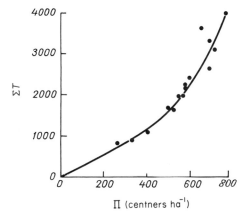

Fig. 125   Relationship between possible productivity and the sum of temperatures.

these data that there is a certain relationship between the productivity and the sum of temperatures above 10°C. This fact confirms the possibility of using summed temperature as an agroclimatic index characterizing the effects of both the radiation regime and the temperature.

At the same time, the nonlinearity of the relationship in Fig. 125 shows that identical changes in the temperature sum in different ranges of its values may produce different effects on the maximum production of plant cover. In addition, the evaluations available point to the fact that the relation between possible production and temperature sums in other regions does not always coincide with the dependence shown in Fig. 125. It therefore seems appropriate to use a composite index that takes into consideration the effect of both temperature and radiation, according to the model set forth in this book, in order to make agroclimatic calculations more accurate.

Of interest is a comparison of the possible productivity of vegetation cover with the value of the radiation balance at the earth's surface. The results of such a comparison, carried out with material for the European part of the USSR, are presented in Fig. 126. For this purpose, the annual values of the radiation balance at the earth's surface under conditions of sufficient moisture (R_0) were used.

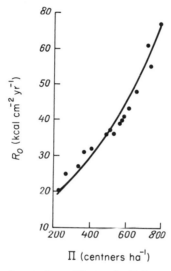

Fig. 126 Dependence of possible productivity on the radiation balance.

The close dependence between the values of possible productivity and radiation balance confirms the idea about the significance of the radiation balance as a determining factor in the development of vegetation (Budyko, 1956). Such a dependence is presumably to be explained by the relation of the radiation balance to the potential value of plant transpiration, as well as by the direct influence of radiation upon photosynthesis in plant cover.

Photosynthesis and the properties of vegetation cover

Let us now discuss the question of the possibility of using the above-stated theory for an explanation of regularities in the formation of the kinds of natural vegetation.

It is known that the varieties of vegetation-cover types in different areas of the globe are caused, to a considerable extent, by the effect of climatic conditions on the development of vegetation.

Numerous investigations aimed at studying the effect of climate on vegetation have been carried out, mainly by empirical methods. This has limited the possibility of explaining the causative mechanism in the action of climatic factors on the properties of vegetation cover. At the present time, it is possible to put the question about the dependence of properties of vegetation on climatic conditions on the basis of general physical regularities that describe the influence of atmospheric factors in the life activity of plants. Such an approach should permit us to estimate theoretically the mean values of such characteristics of the plant cover as the amount of biomass and the productivity in geographical zones corresponding to different climatic conditions.

For this purpose, let us consider the balance of organic mass in plant cover.

In analyzing the organic matter balance in plant cover, we will use the relationship

$$M = \mu S + m, \tag{8.39}$$

where M is the mass of organic matter in a plant cover per unit area occupied by it, S is the leaf-area index, μ is the mass of leaves corresponding to a unit area of leaf surface, and m is the mass of organic matter contained in all plant organs except leaves per unit of area.

The productivity of vegetation cover per unit of area is determined by the formula

$$\Pi = A(S) - B(M), \tag{8.40}$$

where $A(S)$ is photosynthesis in the layer of vegetation as a function of the value of the leaf-area index S, and $B(M)$ is the loss of organic matter for respiration and atrophy of individual plant organs, dependent on the mass of organic matter M.

It is natural to consider that the loss of organic matter in respiration of leaves and their atrophy is proportional to the mass of leaves, that is, equal to $v\mu S$, where v is a coefficient of proportionality.

Then

$$\Pi = A(S) - v\mu S - B(m). \tag{8.41}$$

To establish the function $A(S)$, one should use the physical theory of photosynthesis in vegetation stated above.

Taking into account the character of this dependence, we can establish that the value $\partial A/\partial S$ is positive and decreases monotonically with the increase of

S, approaching zero at high values of the leaf-area index. In this connection, if

$$\left.\frac{\partial A}{\partial S}\right|_{S=S_0} > v\mu,$$

there is a value of the leaf-area index S_0 at which vegetation productivity reaches its maximum. This value of S_0 can be derived from the following condition

$$\left.\frac{\partial A}{\partial S}\right|_{S=S_0} = v\mu. \tag{8.42}$$

It seems probable that as a result of the long evolution of autotrophic plants, directed toward increasing the efficiency of their photosynthetic activity, values of leaf-area index in a natural vegetation cover sufficiently provided with moisture for transpiration are observed that more or less correspond to the optimal value S_0. To test this statement with the aid of the above calculation scheme, the value of S_0 for various climatic conditions was determined from Eq. (8.42). This value turned out to be rather stable, slightly diminished at higher latitudes, and, on the average, equal to 5 for leaf-bearing plants.

Such an evaluation agrees satisfactorily with the leaf-area index values obtained as a result of observations in many natural vegetation covers in regions of sufficient moisture [see "Основы лесной биогеоценологии (The Foundations of Forest Biogeocenology)", 1964], which confirms the hypothesis stated above.

The development of perennial plants continues until they reach their natural maturity, that is, the state when the income of organic matter in the plant cover is compensated by the outgo for respiration and atrophy of both individual plant organs and individual plants. In this case, the following condition is fulfilled:

$$A(S) - v\mu S - B(m) = 0. \tag{8.43}$$

If we assume that $S = S_0$, we find the limiting value of organic mass M_0 that may be accumulated in a vegetation cover that has reached a stationary state, from the equation

$$A(S_0) = B(M_0). \tag{8.44}$$

This equation can be used for a theoretical evaluation of biomass contained in typical vegetation covers of different natural zones in conditions of sufficient moisture.

Following the idea of Davidson and Philip (1958), it is possible to write an equation that will characterize the change of biomass in vegetation over time.

This will permit us to evaluate the rate of accumulation of biomass in the course of the approach of plant cover to a state of natural maturity.

Such an equation has a form that coincides with Eq. (8.41),

$$\frac{dM}{dt} = A(S) - v\mu S - B(m), \tag{8.45}$$

where dM/dt is the rate of change of the amount of biomass through time.

Equations (8.44) and (8.45) have been used by us to evaluate the biomass stock in plant covers of the zone of sufficient moisture in both the stationary state and that changing in time.

Calculations of this sort are complicated by insufficient detail of the available information about the intensity of processes of biomass loss in respiration and atrophy of individual organs of plants, necessary for determination of v and B.

Nevertheless, utilization of the values of these parameters that are available in the literature permits us to calculate by Eq. (8.44) the values of biomass stock in forests of different latitudinal zones, which agree satisfactorily with the materials of a summary by Lavrenko et al. (1955). It should be indicated that such a calculation permits finding out which climatic factors affect the changes in biomass stock, upon a transition from one type of vegetation cover to another.

In particular, it follows from the formulas used that the diminution in the biomass stock in forests with an increase in geographical latitude depends most of all on the reduction in the duration of the growing season, while the effect of lower air temperature during the growing season and that of a change in radiation turn out to be less important.

Calculation by Eq. (8.45) permits establishing the general regularities of change in biomass during the course of development of a perennial vegetation cover. These regularities are characterized by an increase in the rate of biomass accumulation during the first years of existence of the plant cover. In the course of time, this increase changes into a gradual diminution in the rate of accumulation. When the rate of accumulation becomes small, the vegetation cover approaches the state of natural maturity.

Making these calculations has shown that with the aid of Eq. (8.45), it is possible to obtain relations of the biomass stock in forests to their age that are in good agreement with the data of appropriate observations.

This kind of calculation might be compared to the investigations of Khil'mi (1957, 1966), who worked out a method for quantitative calculation of biomass growth in forest, based on dimensional theory and general physical ideas. A comparison of the results of calculations performed by Eq. (8.45) with similar calculations of Khil'mi shows that they yield relations of the biomass stock with time that are similar in form.

In conclusion, we should indicate that for a still broader use of the meteorological theory of photosynthesis, an accumulation of factual material on the parameters determining the growth of biomass in different vegetation covers is necessary. Such material could be obtained in interdisciplinary research expeditions, carried out according to a broad program and utilizing contemporary measuring techniques.

3. Utilization of Solar Energy by Living Organisms

Energetics of the natural vegetation cover

Although, in the course of photosynthesis, plants use a small portion of the energy from incoming solar radiation, this portion is converted into a comparatively stable form of chemical energy, which can be preserved for a long time before it is dissipated, that is, converted into heat. The energy assimilated by photosynthesizing plants is expended for maintenance of almost all the forms of organic life; it is also used in the process of soil formation, and has an influence on many other natural processes.

This energy is of great importance both for agricultural production and also for industrial energetics, which largely uses the photosynthetic products of past geological epochs.

It has already been noted that the effectiveness of natural vegetation cover with regard to assimilation of the energy of solar radiation varies a great deal, depending on the natural conditions. The coefficient of useful utilization of solar energy in photosynthesis, decreasing with inadequate heat or moisture, reaches its maximum values under optimal conditions of the heat and water regimes. The coefficient also depends on the physical and chemical properties of the soil.

For a quantitative study of the utilization of solar energy by natural plant cover, it is necessary to have data on the income of solar radiation and the productivity of the plant cover. During the investigations on the radiation regime at the earth's surface carried out in the Main Geophysical Observatory, maps of photosynthetically active radiation relating to different areas, including world maps (Efimova, 1965, 1969, and elsewhere), were constructed, along with maps of total solar radiation.

To determine the average productivity values of the kinds of natural vegetation cover, one could use data from various summaries, including data of empirical determination of productivity in individual geographical zones. Recently, in papers of Lieth (1964–1965), Bazilevich and Rodin (1967, and others), and other authors, the first maps of vegetation productivity on the continents have been drawn. In pointing to the great importance of these investigations for studying the geographical regularities of the productivity of vegetation cover, we must note that because of the inadequacy of basic data, these maps have been schematized to a considerable extent. Thus, for example, in the more detailed maps by Bazilevich and Rodin, the data of productivity are presented, not by isolines, but in the form of class intervals of productivity values for different geobotanical zones. Application of such maps to studying the spatial distribution of the coefficient of solar-energy assimilation by plants is hampered by the fact that productivity may vary not only with transition from one zone to another but also within each zone.

As a result, a new map of the natural vegetation productivity in the USSR (Budyko and Efimova, 1968) has been constructed to evaluate the utilization of solar energy by vegetation cover.

In designing this map, it was taken into consideration that, as indicated in the previous section, the productivity of natural vegetation under conditions of sufficient moisture depends on the radiation balance at the earth's surface. The relationship between radiation balance and the amount of precipitation is used as an index of moisture conditions.

In accordance with this, a graph was constructed in which empirical values of the annual productivity of natural plant covers (the annual increase of organic matter in the aerial and underground domains of vegetation) are compared with values of radiation balance and precipitation. This graph is shown in Fig. 127, where along the vertical axis are plotted the values of productivity of dry organic matter Π, in centner ha^{-1} for the year, and along the horizontal axis, the ratio of the annual values of the radiation balance R to the amount of heat Lr necessary to evaporate the annual precipitation (the radiative index of dryness). The curves in this graph correspond to different values of radiation balance (in kilocalories per square centimeter per year).

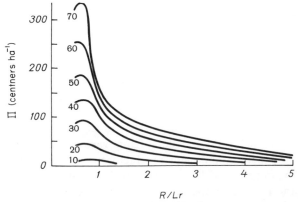

Fig. 127 Dependence of the productivity of natural vegetation cover Π on meteorological factors: the radiative index of dryness (R/Lr) and the net surface of radiative energy.

Although all the data on vegetation productivity that are available in the literature were used to construct this graph, it should be mentioned that such data in lower latitudes (that is, for large R) are very few. This restricts the graph's accuracy for these conditions. It is believed that for middle latitudes, the relations presented in the graph are more reliable.

The system of isolines in the graph agrees well with the concept of the law of geographical zonality set forth in Chapter VI of this book. It is seen from the graph that changes in productivity in relation to the index of dryness are rather similar at different levels of radiation balance. It can be noted that similar relationships between productivity and climatic factors were obtained in the studies of Bazilevich and Rodin (1969), and Drozdov (1969). We will point out the fact that some features of these relationships require additional study. These include the question of the dependence of maximum productivity values at given values of radiation balance on the radiative index of dryness.

It is not easy in Fig. 127 to determine the exact location of the maxima of the curves. In a paper by Armand (1967), it was suggested that such maxima occur under climatic conditions of high and middle latitudes, but that in low latitudes productivity increases without limit as the index of dryness decreases. Bazilevich et al. (1970) came to the conclusion that such maxima exist in all latitudes, the value of the radiative index of dryness corresponding to the maxima increasing with increasing latitude.

For construction of a productivity map by the use of Fig. 127 and material on the radiation balance and the precipitation regime, calculations of productivity at 200 points in the USSR were carried out. On the basis of these data, a map was drawn (Fig. 128). It is apparent from this map that values of annual increase in the natural vegetation cover vary from less than 20 centner ha^{-1} on the islands and Siberian coast of the Arctic Ocean, up to values exceeding 200 centners ha^{-1} on the Black Sea coast of the Caucasus. In the zones of sufficient moisture, an increase of productivity is observed with a shift from north toward south, in accordance with the increase of incoming solar radiation and in the duration of the growing period. A decline in vegetation productivity is observed in regions of insufficient moisture; in the deserts of Central Asia, productivity is reduced to 20 centners ha^{-1} per year.

Comparison of the mapped values of annual productivity of the natural vegetation cover with data from the map by Bazilevich and Rodin shows in the main a satisfactory agreement in characteristics of the annual increase of biomass in the different geobotanic zones. Some differences between the maps in the zones of arid steppes, deserts, and some regions of Eastern Siberia can be explained by the insufficient amount of empirical data for these areas.

Using the constructed map of vegetation productivity and the map of

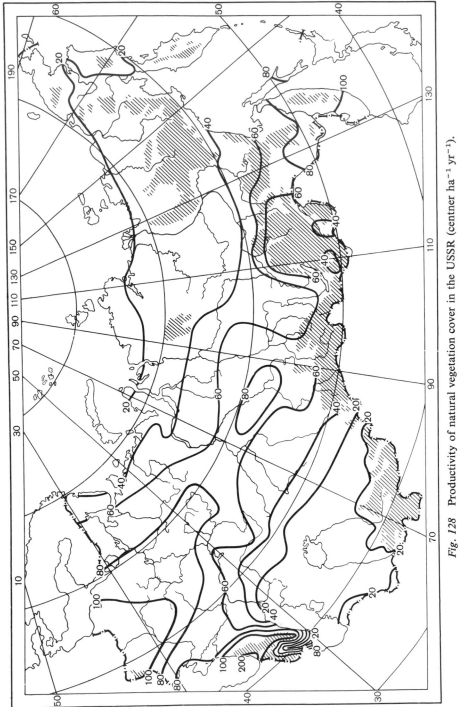

Fig. 128 Productivity of natural vegetation cover in the USSR (centner ha^{-1} yr^{-1}).

photosynthetically active radiation in the growing period (Efimova, 1965), it is possible to calculate what part of the energy of incoming radiation is assimilated in the organic matter formed during the year. Such a calculation has been carried out considering the approximate calorific value of plant organic matter as 4000 cal g^{-1}.

In Fig. 129 is presented a map of the distribution of the energy contained in the annual increase in the organic mass of vegetation, constructed on the basis of data from the above-mentioned calculation. This energy is expressed as a per cent of the energy of photosynthetically active radiation during the growing period. It can be seen from the map that in the annual increase of organic matter, up to 2% of the incoming photosynthetically active radiation is used. The greatest coefficient of utilization of the energy of solar radiation (1.8–2.0%) is observed in the area of the maximum annual increase, namely, the Black Sea coast of the Caucasus. The utilization of energy over almost the whole area of the European USSR is relatively great (1.0–1.2%), with the exception of the arid regions situated in the south and southeast. In the Asian territory of the USSR, about 1% of the energy is used in the central part of western Siberia and in the south of the Khabarovsk district and in Primor'e; in the rest of the area, the annual increase in biomass ranges from 0.4 to 0.8% of the incoming photosynthetically active radiation. In the deserts and semi-deserts of Central Asia, assimilation of energy in the annual increase of biomass reduces to 0.1–0.2%.*

The diminution of the coefficient of solar energy utilization by plants in the eastern regions of our country, as compared to the western, can be explained by the less favorable moisture conditions in many eastern regions and also by a certain reduction in the duration of the growing period that takes place there.

The mean (for the entire area of the USSR) coefficient of assimilation of photosynthetically active solar radiation by the natural vegetation cover equals approximately 0.8%. The value of the analogous coefficient for the total solar radiation will be less by a factor of about 2, that is, equal to 0.4%.

It might be thought that these values are too small to let the process of photosynthesis directly affect the principal components of the heat balance at the earth's surface. In this respect, it is usually considered that photo-synthesis is not a substantial factor affecting conditions of climate and weather.

In recent years, however, it has been established that in the contemporary epoch, climatic conditions are characterized by considerable instability. Consequently, changes in the components of the earth's energy balance

* We should note that these coefficients of solar energy utilization do not coincide with those given at the beginning of the chapter, in which total solar radiation is taken into consideration instead of photosynthetically active radiation.

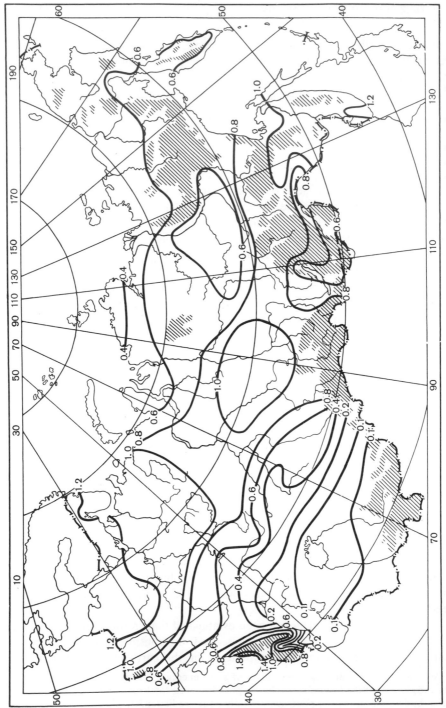

Fig. 129 Utilization of solar energy by vegetation cover [in per cent of the income of photosynthetically active radiation].

amounting to several tenths of one per cent of the incoming solar radiation may have an appreciable effect on the location of ice cover and on the climate of middle and high latitudes (see Chapters 4 and 5 of this book).

From this point of view, the question about the possible influence of the energy of photosynthesis on meteorological processes requires some attention. We note that such an influence is restricted by the comparatively rapid return into the atmosphere of the energy assimilated in the course of photosynthesis, as a result of the general biological circulation converting this energy into heat.

Climatic conditions are therefore affected by the difference between the energy used in photosynthesis and the amount of heat obtained as a result of the decay of organic matter. This difference can make up only a small portion of the energy expenditure in photosynthesis, and its climate-forming importance for the contemporary epoch is probably insignificant. Less clear is the analogous problem concerning periods when a rapid accumulation of organic matter in the earth's crust occurred (for example, during the coal-forming periods). However, even in these conditions, a substantial effect of photosynthesis on the meteorological regime seems unlikely.

There are some cases, however, when such an effect shows in a rather noticeable form—these are the cases of fires that spread over extensive areas of vegetation. Under such conditions, photosynthetic energy accumulated during a long time is converted into heat so rapidly that the value of the additional heat input for a unit area turns out to be many orders greater than the value of energy in solar radiation. As a result, in the area where large forest fires occur, the meteorological regime is suddenly changed, such changes embracing a considerable thickness of the atmospheric air.

Apart from such particular cases, we should point out that vegetation cover produces the greatest effect on climate, not as a result of the solar energy conversion in photosynthesis, but because of the effect of transpiration on the balances of heat and moisture and as a result of change in the aerodynamic roughness of the earth's surface (see Chapter X of this book).

Thus, data on the coefficients of solar energy utilization by vegetation have significance, for the most part, as a characteristic of climatic conditions of the development of vegetation and as an index of the efficiency of different types of vegetation cover.

Transformation of energy in the biological cycle

At present, there exists only an approximate knowledge of the transformation of energy in the planetary biological cycle. We present some of these data below, taking into account the fact that their accuracy is relatively low. The general productivity of autotrophic plants on land and ocean, according to contemporary data, amounts to about 83×10^9 tons yr^{-1} (Duvigneaud and Tanghe, 1967; Bogorov, 1969; Bazilevich et al., 1970, and elsewhere). Almost two thirds of this value, which amounts to about 53×10^9 tons yr^{-1}, is obtained from the vegetation cover on land. Only about 30×10^9 tons yr^{-1} of organic matter is created by the autotrophic plants of the oceans.*

Taking these values into consideration, we find that the mean productivity for a unit area of the land surface is approximately 3.6 tons ha^{-1} yr^{-1}, for the unit area of the ocean surface, 0.8 ton ha^{-1} yr^{-1}, and for the globe as a whole, 1.6 tons ha^{-1} yr^{-1}. Earlier we provided some data which indicated that depending on the climatic and other natural factors, productivity values in various regions of the land vary within wide limits, for example, from several tens of tons on a hectare per year in wet tropical forests to zero in the polar deserts.

The mean productivity for the globe corresponds to an energy expenditure approximately equal to 0.07 kcal cm^{-2} yr^{-1}, that is, about 0.05% of the amount of solar radiation incident on the earth's surface and about 0.1% of the value of photosynthetically active radiation.

The organic matter created by autotrophic plants is assimilated by herbivorous organisms, in which are included many of the animals. As a result, a new form of organic matter is created, which is used then by carnivorous organisms. The biological mass of these organisms also enters the general cycle of organic matter and becomes an item of the nutrition of various living organisms.

The processes of nutrition that interrelate living organisms are processes of energy transmission from some organisms to others. These processes balance the constant energy loss that occurs in the course of vital activity of plants and animals and provides for all the biological functions of living organisms.

Observations have shown that the efficiency of the reproduction of organic matter in its transmission from one organism to another is relatively small. Such a feature is quite clear, because an increase in biomass is only one of many functions of living organisms that require the expenditure of energy for their maintenance. Thus, for example, a considerable quantity of energy is spent in respiration. Many organisms expend energy in the processes of reproduction, movement in space, and so forth.

Above have been presented data showing that the natural vegetation cover uses a small portion of the incoming solar energy for creation of organic matter in the course of photosynthesis. A portion of this organic matter is

* These values relate to the dry mass of organic matter. Data on oceanic productivity are often expressed in the units of wet mass, which is not always mentioned in the available literature.

disbursed by the autotrophic plants themselves for respiration and the atrophy of some parts of a plant in the course of its development. As a result, the net productivity of plants often does not exceed half of the quantity of matter created by photosynthesis.

Herbivorous organisms, consuming the production of autotrophic plants, use for the creation of their own biomass no more than 10% of this production. A similar order of magnitude characterizes the coefficient of utilization of the biomass of herbivorous animals by carnivores [refer to Duvigneaud and Tanghe (1967), and elsewhere]. Thus, the flux of energy going as far as the third trophic level of the biological chain of nutrition decreases by more than a factor of a hundred in comparison with the quantity of energy assimilated by autotrophic plants.

The actual structure of energetic interrelations between different groups of living organisms is usually much more complicated than such a simple scheme. Trophic relations between individual species of plants and animals often have the form of a web that unites different kinds of living organisms into a single energy system.

However, in all cases, the aforementioned regularity is carried out; that is, in transmission of energy from one organism to another, the greater portion of it is lost. In this connection, the energetic relations that unite different groups of plants and animals can be visualized as a stepped pyramid, which rapidly becomes narrower with a transition from one layer to another. The energy flux passing through living organisms in the course of their trophic interaction brings to the organisms closing the chain of nutrition only negligible quantities of energy, when compared to the energy assimilated by autotrophic plants.

The amount of energy transmitted by some living organisms to others corresponds to their productivity, that is, the mass of organic matter created by them. The productivity of different groups of living organisms is associated with their biological mass by complicated relationships. Some of these were considered for autotrophic plants in the preceding section.

Although the available material is insufficient for any kind of accurate evaluation of total biomass of different animals and plants, some examples of such evaluations deserve attention.

Thus, for example, Kovda (1969) considers the general biomass of the lands approximately equal to 3×10^{12} tons, more than 95% of which relates to phytomass and less than 5% to zoomass. The phytomass attains its greatest unit-area value in forest regions, decreasing to zero in deserts.

The biomass of animals per unit of area also varies within wide limits. The most significant component of this biomass is usually the mass of invertebrates, among which the organisms living in the soil are of greatest importance.

The biomass of large animals per unit of area is relatively small. Thus, it follows from Huxley's summary (1962) that in the African savanna, the biomass of large wild animals can reach 15–25 tons km^{-2}, in the forests of middle latitudes, 1 ton km^{-2}, in the tundra, 0.8 ton km^{-2}, and in semidesert, 0.35 ton km^{-2}.

We can evaluate the biological mass of mankind and calculate the consumption of energy in its nutrition much more accurately than can be done for any other groups of animals and plants.

With the contemporary population of the globe exceeding three billion, the biomass of mankind is about 0.2×10^9 tons. On the assumption that each person expends daily on the average about 2.5×10^3 kcal of energy, we find that the total consumption of energy by people comes to approximately 3×10^{15} kcal yr^{-1}.

This value corresponds approximately to the contemporary productivity of agricultural production, which, however, does not provide the population with the necessary quantity of food products in all regions of the globe.

In many trophic chains, man occupies one of the last places, since he consumes both the primary production of autotrophic plants and the biomass created by many herbivores and carnivores. In this connection, his position on the energy pyramid of nutrition mentioned above corresponds to its upper layers, which are much more narrow than the base of the pyramid, which characterizes the productivity of autotrophic plants. It is easy to see from the above data that in the contemporary epoch, man consumes about 0.7% of the primary production of the organic world. Several thousand years ago, the figure was considerably less than 0.1%, and in the near future it is expected to increase greatly.

In correspondence with the development of agriculture necessary for provision of the growing population with food products, the dimensions and form of the pyramid characterizing the energy exchange in the biological cycle on our planet are constantly changing.

Besides consuming an ever greater portion of the primary biological production, man expends a great and still growing amount of additional energy, which represents a new source of heat for our planet. It will be seen from the material contained in Chapter X that this creates a near-future perspective of a considerable change in climate, which, for the first time in the history of the earth, begins to depend substantially on the activity of biological organisms.

REFERENCES

Арманд Д. Л. (1967). Некоторые задачи и методы физики ландшафта. Сб. «Геофизика ландшафта». Изд. «Наука», М.
Armand, D. L. (1967). Some questions and methods in physics of the landscape. *In*

"Geofizika Landshafta (Geophysics of the Landscape)," (D. L. Armand, ed.) pp. 7–24. Izdat. Nauka, Moscow. MGA 19.12-16.

Атлас теплового баланса земного шара. (1963). Под ред. М. И. Будыко. Междуведомственный геофизический комитет, М.

"Atlas Teplovogo Balansa Zemnogo Shara (Atlas of the Heat Balance of the Earth)" (M. I. Budyko, ed.). Akad. Nauk SSSR, Prezidium. Mezhduvedomstvennyi Geofiz. Komitet, Moscow, 1963; Guide to the "Atlas of the Heat Balance of the Earth." U.S. Weather Bur., WB/T No. 106. U.S. Weather Bur., Washington, D.C., 1964.

Базилевич Н. И., Родин Л. Е. (1967). Картосхемы продуктивности и биологического круговорота главнейших типов растительности суши земли. Изв. Геогр. о-ва СССР, № 3.

Bazilevich, N. I., and Rodin, L. E. (1967). Cartographic models of productivity and biological circulation in the principal types of land vegetation of the earth. *Izv. Geogr. Obshchestva SSSR* **99** (No. 3), 190–194, 1967.

Базилевич Н. И., Родин Л. Е. (1969). Географические закономерности продуктивности и круговорота химических элементов в основных типах растительности земли. Сб. «Общие теоретические проблемы биологической продуктивности». Изд. «Наука», Л.

Bazilevich, N. I., and Rodin, L. E. (1969). Geographic regularities in productivity and the circulation of chemical elements in the earth's main vegetation types. *In* "Obshchie Teoreticheskie Problemy Biologicheskoi Produktivnosti" (O. V. Zalenskii, and L. E. Rodin, eds.), pp. 24–33 + maps. Izdat. Nauka, Leningrad; *Sov. Geogr. Rev. Trans.* **12**, No. 1, 24–53 (1971).

Базилевич Н. И., Родин Л. Е., Розов Н. Н. (1970). Географические аспекты изучения биологической продуктивности. Изд. Геогр. о-ва СССР, Л.

Bazilevich, N. I., Rodin, L. E., and Rozov, N. N. (1970). "Geograficheskie Aspecty Izucheniia Biologicheskoi Produktivnosti (Geographical Aspects of Biological Productivity)." Izdat. Geograf. Obshch. SSSR, Mater. V S'ezda, Leningrad. *Sov. Geogr. Rev. Trans.* **12** (No. 5), 293–317 (1971).

Берлянд Т. Г. (1961). Распределение солнечной радиации на континентах. Гидрометеоиздат, Л.

Berliand, T. G. (1961). "Raspredelenie Solnechnoi Radiatsii na Kontinentakh (Distribution of Solar Radiation on the Continents)." Gidrometeoizdat, Leningrad.

Богоров В. Г. (1969). Жизнь океана. Изд. «Знание», М.

Bogorov, V. G. (1969). "Zhizn' Okeana (The Life of the Ocean)." Izdat. Znanie, Moscow.

Будыко М. И. (1949). К теории интенсивности физико-географического процесса. Вопросы географии, вып. 15.

Budyko, M. I. (1949). On the theory of the intensity of physicogeographic processes. *Vop. Geogr.* **15**.

Будыко М. И. (1956). Тепловой баланс земной поверхности. Гидрометеоиздат, Л.

Budyko, M. I. (1956). "Teplovoi Balans Zemnoi Poverkhnosti." Gidrometeoizdat, Leningrad; "Heat Balance of the Earth's Surface," translated by N. A. Stepanova. U.S. Weather Bur., Washington, D.C., 1958. MGA 8.5-20, 13E-286.

Будыко М. И. (1964). К теории влияния климатических факторов на фотосинтез. ДАН СССР, т. 158, № 2.

Budyko, M. I. (1964). A contribution to development of a theory of the influence of climatic factors on photosynthesis. *Dokl. Akad. Nauk SSSR* **158**, No. 2, 331–334; *Dokl. Acad. Sci. USSR Earth Sci. Sect.* **158**, 1–3 (1965).

Будыко М. И. (1968). О происхождении ледниковых эпох. Метеорология и гидрология, № 11.

Budyko, M. I. (1968). On the origin of glacial epochs. *Meteorol. Gidrol.* No. 11, 3–12. MGA 20.11-383.

Будыко М. И., Гандин Л. С. (1964). Об учете закономерностей физики атмосферы в агрометеорологических исследованиях. Метеорология и гидрология, № 11.

Budyko, M. I., and Gandin, L. S. (1964). Agrometeorological studies taking into account the laws of atmospheric physics. *Meteorol. Gidrol.* No. 11, 3–11. MGA 16.7–85.

Будыко М. И., Гандин Л. С. (1965). К теории фотосинтеза в слое растительного покрова. ДАН СССР, т. 164, № 2.

Budyko, M. I., and Gandin, L. S. (1965). On the theory of photosynthesis in a layer of plant cover. *Dokl. Akad. Nauk SSSR* **164**, No. 2, 454–457; *Dokl. Bot. Sci.* **163–165**, 122–125 (1966).

Будыко М. И., Гандин Л. С. (1966). Влияние климатических факторов на растительный покров. Изв. АН СССР, сер. геогр., № 1.

Budyko, M. I., and Gandin, L. S. (1966). Influence of climatic factors on plant cover. *Izv. Akad. Nauk SSSR Ser. Geogr.* No. 1, 3–10. MGA 17.8-65.

Будыко М. И., Гандин Л. С., Ефимова Н. А. (1966а). Применение физических методов для разработки агроклиматических показателей. Метеорология и гидрология, № 5.

Budyko, M. I., Gandin, L. S., and Efimova, N. A. (1966a). The use of physical methods in working out agroclimatic indices. *Meteorol. Gidrol.* No. 5, 3–10. MGA 17.11-74.

Будыко М. И., Гандин Л. С., Ефимова Н. А. (1966б). Влияние климатических факторов на продуктивность растительного покрова. Сб. «Современные проблемы климатологии». Гидрометеоиздат, Л.

Budyko, M. I., Gandin, L. S., and Efimova, N. A. (1966b). Effect of climatic factors on the productivity of plant cover. *In* "Sovremennye Problemy Klimatologii (Contemporary Problems of Climatology)" (M. I. Budyko, ed.), pp. 312–320. Gidrometeoizdat, Leningrad. MGA 18.12-64.

Будыко М. И., Ефимова Н. А. (1968). Использование солнечной энергии природным растительным покровом на территории СССР. Ботанический журнал, т. 23, № 10.

Budyko, M. I., and Efimova, N. A. (1968). The utilization of solar energy by the natural vegetation cover in the USSR. *Bot. Zh.* **23**, No. 10.

Винберг Г. Г. (1948). Эффективность утилизации солнечной энергии планктоном. Природа, № 12.

Vinberg, G. G. (1948). Efficiency of utilization of solar energy by plankton. *Priroda* (*Moscow*) No. 12.

Гандин Л. С.. Менжулин Г. В., Усов В. Б. (1969). Расчет влияния метеорологических и биоклиматических факторов на фотосинтез с помощью электронной вычислительной машины. Сб. «Общие теоретические проблемы биологической продуктивности». Изд. «Наука», Л.

Gandin, L. S., Menzhulin, G. V., and Usov, B. V. (1969). Calculation of the effect of meteorologic and bioclimatic factors on photosynthesis by means of electronic computers. *In* "Obshchie Teoreticheskie Problemy Biologicheskoi Produktivnosti" (O. V. Zalenskii and L. E. Rodin, eds.), pp. 174–181. Izdat. Nauka, Leningrad.

Дроздов А. В. (1969). Продуктивность зональных наземных растительных сообществ и показатели водно-теплового режима территории. Сб. «Общие теоретические проблемы биологической продуктивности». Изд. «Наука», Л.

Drozdov, A. V. (1969). The productivity of zonal terrestrial plant communities and the moisture and heat parameters of an area. *In* "Obshchie Teoreticheskie Problemy Biologicheskoi Produktivnosti" (O. V. Zalenskii and L. E. Rodin, eds.), pp. 33–39. Izdat. Nauka, Leningrad; *Sov. Geogr. Rev. Trans.* **12**, No. 1, 54–61 (9171).

Ефимова Н. А. (1965). Распределение фотосинтетической активной радиации на территории Советского Союза. Труды ГГО, вып. 179.

Efimova, N. A. (1965). The distribution of photosynthetically-active radiation in the Soviet Union. *Tr. Gl. Geofiz. Observ.* **179**, 118–130. MGA 17.7-267.

Ефимова Н. А. (1968). Основные особенности метеорологического режима на полях озимой пшеницы и озимой ржи. Труды ГГО, вып. 229.

Efimova, N. A. (1968). Principal characteristics of the meteorological regime on fields of winter wheat and winter rye. *Tr. Gl. Geofiz. Observ.* **229**, 23–36. MGA 20.5-33.

Ефимова Н. А. (1969). Географическое распределение сумм фотосинтетически активной радиации. Сб. «Общие теоретические проблемы биологической продуктивности». Изд. «Наука», Л.

Efimova, N. A. (1969). Geographical distribution of the sums of photosynthetically-active radiation. *In* "Obshchie Teoreticheskie Problemy Biologicheskoi Produktivnosti," (O. V. Zalenskii and L. E. Rodin, eds.), pp. 160–164. Izdat. Nauka, Leningrad; *Sov. Geogr. Rev. Transl.* **12**, No. 1, 66–74 (1971).

Ковда В. А. (1969). Проблема биологической и хозяйственной продуктивности суши. Сб. «Общие теоретические проблемы биологической продуктивности». Изд. «Наука», Л.

Kovda, V. A. (1969). The problem of biological and economic productivity of the earth's land areas. *In* "Obshchie Teoreticheskie Problemy Biologicheskoi Produktivnosti" (O. V. Zalenskii and L. E. Rodin, eds.), pp. 8–24. Izdat. Nauka, Leningrad; *Sov. Geogr. Rev. Transl.* **12**, No. 1, 6–24 (1971).

Лавренко Е. М., Андреев В. Н., Леонтьев В. Л. (1955). Профиль продуктивности надземной части природного растительного покрова СССР. Ботанический журнал, т. 10, № 3.

Lavrenko, E. M., Andreev, V. N., and Leont'ev, V. L. (1955). The profile of productivity of the above-ground parts of natural vegetation of the USSR. *Bot. Zh.* **10**, No. 3.

Любименко В. Н. (1935). Фотосинтез и хемосинтез в растительном мире. Сельхозгиз, Л.

Liubimenko, V. N. (1935). "Fotosintez i Khemosintez v Rastitel'nom Mire (Photosynthesis and Chemosynthesis in the Plant World)." Sel'khozgiz, Leningrad.

Максимов Н. А. (1926). Физиологические основы засухоустойчивости растений. Изд. ВИПБиНК, Л.

Maksimov, N. A. (1926). "Fiziologicheskie Osnovy Zasukhoustoichivosti Rastenii (Physiological Basis of Drought-Resistance in Plants)." Izdat. Vses. Inst. Prikl. Bot., Leningrad.

Максимов Н. А. (1944). Развитие учения о водном режиме растений от Тимирязева до наших дней. Изд. АН СССР, М.

Maksimov, N. A. (1944). "Razvitie Ucheniia o Vodnom Rezhime Rastenii ot Timiriazeva do Nashikh Dnei (Development of the Study of the Water Regime of Plants from Timiriazev to Our Day)." Izdat. Akad. Nauk SSSR, Moscow.

Ничипорович А. А. (1963). О путях повышения производительности фотосинтеза растений в посевах. Сб. «Фотосинтез и вопросы продуктивности растений». Изд. АН СССР, М.

Nichiporovich, A. A. (1963). Means of increasing photosynthetic productivity of plants in fields. *In* "Fotosintez i Voprosy Produktivnosti Rastenii" (A. A. Nichiporovich, ed.), pp. 5–37. Izdat. Akad. Nauk SSSR, Moscow.

Основы лесной биогеоценологии. (1964). Под ред. В. Н. Сукачева и Н. В. Дылиса. Изд. «Наука».

"Osnovy Lesnoi Biogeotsenologii (The Foundations of Forest Biogeocenology)" (V. N. Sukachev and N. V. Dylis, eds.). Izdat. Nauka, Moscow, 1964.

Росс Ю. К. (1964). К математической теории фотосинтеза растительного покрова. ДАН СССР, т. 157, № 5.

Ross, Iu. K. (1964). Toward a mathematical theory of photosynthesis of plant cover. *Dokl. Akad. Nauk SSSR* 157, No. 5, 1239–1242; *Dokl. Bot. Sci.* 157–159, 140–143 (1965).

Росс Ю. К., Бихеле З. (1968—1969). Расчет фотосинтеза растительного покрова. I. Сб. «Фотосинтез и продуктивность растительного покрова.» Тарту. II. «Фотосинтетическая продуктивность растительного покрова.» Тарту.

Ross, Iu. K., and Bikhele, Z. (1968–1969). Calculation of photosynthesis of plant cover, I. *In* "Fotosintez i Produktivnost' Rastitel'nogo Pokrova" (L. Nil'son, ed.), pp. 75–100 (Engl. abstract). Akad. Nauk Estonskoi SSR, Inst. Fiz. Astron., Tartu, 1968; II. *In* "Fotosinteticheskaia Produktivnost' Rastitel'nogo Pokrova" (Kh. Moldau, ed.), pp. 5–43 (Engl. abstract). Akad. Nauk Estonskoi SSR, Inst. Fiz. Astron., Tartu, 1969.

Хильми Г. Ф. (1957). Теоретическая биогеофизика леса. Изд. АН СССР, М.

Khil'mi, G. F. (1957). "Teoreticheskaia Biogeofizika Lesa." Izdat. Akad. Nauk, Moscow; "Theoretical Forest Biogeophysics." OTS 61-31089. Isr. Program Sci. Transl., Jerusalem, 1962.

Хильми Г. Ф. (1966). Основы физики биосферы. Гидрометеоиздат, Л.

Khil'mi, G. F. (1966). "Osnovy Fiziki Biosfery (Principles of the Physics of the Biosphere)." Gidrometeoizdat, Leningrad. MGA 18.2-6.

Davidson, I. L., and Philip, I. R. (1958). Light and pasture growth. *In* "Climatology and Microclimatology," *Proc. Canberra Symp., 1956*, UNESCO Arid Zone Res., No. 11, 181–187. 1958.

Duncan, W. G., Loomis, R. S., Williams, W. A., and Hanau, R. (1967). A model for simulating photosynthesis in plant communities. *Hilgardia* 38.

Duvigneaud, P., and Tanghe, M. (1967). "Ecosystèmes et Biosphere." Bruxelles.

Huxley, I. (1962). Les bases écologiques en Afrique Orientale, *Endeavour* 21, No. 82.

Lieth, H. (1964–1965). Versuch einer kartographischen Darstellung der Produktivität der Pflanzendecke auf der Erde. *In* Geogr. Taschenbuch (E. Meynen, ed.), pp. 72–80. Wiesbaden, F. Steiner Verlag.

Monsi, M., and Saeki, T. (1963). Über den Lichtfaktor in den Pflanzengesellschaften und seine Bedeutung für die Stoffproduktion. *Jap. J. Bot.* 14, No. 1.

Monteith, J. L., Szeicz, G., and Yabuki, K. (1964). Crop photosynthesis and the flux of carbon dioxide below the canopy. *J. Appl. Ecol.* 1.

Monteith, J. L. (1965). Light distribution and photosynthesis in field crops. *Ann. Bot.* (London) 29, No. 113.

Rabinowitch, E. (1951). "Photosynthesis and Related Processes." Vol. 2, Wiley (Interscience), New York. (Русский перевод: Е. Рабинович. Фотосинтез, т. 2. ИЛ, 1953.)

Uchijima, Z. (1966). An improvement of semi-empirical methods of evaluating the total photosynthesis of a plant community. *Nogyo Kisho* 22, No. 1.

de Wit, C. T. (1965). Photosynthesis of leaf canopies. Landbouwhogeschool, Centrum voor Landbouwpublikaties. (Verslagen van landbouwkundige onderzoekingen, No. 663.)

IX

Change of Successive Faunas

1. Critical Epochs of Geological History

It has been established in numerous paleontological investigations that the contemporary animal world has appeared as a result of a long evolution. During the course of this evolution, along with relatively slow changes in the animal world, abrupt changes in faunas repeatedly took place, for example, at the end of the Silurian period (when many groups of invertebrates became extinct), at the end of the Paleozoic era (when several groups of invertebrates, fish, and amphibians vanished), and at the end of the Mesozoic era (the extinction of some groups of invertebrates and many reptiles).

The disappearance of these animals was accompanied by a rapid development of new faunas, whose representatives filled the vacant ecological niches.

From the data of the geological chronicle, it is difficult to establish the duration of the epochs during which abrupt changes in the animal world occurred. It is known, however, that they were comparatively short, and that is why they are usually referred to as critical epochs of geological history.

The question concerning the causes of the extinction of large groups of animals during the critical epochs, which has great importance for clarification of the general regularities of change in successive faunas, has been discussed in numerous investigations.

In the works of Cuvier, who was one of the founders of paleontology, done at the beginning of the 19th century, the change of successive faunas during the history of the earth was explained by repeated catastrophes that annihilated the animals of remote eras. In his book "Discours sur les

révolutions de la surface du globe" (1812), Cuvier wrote: "Life on our planet
was more than once shaken by frightful events. Innumerable living creatures
fell victims of catastrophes."

As is well known, Cuvier's opinions were later rejected under the influence
of the work of Lyell and Darwin. Proceeding from the principle of uniformitarianism that explains the changes in the structure of the earth's crust by
the activity of factors now existing, Lyell and his followers came to consider
the theory of cataclysms useless for geological research. The theory of
biological evolution by Darwin, created not without influence of the uniformitarian viewpoints of Lyell, explained the change of different faunas in the
geological past rather by the effect of the natural selection under stable or
slowly varying conditions than by the effect of catastrophes.

In subsequent works by Kovalevskii and other investigators, numerous
paleontological data were collected, and they confirmed the leading role,
studied by Darwin, of the mechanism of biological evolution in the formation
of the animal world during remote epochs.

Accepting that the analysis of Darwin's concept explains the general
regularities of biological evolution, the question should still be raised concerning the possible effect on the change of successive faunas, along with the
slow action of natural selection, of rapid changes caused by action on the
animal world of catastrophic shifts in climatic conditions.

The statement of this question arises from the necessity of taking into
account the enormous time scales of the periods of development of nature
in the geological past, which cannot be compared with the scale of those
accessible to the immediate observation of man.

It must be borne in mind that possible deviations of the indices of intensity
of many natural processes from the norm increase with an increase in the
time period under consideration. Thus, for example, disastrous earthquakes
are hardly probable in short intervals of time but quite probable over a
sufficiently long period.

From a general point of view, therefore, it seems natural to suppose that
during the long geological history of the earth, some manifestations of such
major anomalies in the characteristics of the natural processes would appear
that have not been observed during the comparatively short time of the
existence of mankind and especially during the very short period in which man
has been studying Nature around him. During recent years, such a viewpoint
has been time and again expressed in the papers of geologists (Nalivkin,
1969, and elsewhere).

Let us discuss the possibility of using this idea for studying the problem of
the change of successive faunas.

It is known from the data of paleontological investigations that the process
of extinction of large taxonomic groups of animals (orders, suborders, and

families) that have disappeared is characterized by the fact that groups of animals, that were different in biological relations and occupied quite different ecological niches, often became extinct together during periods of time that are short from the point of view of geological history. It follows from statistical considerations that such a phenomenon cannot be the result of a struggle for existence under unvarying external conditions.

As an example, let us consider the known case of simultaneous extinctions of large groups of animals that took place at the end of the Cretaceous period. In that time, of the existing ten orders of reptiles, five orders disappeared, including the land dinosaurs (two orders), the flying pterosaurs, and also the water-dwelling ichthyosauri and plesiosauri. The five orders included 35 families, containing very many species (Colbert, 1965).

Let us assume that the mean duration of the time of existence of a reptile order that became extinct in the Cretaceous period was approximately 100 million years, and let us consider that the time of disappearance of the order can be determined with accuracy to five million years.

The probability of a chance coincidence during five million years of the extinction of five orders out of ten, calculated by the Poisson formula, turns out approximately equal to $\frac{1}{10000}$. Such an extremely small value indicates that the coincidence of the extinctions of these groups of reptiles was caused by certain changes in the natural environment, rather than happening by chance.

A similar calculation could be carried out to evaluate the probability of the extinction in a brief time of several families comprised in the same order, and only weakly connected with each other in terms of mode of life. The probability of such an event under stable conditions of the environment turns out to be extremely low.

In examining paleontological data, it is not difficult to ascertain that in most cases, large taxonomic subdivisions of the animal world disappeared, not one by one, but in relatively numerous groups. Thus, for example, most of the orders and suborders of reptiles and amphibians that have become extinct disappeared during three critical epochs of geological history, namely, at the ends of the Permian, the Triassic, and the Cretaceous periods. It follows from the above calculation that such coincidences would have been hardly probable under constant or slowly changing external conditions, even if the duration of these critical epochs extended over several million years.

The conclusion about the impossibility of explaining the disappearance of many large groups of animals by the struggle for existence under stable external conditions follows not only from the above calculation but also from some qualitative considerations.

It has been repeatedly pointed out in the paleontological literature that the mammals came to occupy the ecological niches belonging to reptiles of the

Mesozoic era, not in the course of competition with them, but only after their extinction, when the niches became vacant.

Among particular examples of this sort, we will mention the interesting case of the phytosaur extinction that occurred at the end of the Triassic. These reptiles suddenly disappeared, vacating an ecological niche that afterwards was occupied by crocodiles, which appeared later and originated from the same initial forms as the phytosaurs, and were very similar to them. Explanation of such examples without consideration of temporal changes in natural conditions presents difficulties.

Thus, in order to understand the reasons for great changes of fauna in the geological past, it is necessary to consider not only the effect of purely biological causes but also the action of additional factors associated with sudden changes in environmental conditions.

This viewpoint has been expressed in papers on historical geology (Strakhov, 1937) and hydrobiology (Lindberg, 1948), and in a number of other studies.

In studies dedicated to the problem of the extinction of various animal groups, a great number of hypotheses about changes in the natural conditions that furthered the extinction process has been offered. We will not discuss here the considerations in favor of one or the other hypothesis, since the qualitative character of these considerations does not permit making any final conclusions about their validity.

Here we will consider one of the possible mechanisms of the effect of environment on biological evolution, the significance of which can be evaluated by the use of the results of quantitative calculations.

Among the external factors affecting biological organisms, the influence of climate has the most general character. This influence extends to all spheres inhabited by living creatures and exerts a profound influence on them.

It is well known that the climatic variations that took place in the past led to significant changes in the location of animals and plants on our planet. Less clear is the question, to what degree these changes affected biological evolution, although the existence of this relationship is considered to be more or less universally recognized.

Leaving to one side the task of investigating the effect that comparatively slow changes in climate, caused by such factors, for example, as change of relief and displacement of coastlines of the continents, had on the evolution of animals and plants, let us turn to the poorly investigated problem of the significance for biological evolution of short-term but sharp fluctuations of climate.

The possibility of investigating such fluctuations becomes apparent as a result of studies in which the variability of solar radiation incident on the earth's surface has been established. This variability is a consequence of the instability of atmospheric transparency, depending essentially on the amount of dust entering the atmosphere after volcanic eruptions (Budyko, 1969).

In Chapter V of this book, reference was made to the variability in the number of volcanic eruptions in time and to the temperature fluctuations caused by volcanic activity and associated with this variability.

Although the effect of single eruptions on the temperature of the earth is comparatively small, because of the limited amount of dust penetrating the atmosphere after each eruption, it is evident that the earth's temperature will be changed much more powerfully when many explosive eruptions coincide within a short interval of time. The possibility of such coincidences for long periods of time, which is a consequence of general statistical laws, grows appreciably with fluctuations of volcanic activity. Analogously, the greatest amount of dust thrown out into the atmosphere during one volcanic eruption will increase with the lengthening of the period under consideration for the same reason as does the greatest frequency of eruptions.

Calculation of the greatest amount of dust that can be ejected into the atmosphere during volcanic eruptions in a short period of time involves a number of difficulties.

A preliminary evaluation of this amount can be carried out with material from the summary by Lamb (1969), who compiled a table of explosive eruptions that took place in the 18th to 20th centuries. Lamb included in this table an evaluation of the quantity of dust that entered the atmosphere after each eruption, and presented it in the form of a scale on which all the values were compared with the amount of dust injected during the eruption of Krakatoa in 1884. This value was assumed equal to 1000 arbitrary units.

Analysis of the data from Lamb's summary shows that the amount of dust injected into the atmosphere in each decade varies within wide limits. The maximum magnitude of this value grows with an increase in the general duration of a period of time, that is, with an increase in the number of decades under consideration.

This dependence can be expressed in the form of a simple empirical formula

$$N = a \log(T/t), \tag{9.1}$$

where N is the greatest amount of dust injected into the atmosphere in the interval of time t during a period of duration T; a is a coefficient equal to 3000.

This formula can be used for the values of T that are much greater than t.

It follows from Eq. (9.1) that the greatest amount of dust injected into the atmosphere during a decade ($t = 10$) for $T = 300$ equals 4400, which agrees well with the greatest value in Lamb's summary.

If we use this formula as an extrapolation to greater intervals of time, we find that for $T = 10^4$, $N = 9000$, and for $T = 10^7$, $N = 18,000$ [units].

Thus, for long periods of time, a coincidence of volcanic eruptions is possible during a decade producing ejected dust equivalent in amount to nine or even eighteen eruptions of Krakatoa.

One should not exaggerate the reliability of this estimate, derived by a method of extrapolation. Still, we might suggest that the above values are characterized by underestimation rather than overestimation of the greatest decadal quantity of dust from volcanic eruptions penetrating the atmosphere.

The logarithmic dependence assumed in Eq. (9.1) follows from statistical laws characterizing the coincidence of events that are not interconnected.

It is, however, well known that the eruptions of individual volcanoes cannot be considered as random events independent of each other, because the level of volcanic activity changes substantially during various geological epochs. Thus, for example, from the work of Ronov (1959), it follows that during various geological periods, volcanic activity differed by a factor of several times. It is evident that in the presence of general changes in volcanic activity, an assessment of the frequency of coincidence of eruptions that is based on the idea of their independence must be underestimated.

In this respect, it should be indicated that, although Lamb considers the data on volcanism in recent centuries characteristic of a period with a relatively high level of volcanic activity, long periods of time with far greater volcanic activity occurred in the geological past. Consequently, for these intervals, the evaluations of dust amount obtained from Lamb's summary cannot be overestimated.

Let us examine the question of how the earth's temperature changed with the coincidence of many volcanic eruptions.

If, during a decade, ten eruptions comparable to that of Krakatoa took place, then the mean diminution of direct radiation in that time, according to the data from Chapter V, would be at least 10–20%, since the rate of dust input into the stratosphere during this period would be no less than its rate of fallout. In this situation, global radiation would decrease by 2–3%, and the mean temperature of the earth's surface would drop by 3–5 C°.

With the coincidence of twenty volcanic eruptions during a decade, the radiation regime would change more strongly. Estimates by the formulas of atmospheric optics show that in this case, total radiation would decrease by no less than 5%. Such a decline of radiation would lead to a drop in the mean temperature of the earth's surface by 5–10 C°, this cooling extending both to the atmosphere and the upper layer of ocean water.

Notwithstanding the approximate character of the data presented here, it can be inferred from them that volcanic eruptions from time to time have caused short-term but appreciable drops in temperature, which spread over the whole planet.

It is important to note that the probability of abrupt short-term drops in temperature increased greatly in epochs of active mountain-formation, when volcanism became stronger. Under such conditions, the lowering of temperature may presumably have been greater than the evaluations given above.

Without doubt, such short-term drops in temperature would have an enormous effect on various forms of organic life.

As was pointed out in Chapter VII of this book, a definite thermal zone of existence is characteristic of all living organisms without any exceptions, this zone being in many cases quite narrow. A sudden drop in temperature lasting several years or decades would lead to the extinction of many animal and plant species, first of all those that lived under climatic conditions close to the lower boundary of their thermal zone of existence. If the temperature drop over the whole planet permitted preservation of one or another species, even if only in the warmest regions, then, after cessation of a temperature drop, appropriate plants and animals could colonize their former areas. If the cooling trend was sufficiently great in the warmest areas also, then the species or groups of species under consideration would disappear completely.

In turning to specific ways in which sharp drops in temperature affect the vital activity of different organisms, we must point out that this action would have been highly diverse.

For each organism the significance of a lowering in temperature can be established: (a) leading immediately to its death; (b) reducing its activity to the limits where it perishes in the course of the struggle for existence; (c) reducing the organism's resistance against infectious diseases, as a result of which it falls their inevitable victim; (d) disturbing the process of reproduction.

The values of the decreases in temperatures corresponding to these conditions may be different, but even the smallest of them would have proved sufficient for extinction of an animal species under consideration.

Among the cases of the simultaneous disappearance of large groups of animals that took place in the past, special interest attaches to the outstanding scale of the extinction of reptiles and amphibians at the end of the Triassic, and the still more enormous extinction of reptiles at the end of the Cretaceous period.

Turning to consider the peculiarities of these two moments in geological history, we must first of all emphasize that both of them took place in epochs of intensive mountain formation, when, because of an awakening of volcanic activity the probability of simultaneous eruption of a large number of volcanoes was the greatest.

It should be borne in mind that a significant general intensification of volcanism not only increased the probability of initiating an especially large temperature drop but also heightened the probability of the appearance of a series of such drops, which could be clustered during hundreds of thousands or millions of years.

It is well known that an important characteristic of reptiles and amphibians is their absence of heat regulation, which makes them especially sensitive to the temperature regime.

The climate of the Mesozoic era was characterized by a weakly marked thermal zonality, a higher temperature in low latitudes as compared with the contemporary epoch, and a much higher temperature in extratropical areas, which created favorable conditions for the existence of animals without heat regulation (poikilothermal) over the entire earth.

Another situation took place at the end of the Paleozoic era, when thermal zonality was intensified from time to time, which presumably caused difficulties for poikilothermal animals. An interesting indication of this appeared in unique adaptations characteristic of some reptiles of the Permian period (dimetrodon, edaphosaur). These reptiles had an enormous crest on their backs, which, according to the views of some paleontologists (Romer, 1945), they used for heating their bodies at low temperatures. Setting the crest perpendicular to the sun's rays, these reptiles could absorb an additional amount of heat sufficient for supporting further physical activity. We note that a quantitative calculation of heat balance of the reptiles' bodies by the method set forth in Chapter VII shows that such an adaptation enabled them to raise their mean body temperature by several degrees, a value that was quite substantial under conditions of an inadequately warm climate.

The absence of this device in the Mesozoic reptiles is one of the indications of the existence of a comparatively warm climate in all latitudes in that era. Sudden large drops in temperature should have sharply affected the poikilothermal animals of that time.

The reptiles existing now represent a remnant of the rich and varied fauna of the Mesozoic era that survived after the extinction of the overwhelming majority of the large and many small forms of this fauna. We have every reason to consider that contemporary reptiles are capable of greater endurance in relation to low temperatures than those animals that became extinct; therefore, their ecology can give an idea of the upper limit of the endurance of reptiles in relation to cold.

Zoogeographic research has shown that the existing reptiles are, in the main, tropical and subtropical forms, since the great majority of their species is concentrated in the low latitudes. The comparatively few reptiles living outside this zone are active only during the warm season, and in various ways protect themselves against chilling in the cold periods. Diurnal rhythms are characteristic of the activity of many reptiles, their activity usually ceasing during the coldest hours of the twenty four.

The papers of Bogert (1959) and his collaborators, who have studied the ecology of reptiles, established the enormous effect on their activity of the necessity to maintain a definite body temperature. When reptiles experience a shortage of heat, they tend to warm themselves in the sun's rays or near the heated surface of the earth. In cases of cooling, some lizards change their color in order to increase the absorption of solar radiation.

Using the data of laboratory and field observations, it is possible to conclude with confidence that the lowering of the mean temperature in the habitat of many reptiles by a value of approximately 10° must lead to their death.

For this reason, the ecology of an animal belonging to the oldest of the surviving reptiles, namely, the rhynchocephalians, is interesting. The only species in this order is the tuatara (Sphenodon or Hatteria), now inhabiting several small islands of New Zealand. The existence of this animal under the cool climatic conditions of New Zealand is sometimes considered as an evidence of the relative endurance of ancient reptiles to low temperatures (Bellairs and Carrington, 1966).

However, this conclusion is based on a wrong notion of the New Zealand climate. The main feature of this pronounced marine climate is the absence of significantly cold weather in the course of the year, which ought to be considered rather a favorable factor for poikilothermal animals.

In investigations, it was established that maturing of an embryo in the tuatara egg occurs very slowly and lasts for about fifteen months, the development of the embryo ceasing in the colder time of the year. Such a long development considerably increases the risk of destruction of the few tuatara eggs by other animals, which indicates the difficulty of survival of archaic reptile types at insufficiently high temperatures. It is evident that even a moderate drop in temperature would make the development of tuatara eggs impossible and lead to the extinction of this species.

Turning to the possible effect of a severe drop in temperature on poikilothermal animals of the Mesozoic era, it should be pointed out that at present it is difficult to reconstruct the precise criteria that determined the sensitivity of different fossil reptiles to cold, and caused the extinction of some forms and the survival of others. We might only suggest that a drop in temperature must have been especially disastrous for large animals, and also for oceanic species, which, at the times of strongest cooling, could not shelter in warmer refuges, as contemporary reptiles do.

This suggestion agrees well with the fact of an almost complete extinction of large land reptiles and also of both orders of marine reptiles at the end of the Upper Cretaceous.

Although the possibility of preservation of relatively small forms of the land reptiles was increased thanks to their ability to find refuges, it can be considered that the survival of some reptile groups after severe cooling took place only in limited warmest areas.

It is quite clear that harsh cooling was much less dangerous for animals that possessed heat regulation, that is, for mammals and birds. It is well known that these animals succeeded in making the transition from the Cretaceous to the Tertiary period and then occupied all the ecological niches vacated by the now extinct reptiles.

Worth mentioning is the question concerning the extent to which the extinction of reptiles in critical moments of their history was really simultaneous. Although analysis of the available paleontological material runs into great difficulties owing to the unreliability of dating different sediments, we still have the impression that the disappearance of various species of reptiles at the end of the Upper Cretaceous relates to relatively close but not coinciding periods of time.

This conclusion could be in agreement with the concept of the effect of harsh short-term cooling on the extinction of reptiles, if we took into account the aforementioned probability of the appearance of a series of short-term drops in temperature during periods of intensified volcanism. The first cooling would be able to destroy the animals least adjusted to cooling, and the subsequent drops to cause extinction of other groups, weakened by the previous cooling.

Let us look at the question as to what extent this concept permits us to overcome the difficulties of explaining the extinction of Mesozoic reptiles that have been mentioned in the existing investigations. For this purpose, we will discuss the considerations of Colbert, who, in the final section of his book "The Age of Reptiles" (1965, p. 203), sets forth contemporary attitudes towards this problem.

In discussing the probability of the effect of catastrophic change in environmental conditions on reptile extinction, Colbert writes: "Did some great event take place that wiped out these reptiles ? If so, why should a great catastrophe be so selective—why should it have caused the extinction of five orders of reptiles and allowed the continuation of five others ? Why should all families and genera and species belonging to these five orders have disappeared completely ? Moreover, if it was a physical catastrophe of some sort, why is it not recorded in the rocks? The continuity of sediments to be seen in certain localities as Cretaceous beds are succeeded by Tertiary beds indicates an orderly world in those distant days, like the orderly world we know. And indeed this is an expression of the principle of uniformitarianism, so important to the science of geology. From all of the records of the rocks, the world around, there is ample reason to think that earth processes and life processes in the past were as they are today; that events of past ages must be explained by the forces which we see acting in nature at the present time. There is no place for world-wide catastrophes in the world of the past or of the present if the principle of uniformitarianism has any validity."

Colbert further points out that at the end of the Cretaceous period, the Laramide Revolution, associated with the formation of several present-day mountain systems, took place. He believes that such a change in the natural environment was slow enough so that the reptiles could adapt themselves to it in the course of evolution. Colbert believes that the difference between the climates of the Upper Cretaceous and the Lower Tertiary periods was quite small and could not have been the cause of the extinction of reptiles. In discussing the question of the possible importance of a temperature change during the transition from the Cretaceous to the Tertiary period, Colbert principally gives attention to the hypothesis of an abrupt rise in temperature in that time, and points out the difficulty of the agreement of this hypothesis with the fact of extinction of some groups of reptiles and survival of others. He expresses special uncertainty about the possible effect of temperature fluctuations on the extinction of sea animals, in view of the great thermal inertia of the ocean.

Colbert also rejects such hypotheses about possible causes of the extinction of reptiles as the suggestion of their competition with Cretaceous mammals that could destroy the reptiles' eggs, the idea of the effect of irradiation on the reptiles, and several others. In conclusion, he suggests that the extinction of reptiles was explicable by a combination of complicated effects, whose real nature, perhaps, will never be clarified.

From our point of view, this pessimistic conclusion can be considered to be well grounded when studying this problem on the basis of only paleontological data, without using the methods and materials of adjacent disciplines. Utilization of paleoclimatological data permits us to overcome the difficulties mentioned by Colbert and to answer the questions he has raised.

Thus, for example, it follows from the above concept that for the periods comparable in duration with the Mesozoic era, sharp lowerings of temperature must have occurred, with undoubted disastrous effects on animals without heat regulation. Such lowerings were most probable during epochs of active volcanism, when the extinction of reptiles also took place. The calculations that have been made show that with those cooling trends, a considerable chilling of the upper layers of the ocean would have occurred, which might lead to extinction of marine species.

Because of their short duration, such cooling events could not leave direct traces in geological deposits, though their effect on the organic world was disastrous in the full sense of the word.

It has been pointed out that the qualitative regularities of the extinction process, as a result of which only land reptiles and essentially small forms survived, agree well with the probable consequences of a brief cooling. It can also be considered that the extinction of all the representatives of some orders and the survival of some representatives of other orders must indicate, to some extent, differences in the endurance of different orders under cooling conditions. The presence of direct connections between the evolutionary processes of reptiles, as found in different orders, and their relation to thermal conditions, seems entirely natural.

We are bound to agree with one of the difficulties in the explanation of reptile extinction indicated by Colbert, namely, the difficulty of the compatibility between this explanation and the concept of uniformitarianism mentioned by him.

In this connection, we must note that the only element of this concept possessing an absolute character is the conservation in all geological epochs of the action of fundamental physical and chemical laws and their direct consequences. Regularities in development of geological, geographical, and biological processes that do not follow from the laws of the exact sciences and represent empirical generalizations do not have any absolute value. In specific historical conditions, they may change substantially. This idea, grounded in contemporary geological investigations, does not mean negation of the possibility of applying the uniformitarian approach to the study of our planet's past. However, a thorough test of the validity of methods based on the principle of uniformitarianism is necessary when they are applied to investigation of processes of the remote past.

Returning to the problem of the effect of short-term drops in temperature on biological evolution, it seems possible to consider them to be one of the important reasons for the change of successive faunas in the geological past.

This conclusion does not mean, however, a return to Cuvier's concept. Contrary to his views, we consider it certain that the change of successive faunas depended not only on catastrophic changes in natural environment but also on the permanent influence of natural selection under more or less stable conditions of environment. Climatic catastrophes might in this connection be a factor accelerating the tempo of biological evolution.

2. The Change of Fauna at the End of the Pleistocene

In noting the probability of the effect of climatic fluctuations on change of successive faunas in the critical epochs of geological history, we should look at the possibility of significant changes in the animal world that do not depend on fluctuations in climatic conditions.

From this point of view, great interest attaches to the last change in fauna before the contemporary epoch, which took place at the end of the Pleistocene, shortly before the ending of the Würm glaciation.

This was a time of significant changes in the composition of the animal world in extratropical areas. Thus, in Europe, among the once widely distributed animals that became extinct were large herbivores such as the mammoth, the woolly rhinoceros, a steppe variety of the aurochs, and the giant Irish deer, and also some large carnivores such as the cave lion and cave bear. In addition, surviving animal species underwent changes in distribution; large herds of reindeer, for example, disappeared from western and central Europe.

Similar changes in the animal world also occurred at that time in Asia and North America.

The reason for this significant change in the fauna of middle latitudes at the end of the Pleistocene has been discussed in a number of investigations.

Many authors suppose that the reasons are associated with the climatic changes that took place in the time under consideration. This viewpoint was expressed, in particular, in a monograph by Axelrod (1967) and in several earlier works. In opposition to this, some investigators consider that the extinction of animals at the end of the Pleistocene is a result of the activity of primitive man.

Even in the 19th century, some authors expressed the opinion that primitive man could have exterminated the mammoth and certain other species of animal. In the contemporary literature, this viewpoint is supported by Pidoplichko (1963, and elsewhere), who, however, ties it with a concept of antiglacialism which is open to argument.

Extensive material that confirms the important role of human activity in the extinction of animals at the end of the Pleistocene is contained in the papers of Martin (1958, 1966, 1967, and others). He considers that primitive man had a determining influence on the disappearance of many animals, not only in middle but also in tropical latitudes.

It must be indicated, however, that most authors doubt that human activity at such an early stage could have played a major role in the disappearance of large and widely distributed animals.

A review of the literature contained in a monograph by Butzer (1964) notes that the animals that became extinct were distinguished by a high degree of specialization and therefore could not adapt themselves to changes in the natural environment in the late Würm. Butzer also calls attention to the fact that the disappearance of large herbivores at the end of the Pleistocene was accompanied by the extinction of certain carnivores that had not been the object of mass hunting by primitive man. In addition, Butzer notes that not all the European ungulates of that period became extinct and that large herds of large herbivores have survived until recently in tropical countries. These animals continue to live and multiply, despite intensive hunting by the local population. In Butzer's view, all these considerations contradict the possibility that man may have exterminated several species of animals at the end of the Upper Paleolithic.

Butzer acknowledges, however, that the presence of remains of mass killings of large animals at many Upper Paleolithic sites suggests the possibility that man may have played a certain role in affecting the total biomass balance of the now extinct animals.

Discussing the question of the reasons for the extinction of mammoths, Colbert wrote: "Why did the mammoths become extinct? This question, like so many of the questions having to do with problems of extinction, is extremely difficult to answer. In fact, it is probable that we shall never know the real reason for the disappearance of mammoths a few thousand years ago, after their successful reign through Pleistocene time. Very likely the extinction of the mammoths was the result of complex causes. Man may have had something to do with it, but we can hardly believe that primitive men were of prime importance in bringing an end to these numerous, widely distributed, and gigantic mammals." (Colbert, 1955, p. 416).

It should be noted that the discussion of the causes of substantial change in the animal world of Europe at the end of the Upper Paleolithic has been limited in the available literature to qualitative considerations, which cannot be easily proved or refuted without attempts at a quantitative treatment of the problem. It can be shown, for example, that the high degree of specialization of the animals that became extinct at the end of the Upper Paleolithic did not interfere with their existence during the abrupt changes in the natural environment that occurred repeatedly during the Pleistocene.

The fact that large carnivores became extinct at the same time as large herbivores does not prove the absence of man's role in the process, because the extinction of the carnivores may be explained in terms of the disturbance of their system of nutrition as the relevant herbivores became extinct both from natural causes and as a result of man's activity.

Nor is it so obvious that the preservation of herds of large herbivores in the tropics necessarily excludes the possibility that similar animals may have been exterminated by hunters in Europe in the Upper Paleolithic.

We should note that the period of time when this extinction of animals occurred was comparatively short and lasted for no more than several tens of thousands of years. It is seen from the material set forth in the previous section that for such an interval of time, large-scale coolings covering extensive areas are unlikely.

In the absence of any pronounced short-term fluctuations of climate in the epoch under consideration, substantial but slow changes in climatic conditions proceeded, which were associated with the evolution of continental glaciations. Such changes would lead to a gradual displacement of natural zones, which undoubtedly affected the geographical distribution of animals in extratropical latitudes. Less clear is the effect of slow climatic changes on the extinction of many animal species.

We will try to consider the question of the possible effect of man's activity on the extinction of animals at the end of the Pleistocene on a quantitative basis, taking account of the basic factors that influence animal numbers.

If this calculation confirms a substantial effect of this activity on the extinction process, then the significance of other factors, climatic changes included, could be considered secondary.

Changes in fauna at the end of the Pleistocene corresponded to the culture of the end of the Old Stone Age, the Paleolithic. The Upper Paleolithic began in Europe 30,000 to 40,000 years ago, during the epoch of the last Würm glaciation. It was at that time that present-day man first appeared in Europe, replacing the previous Neanderthal race and using an improved technique of working stone and bone weapons to create an effective system of mass hunting of large herbivorous animals. The Upper Paleolithic also witnessed a substantial increase in the population of Europe, a rise in the level of material culture, and the first successes in the development of the graphic arts, as reflected particularly in the well-known animal drawings in the caves of France and other European countries. The Upper Paleolithic ended 10,000 to 13,000 years ago, shortly before the complete ending of the Würm glaciation.

The end of the Upper Paleolithic was associated with substantial changes in the way of life of Europe's population, marked by a spreading of Mesolithic culture, in which new stoneworking techniques made their appearance, but some achievements of the Upper Paleolithic culture, such as the art of rock painting, were to some extent lost.

It is likely that the end of the Upper Paleolithic marked a major turning point in the early history of mankind. This turning point was evidently related to the cessation of mass hunting of large herbivores, which had been the main source of supply of food and other essentials for Upper Paleolithic man. The end of this supply led to a search for new means of existence.

We will present here a calculation model, by means of which, with the aid of the data of some paleogeographical and biological investigations, one could find out how hunting during the Upper Paleolithic affected the number of hunted animals (Budyko, 1967).

This model is founded on an equation characterizing the changes in the numbers of a given animal species with time

$$\frac{dn}{dt} = \alpha n - \beta n, \tag{9.2}$$

where n is the number of animals per unit area, dn/dt is the rate of change in the number with time, α is the relative growth of numbers as a result of births, and β is the relative decline of numbers as a result of mortality during the unit of time.

The parameters α and β may depend on the magnitude of n, the actual dependences varying with different species of animals.

The use of computations based on Eq. (9.2) and field-work data show that the numbers of individual animal species may fluctuate widely under natural conditions. These fluctuations, with periods comparable in order of magnitude to the lifetime of one generation of the animals, can be explained by changes in the food regime reflecting differences in meteorological conditions from year to year, by outbreaks of epidemics, and by the complex interplay between the numbers of herbivores and carnivores, which, as shown by Volterra, have in some cases the character of autofluctuations (Severtsev, 1941; Laek, 1954; and elsewhere).

At the same time, the mean number of a given species, over a long period of time that is much greater than the mean lifetime of the animals, tends to be more or less constant, under constant average external conditions. Changes in this mean number may arise either as a result of changes in natural conditions or in conjunction with the evolutionary development of the species studied or of other species interacting with it (Severtsev, 1941; Shmal'gauzen, 1946).

These regularities in the changes in animal populations are greatly altered whenever the animals are systematically hunted. In that case, Eq. (9.2) takes the form

$$\frac{dn}{dt} = \alpha n - \beta_1 n - g, \tag{9.3}$$

where g is the number of animals exterminated by hunters during a given period.

It is obvious that in this case, the coefficient β_1, designating animal mortality from natural causes, will, all other things being equal, be smaller than coefficient β because the Paleolithic hunters could more easily kill sick or weakened animals than healthy, strong ones.

Since the products of the hunt were the main sources of food for Upper Paleolithic man in Europe, we can assume that $g = \gamma m$, where m is the human population per unit area, and γ is the relative amount of biomass of the hunted animal that is consumed by one person during the given period of time (the ratio of the weight of the consumed biomass to the mean weight of one animal).

Equation (9.2) thus takes the form

$$\frac{dn}{dt} = \alpha n - \beta_1 n - \gamma m. \tag{9.4}$$

It should be noted that in computing the decline in animal numbers resulting from systematic hunting, we cannot, for a number of reasons, make use of the "collision principle" proposed by Volterra for the study of the carnivore–herbivore relationship.

In accordance with this principle, the number of exterminated animals is considered proportional to their quantity, which is a natural assumption for small animals that can escape from pursuit. We can assume that man equipped with the technique of mass hunting could in all cases seek out his prey within his territory, especially such large animals as mammoths, which lived in open tundra and steppe. For this reason, the magnitude of γm in Eq. (9.4) should be considered independent of n as long as the hunted animals continue to remain within the tribal territory in numbers sufficient to meet the current requirement of the tribe.

In computing changes in the numbers of large herbivores during the Upper Paleolithic, we must also consider changes in human population during that period. These changes are obviously given by an equation similar to Eq. (9.2), namely,

$$\frac{dm}{dt} = am - bm, \tag{9.5}$$

where a and b are, respectively, the coefficients of human birth and mortality.

These coefficients depend on a whole series of factors, but in view of the absence of data, we will have to limit ourselves to a rough estimate of the mean value of the difference between these coefficients, $c = a - b$, which we will consider not to be a function of either time or population density.

In that case, Eq. (9.5) yields

$$m = m_0 e^{ct}, \tag{9.6}$$

where m is the human population at time t, and m_0 is the population at the beginning of the given period.

Certain ideas concerning the population density in Europe at the beginning and end of the Upper Paleolithic can be reached on the basis of available ethnographic studies relating to tribes at different levels of historical development.

Using such a method, various authors have estimated the population density of Europe at the end of the Upper Paleolithic at 5–50 persons per 100 km². These magnitudes should be compared with the far lower density of a population that does not possess the capability of mass hunting, namely, an average of one person per 100 km² [see Braidwood and Reed (1957), Butzer (1964), and others].

If we assume that a corresponding population increase took place during the Upper Paleolithic, which lasted about 25,000 years, we can use Eq. (9.6) to obtain a value for c ranging from 0.64×10^{-4} to $1.56 \times 10^{-4} \, \text{yr}^{-1}$.

Such coefficients of natural increase, extremely low from the present point of view, are typical of the early periods of human history. They are in close agreement with the short average lifetime of Upper Paleolithic man established from skeleton finds.

We will now calculate the change in numbers of one of the species of large herbivores that inhabited the European tundra during the Upper Paleolithic.

If that species predominated in the given terrain in relation to other species of herbivores, it could use most of the available fodder resources, which, in the tundra, are adequate to support animal numbers approximately equivalent to 800 kg of biomass per square kilometer (see Chapter VIII).

This magnitude determines the upper limit of the possible number of these animals. We can assume that in the case of animals such as the mammoths, whose numbers did not depend greatly on the activity of carnivores, such a limit could be achieved under favorable conditions.

Let us now see how the numbers of mammoths would have changed after the beginning of mass hunting by man. To make this calculation, we have to solve an equation obtained from Eqs. (9.4) and (9.6),

$$\frac{dn}{dt} = \alpha n - \beta_1 n - \gamma m_0 e^{ct}. \tag{9.7}$$

Multiplying all members of the equation by the average weight of each animal, we give it the form

$$\frac{dN}{dt} = \alpha N - \beta_1 N - \Gamma m_0 e^{ct}, \tag{9.8}$$

where N is the biomass of the studied animals per unit area, dN/dt is the rate of change of that biomass with time, and Γ is the biomass of hunted animals consumed by one person per year.

This equation must be solved for the initial condition $N = N_0$ at $t = 0$, which corresponds to the animal biomass at the beginning of the Upper Paleolithic, equal to the limit imposed by existing fodder conditions.

To simplify the computation in view of the difficulty of estimating coefficient β_1, we will assume that when $\Gamma m_0 e^{ct}$ is less than αN, the right-hand side of Eq. (9.8) will equal zero, that is, the mean animal numbers will not change if losses from hunting are less than the increase in biomass. If the term $\Gamma m_0 e^{ct}$ increases to values equal to or greater than αN_0, we shall ignore the term $\beta_1 N$ and use Eq. (9.8) in the form

$$\frac{dN}{dt} = \alpha N - \Gamma m_0 e^{ct}. \tag{9.9}$$

It is obvious that both of these simplifications will yield a somewhat lower rate of decline of animal numbers as compared with reality.

If we now designate by τ the period of time during which hunters do not greatly affect the numbers of the hunted animals, we can obtain that magnitude from the equation

$$\Gamma m_0 e^{c\tau} = \alpha N_0, \tag{9.10}$$

whence we find that

$$\tau = \frac{1}{c} \ln \frac{\alpha N_0}{\Gamma m_0}. \tag{9.11}$$

To determine the period of time during which the number of mammoths declines all the way to complete extinction, it is necessary to solve Eq. (9.9).

Assuming that $N = N_0$ at $t = \tau$, we can calculate how the reserve of biomass of the studied animals changes with time:

$$N = \frac{\Gamma m_0}{\alpha - c} e^{ct} + e^{c(t-\tau)} \left[N_0 - \frac{\Gamma m_0}{\alpha - c} e^{c\tau} \right]. \tag{9.12}$$

By using this formula, we can calculate the period of time in which the magnitude N becomes zero, which would signify the extinction of the given species of animal.

In making computations with these formulas of the rate of change of numbers of mammoths during the Upper Paleolithic, we must also know the magnitude of the coefficients α and Γ, in addition to the parameters already derived above. The first of these characterizes the ratio of the number of mammoths born in a given year to the total size of the herd. For modern elephants, this coefficient is equal to 0.05.

The coefficient Γ can be estimated roughly on the basis of ethnographic data for northern tribes that subsisted mainly on the products of the hunt of large animals. Bearing in mind that Γ stands not only for direct food consumption, but also for other household uses and nonproductive losses, we can estimate Γ roughly at 500–1000 kg yr^{-1} per person.*

Taking the mean magnitude of $\Gamma = 750$ kg yr^{-1} and assuming on the basis of earlier estimates that $N_0 = 800$ kg km^{-2} and $m_0 = 0.01$ km^{-2}, we used the equations above to calculate the rate of change of the mammoths for two values of the coefficient c: 0.64×10^{-4} and 1.56×10^{-4} yr^{-1}.

Computation of magnitude τ by Eq. (9.11) shows that mammoth numbers changed relatively little over a period of 10,000–25,000 years (depending on

* In an interesting paper by Bibikov (1969), in which the author agrees with the principal conclusions resulting from the calculation given here, such an estimation of biomass expenditure is considered slightly overestimated. Although we agree that the actual consumption of meat and fat of animals was noticeably less than the given value, we consider this estimate possible in view of the fact that biomass would be inevitably expended for household uses (grease, skin, bones of animals) and nonproductive losses associated, in particular, with the difficulties of long storage.

the adopted value of c) after the beginning of mass hunting. Then, however, computation by Eq. (9.11) shows that mammoth numbers began to decline rapidly and that within a few centuries after the end of the period of stability, the mammoth became extinct.

It must be borne in mind in any evaluation of the results of this computation that the approximate character of the values of the parameters tends to limit its accuracy. However, an analysis of the equations shows that significant changes in the magnitudes of the parameters do not affect the general regularities of the process and do not alter the basic conclusion that large animals of the mammoth type could have become extinct during a period of time of the order of the length of the Upper Paleolithic.

It is easily understood that this conclusion will not change if we replace the above dependence of population number on time by a simpler linear relationship. We should note that the conclusion reached would also be corroborated for conditions in which the animal species discussed (for example, the mammoth) makes up only a portion of the herbivores living on the available fodder base. For this purpose, one need only assume that the relationship between the biomass of a given species to the total biomass of hunted animals corresponds approximately to a similar relationship for the biomass of animals killed by hunters.

Moreover, the latter conclusion could be obtained without complicated computations simply by comparing available information on the biomass balance of large herbivores of Europe during the Upper Paleolithic. Of basic importance here is a comparison between the annual magnitude of biomass growth and the human population within the given territory.

If, say, in the case of the mammoth, this growth of biomass did not exceed 4000 kg per 100 km², it is obvious that this increase, even if used entirely by hunting tribes, was adequate to support a population with a density of not more than a few persons per 100 km². It is clear, however, that, having reached this density limit, the population still continued to grow, since it continued to be supplied for a long time with food not only from the increase in biomass, but in part also from the basal herd of the hunted animals.

As a result, the growth of biomass gradually declined, and the size of the herd dwindled to complete extinction, corresponding with the results of the calculation above.

It may be thought that after man had exterminated the mammoths in most of the territory they once occupied, the last herds might have found refuge in uninhabited sections of northern Asia. However, the existence of large herbivores in areas with such a rigorous climate could have been supported by fodder resources only in periods of relative warming. Any climatic fluctuation in the direction of cooling would have led to extinction of the mammoths in these areas too.

Using the equations derived above, it is possible to explain why primitive man was able to exterminate the mammoths but was not able to exterminate the related elephants, which until recently have been so numerous in many tropical regions.

Equation (9.11) shows that the period of preservation of a hunted animal species depends on the possible stock of biomass N_0 and on the relative magnitude of consumption Γ of that biomass by the hunting tribes. According to available data (see Chapter VIII), the biomass of large herbivorous animals in tropical savannas is at least ten times larger than the corresponding magnitude in the tundra. Furthermore, the diet of primitive man in tropical latitudes could include far more plant products than the food of the Paleolithic hunters of Europe, which was necessarily limited to the products of the hunt. Assuming that the magnitude of Γ for tropical hunters was at least half of the value we used for the Upper Paleolithic in Europe and taking a magnitude of N_0 corresponding to savanna conditions, we can use Eq. (9.11) to show that the magnitude of τ for the tropics would have to be roughly three times greater than the value we obtained for Paleolithic Europe. The population of elephants, on the assumption of continuous hunting, could thus maintain itself at a high level for tens of thousands of years after the extinction of the mammoths.

Our theory enables us to explain why only the largest of the herbivorous animals of the Upper Paleolithic in Europe became extinct. Since the upper limit of the numbers of any species was determined by the fodder resources of the given geographic zone, the magnitude of the biomass increase depended primarily on the birth-rate coefficient α. We know that this coefficient is smallest for the largest animals and increases with a decline of animal size. The animals most vulnerable to the hunters of the Upper Paleolithic were thus those species of large herbivores whose biomass increase per unit area was the smallest. The cause of the biological catastrophe affecting these species was quite simple.

In the course of evolution, the increase in body size of the herbivores freed them to a certain extent from the threat of attack by carnivores, and the elimination of this important factor in the decline of animal numbers made possible and advisable a significant reduction of the birth rate. When Upper Paleolithic man started to hunt these animals, he performed the same role that wolves and other carnivores play in the case of smaller herbivores. However, while the smaller herbivores were able to replenish their losses by a high birth rate, the larger herbivores were deprived of this possibility, and the extinction of these animals was only a question of time as soon as they were exposed to hunting, against which they were not adapted by their evolutionary development.

It should be noted that such an explanation of the reason for the predominant extinction of large animals at the end of the Pleistocene differs from one given by Simpson (1944), who held that large animals with their less frequent succession of generations found it more difficult to adapt to the changing natural conditions of the period.

It may be supposed that the actual period of time that elapsed from the start of mass hunting to the beginning of extinction of the large herbivores in some parts of Europe was significantly shorter than the magnitude we derived by our equations. This is related to the assumptions we made in the computations and to the fact that we ignored fluctuations in animal numbers from natural causes, that is, as a result of epizootics and especially changes in the fodder supply, which could be quite substantial during the late Würm.

Such fluctuations could have shortened the process of extinction of a large herbivore in a particular area by many thousands of years, especially if we consider that the replenishment of a species by migration from other areas was made difficult by the continued hunting of large herbivores by Upper Paleolithic man.

From this point of view, the largest animals with the lowest birth rate would be expected to be the first to become extinct under conditions of intensive hunting. Their extinction could have stimulated a temporary increase in the numbers of smaller herbivores by making available additional fodder resources. But further intensification of hunting could have led also to the extinction of species with a higher birth rate, as happened, for example, with the wild reindeer in parts of Western Europe. It should be added that, in the case of the smaller animals, losses from hunting by man were supplemented by substantial losses from predators that weakened the stabilizing effect of the higher birth rate for preservation of the species.

Certain other consequences of our calculation model also require discussion.

The process of reduction of numbers of the hunted animals, slow at first, gradually accelerated, and the last still relatively numerous herds were exterminated quite rapidly. In addition, as the total numbers declined but long before complete extermination of a given species, the hunted animals must have disappeared for more or less extensive periods of time from some areas as a result of natural fluctuations in numbers, the migration of individual herds, and so forth.

As the population of Paleolithic Europe was steadily increasing, the existence of that population, being based on mass hunting, was thus increasingly threatened by a shortage of animals. This explains the exceptional attention that man of the Upper Paleolithic devoted to representations of animals, to which he attributed a magic character and which were supposed to help restore the disappearing herds. But as intensive hunting continued, the general process of extermination of large herbivores accelerated further and its last phase passed especially rapidly; this placed the hunting tribes in a difficult situation, because they were not given sufficient time to make the gradual transition to other means of existence.

It may be supposed, therefore, that the transition to the Mesolithic was a period of hardship for primitive man, possibly associated with a temporary decline in population.

As is well known, the end of the Paleolithic in the middle latitudes of North America was also accompanied by the extinction of large animals, which would tend to support the causal relationship of these phenomena. It is also quite likely that significant changes in natural conditions at the end of the Paleolithic created additional difficulties for the existence of the hunted animals and speeded a process already under way.

It may thus be supposed that the end of Paleolithic culture in Europe was to a certain extent a result of the insoluble conflict between man's capability of hunting large animals, thus assuring a temporary abundance of food and permitting an increase in population, and the limitation of the natural resources for that hunting, which after a certain period of time became exhausted.

We note in conclusion that, as the material of this chapter shows, climatic factors greatly affected the change of successive faunas during many millions of years. Later, man's activity played a determining role in changes of the animal world. While this activity caused noticeable changes in the composition of the animal world in the epoch of the Old Stone Age, the action of man in our own time exerts a constantly growing influence on the fauna of the globe.

REFERENCES

Бибиков С. Н. (1969). Некоторые аспекты палеоэкономического моделирования палеолита. Советская археология, № 4.

Bibikov, S. N. (1969). Some aspects of paleoeconomic modeling of the Paleolithic. *Sov. Arkheol.* No. 4.

Будыко М. И. (1967). О причинах вымирания некоторых видов животных в конце плейстоцена. Изв. АН СССР, сер. геогр., № 2.

Budyko, M. I. (1967). On the causes of extinction of several species of animals at the end of the Pleistocene. *Izv. Akad. Nauk SSSR Ser. Geogr.* No. 2, 28–36; *Sov. Geogr. Rev. Transl.* 8 (No. 10), 783–793 (1967).

Будыко М. И. (1969). Изменения климата. Гидрометеоиздат, Л.

Budyko, M. I. (1969). "Izmeneniia Klimata (Changes of Climate)." Gidrometeoizdat, Leningrad. MGA 21.4–323; *Sov. Geogr. Rev. Trans.* 10, 429–457 (1969).

Линдберг Г. У. (1948). О влиянии смены фаз трансгрессий и регрессий на эволюцию рыб и рыбообразных. ДАН, т. 63, № 1.

Lindberg, G. U. (1948). The influence of phase shifts in transgression and regression on the evolution of fishes and fish-like animals. *Dokl. Akad. Nauk SSSR* 63, No. 1.

Наливкин Д. В. (1969). Ураганы, бури и смерчи. Изд. «Наука», Л.

Nalivkin, D. V. (1969). "Uragany, Buri i Smerchi (Hurricanes, Storms, and Tornadoes)." Izdat. Nauka, Leningrad.

Пидопличко И. Г. (1963). Современные проблемы и задачи изучения истории фаун и среды их обитания. Сб. «Природная обстановка и фауны прошлого», вып. 1. Изд. АН УССР.

Pidoplichko, I. G. (1963). Contemporary problems and questions in the study of the history of fauna and their environments. *Prirodnaia Obstanovka i Fauny Proshlogo* **1**. Izdat. Akad. Nauk Ukrain. SSR, Kiev.

Ронов А. Б. (1959). К послекембрийской геохимической истории атмосферы и гидросферы. Геохимия, № 5.

Ronov, A. B. (1959). On the post-Cambrian geochemical history of the atmosphere and hydrosphere. *Geokhimiya* No. 5.

Северцев С. А. (1941). Динамика населения и приспособительная эволюция животных. Изд. АН СССР, М.

Severtsev, S. A. (1941). "Dinamika Naseleniia i Prisposobitel'naia Evoliutsiia Zhivotnykh (Population Dynamics and Adaptive Evolution of Animals)." Izdat. Akad. Nauk SSSR, Moscow.

Страхов Н. М. (1937). Историческая геология, т. I.

Strakhov, N. M. (1937). "Istoricheskaia Geologiia (Historical Geology)," Vol. 1, Gos. Uchebno-Pedagog. Izdat., Moscow.

Шмальгаузен И. И. (1946). Факторы эволюции. Изд. АН СССР, М.

Shmal'gauzen, I. I. (1946). "Faktory Evoliutsii (Factors of Evolution)." Izdat. Akad. Nauk SSSR, Moscow.

Axelrod, D. I.   (1967). Quaternary extinctions of large mammals. *Univ. Calif. Publ. Geolog. Sci.*, **74**.

Bellairs, A., and Carrington, R. (1966). "The World of Reptiles." Chatto & Windus, London.

Bogert, C. M. (1959). How reptiles regulate their body temperature. *Sci. Amer.* **200**, No. 4.

Braidwood, R. I., and Reed, C. A. (1957). The achievement and early consequences of food production. *Cold Spring Harbor Symp. Quant. Biol.* **22**.

Brooks, C. E. P. (1950). "Climate Through the Ages." Rev. ed. E. Benn, London. (Русский перевод: К. Брукс. Климаты прошлого. ИЛ, М., 1957.)

Butzer, K. W. (1964). "Environment and Archeology." Aldine, Chicago; Methuen, London.

Colbert, E. N. (1955). "Evolution of the Vertebrates." Wiley, New York; Chapman and Hall, London.

Colbert, E. N. (1965). "The Age of Reptiles." Weidenfeld and Nicolson, London.

Cuvier, G. (1812). "Discours sur les révolutions de la surface du globe." Discours préliminaire. *In* "Recherches sur les ossemens fossil es de quadrupedes," Péterville, Paris. (Русский перевод: Ж. Кювье. Рассуждение о переворотах на поверхности земного шара. Медгиз, М.—Л., 1937.)

Laek, D. (1954). "The Natural Regulation of Animal Numbers." Oxford Univ. Press, London and New York. (Русский перевод: Д. Лэк. Численность животных и ее регуляция в природе. ИЛ. М., 1957.)

Lamb, H. H. (1969). Activité volcanique et climat. *Rev. Gèogra. Phys. Géol. Dyn.* **11**, No. 3.

Martin, P. S. (1958). Pleistocene ecology and biogeography of North America. *Amer. Assoc. Advan. Sci.*, *Publ.* **51**.

Martin, P. S. (1966). Africa and Pleistocene overkill. *Nature (London)* **212**, No. 5060.

Martin, P. S. (1967). Pleistocene overkill. *In* "Pleistocene Extinctions" (P. S. Martin and H. E. Wright, Jr., eds.). *Proc. Congr. Int. Assoc. Quart. Res., 7th, Boulder and Denver, 1965.* **6**, 75–120. Yale Univ. Press, New Haven and London.

Romer, A. S. (1945). "Vertebrate Paleontology." Univ. Chicago Press, Chicago.

Simpson, G. G. (1944). "Tempo and Mode of Evolution." Columbia Univ. Press, New York (Русский перевод: Д. Г. Симпсон. Темпы и формы эволюции. ИЛ, М., 1948.)

X

Man and Climate

1. Man's Impact on Climate

Man's influence on climate began to show up several thousand years ago in conjunction with the development of agriculture. In many regions, forest vegetation was destroyed for cultivation of the earth, which led to an increase of wind speed near the earth's surface, change in the regimes of temperature and humidity of the lower layer of air, and also to change in the regimes of soil moisture, evaporation, and run-off. In relatively dry regions, destruction of forests was often accompanied by intensification of dust storms and destruction of soil cover, which appreciably changed natural conditions in those areas.

Still, the destruction of forest, even over extensive areas, probably has a limited effect on large-scale meteorological processes. Diminution of the roughness of the earth's surface and some changes in evaporation over deforested lands alter the precipitation regime slightly, though this alteration is relatively small if forest is replaced by other types of vegetation cover (Drozdov and Grigor'eva, 1963).

Complete destruction of vegetation on a given area, which has taken place repeatedly in the past as a result of man's economic activity, can affect precipitation more substantially. Such cases, in particular, occurred after forests in mountain regions with poorly developed soil cover were cut down. In these conditions, erosion rapidly destroys soil that is unprotected by forest, and as a result, further existence of a developed vegetation cover becomes impossible. A similar situation arises in some areas of arid steppe where

463

the natural plant cover, destroyed as a result of unlimited pasturing of agricultural animals, does not regenerate, so that these areas turn into deserts.

Since the earth's surface without vegetation cover is strongly heated by solar radiation, the relative humidity of the air over it decreases, which heightens the level of condensation and can diminish the amount of precipitation. It is likely that such a mechanism is significant for an explanation of the aforementioned cases in which natural vegetation in arid regions does not regenerate after it has been destroyed by man.

Another way in which man's activity influences climate is associated with the application of artificial irrigation. In arid regions, irrigation has been used for many millennia, beginning with the eras of very ancient civilizations that sprang up in the Nile Valley and between the Tigris and Euphrates Rivers.

Application of irrigation changes the microclimate of irrigated fields radically. Because of the considerable increase of heat expenditure for evaporation, the temperature of the earth's surface becomes lower, which leads to a drop in temperature and a rise in relative humidity of the lower layer of air. Such a change in meteorological regime, however, rapidly fades out beyond the limits of the irrigated fields. Therefore, irrigation results only in change of the local climate and has little influence on large-scale meteorological processes. This question will be discussed below in greater detail.

Other kinds of human activity in the past did not have any noticeable effect on the meteorological regime of extensive areas, and as a result, climatic conditions on our planet were essentially determined, up to recently, by natural factors.

This situation began to change by the middle of the 20th century, owing to a rapid growth in population and especially to acceleration of the general development of technology and energy.

Contemporary man's impact on climate can be divided into two groups. The first relates to a directed influence upon the hydrometeorological regime, and the second to an influence that is a side-effect of man's economic activity.

The first group includes, in particular, measures for management of the water regime of the earth's surface and for management of vegetation cover, a practice that is now rapidly expanding.

Water-regime management

Measures for managing the water regime that most affect climate include irrigation, drainage of wetlands, and construction of storage reservoirs. Let us discuss more thoroughly the physical mechanism of changes in meteorological regime with irrigation (Budyko, 1956).

With irrigation under climatic conditions of dry steppe, semidesert, and desert, a substantial increase occurs in the radiation balance, which may reach several tenths above its initial value.

The increase in radiation balance is, on the one hand, explained by an increase of the amount of short-wave radiation absorbed due to decrease in albedo, which, for moist soil covered by more or less luxuriant vegetation, is appreciably less than the usual albedo values of the surfaces of desert and semidesert. On the other hand, the lowering of temperature of the underlying surface and the rise in humidity of the lower layer of air resulting from irrigation ensure a decline of net long-wave radiation, which also increases the radiation balance.

Irrigation under conditions of an arid climate leads to a sharp increase in the heat converted in evaporation, the value of which is determined principally by the average irrigation. With ordinary amounts of irrigation, an increase of heat converted in evaporation as a rule exceeds the increase in the radiation balance. As a consequence, the value of the outgo of sensible heat is noticeably decreased, and at sufficiently large applications of irrigation water, it amounts to negative values, corresponding to the direction of the mean sensible-heat flux from the atmosphere to the underlying surface. This is evident in the appearance of temperature inversions in daytime.

Thus, under arid-climate conditions, irrigation considerably reduces both the sensible-heat flux (which can even change sign) and the flux of heat transferred by emission of long-wave radiation. With irrigation of sufficiently large areas, this can lead to noticeable changes in the conditions of air-mass transformation on that area.

As a typical example of change in the components of the heat balance with irrigation, we will give here a model of change in heat balance for average summer conditions in the southern part of the lower Povolzh'e at an irrigation application of $10 \text{ g cm}^{-2} \text{ month}^{-1}$, that is, $1000 \text{ m}^3 \text{ ha}^{-1} \text{ month}^{-1}$ (Fig. 130). In this figure, all the numerical magnitudes, which are measured in kilocalories per square centimeter, are rounded to whole numbers.

It can be seen from the data presented in the model that in this case, irrigation ensures an increase in radiation balance of the order of 40%. This results from an appreciable decrease in the values of albedo and net long-wave radiation.

A considerable increase of the heat converted for evaporation in the case in question is the reason that the outgo of sensible heat from the underlying surface to the atmosphere becomes zero. It also leads to a decrease to one half in the sum of sensible-heat outgo and net long-wave radiation.

Similar regularities are apparent from observational data obtained in Pakhta-Aral (Central Asia). The results of these observations, presented in Figs. 131 and 132, permit the heat-balance components of an irrigated oasis

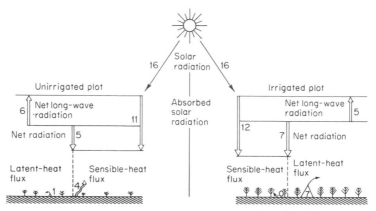

Fig. 130   Effect of irrigation on components of the heat balance in the lower Povolzh'e (components of the radiation and heat balances in kcal cm^{-2} month^{-1}).

to be compared in the diurnal march with those relating to the surrounding semidesert (July). In both figures, the data for the oasis are shown by a solid line and for the desert by a broken line.

The data of Figs. 131 and 132 show an appreciable increase of the radiation balance R in the oasis as compared to the semidesert, and also a great heat outgo for evaporation from the irrigated fields. (In the semidesert, evaporation in the period in question is practically zero.) In accordance with this, as is seen from Fig. 132, the sensible-heat flux P in the desert by day far exceeds that in the oasis, and has the opposite sign. Heat turnover in the soil under the given conditions changes comparatively little under the influence of irrigation.

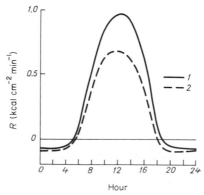

Fig. 131   Diurnal march of the radiation balance in an irrigated oasis and semidesert 1—oasis, 2—semidesert.

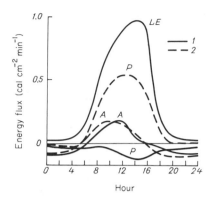

Fig. 132 Diurnal march of the components of the heat balance in an irrigated oasis and semidesert. 1—oasis, 2—semidesert.

As noted above, irrigation substantially affects the thermal regime. In deserts and dry steppes, because of the small magnitudes of heat outgo for evaporation, solar radiation absorbed by the earth's surface is mainly expended in heating the atmosphere by means of the turbulent sensible-heat flux and long-wave emission. Under such conditions, very high temperatures of the active surface are observed.

To determine these temperatures, we can use the heat-balance equation in this form (see Chapter VII):

$$R_0 - 4\delta\sigma T^3(T_w - T) = \rho c_p D(T_w - T) + LE + A, \qquad (10.1)$$

where R_0 is the radiation balance at the earth's surface determined by calculating net long-wave radiation from the air temperature; $4\delta\sigma T^3(T_w - T)$ is the difference in net long-wave radiation derived from the temperature of the active surface T_w and from the air temperature T (δ is emissivity and σ is the Stefan–Boltzmann constant); $\rho c_p D(T_w - T)$ is the sensible-heat flux from the earth's surface to the atmosphere (ρ is the air density, c_p is the heat capacity of the air at constant pressure, D is the integral coefficient of turbulent diffusion); LE is the heat outgo in evaporation (L is the latent heat of vaporization, E is the evaporation); and A is the heat inflow to the soil.

It follows from Eq. (10.1) that

$$T_w - T = \frac{R_0 - LE - A}{\rho c_p D + 4\delta\sigma T^3}. \qquad (10.2)$$

Since the values LE and A under these conditions are far less than R_0, then the value $T_w - T$ in daytime may be very large. Calculations by Eq. (10.2) show that it may be equal to 10–20°.

The great differences of $T_w - T$ correspond to large heat fluxes from the earth's surface to the atmosphere. As a result of heating the lower layer of air, its temperature rises and relative humidity drops. The drop in relative humidity in turn contributes to the reduction of precipitation.

Irrigation of arid territories produces a considerable change in the water balance of the soil. Because of irrigation, evaporation increases sharply, the growth being equal to the irrigation application minus the outflow of irrigation water in percolation.

Accordingly, the heat outgo for evaporation increases considerably, which leads to a considerable drop in the temperature of the active surface.

Taking into account the fact that changes in the air temperature observed with irrigation are far less than those in active-surface temperature, we can derive a formula for determining active-surface temperature when irrigation water is applied:

$$T_w - T_w' = \frac{(R_0 - R_0') - (LE - LE')}{\rho c_p D + 4\delta\sigma T^3},$$ (10.3)

where the values relating to conditions of the irrigated area are designated by primes and those for conditions of the unirrigated area are not primed. In deriving Eq. (10.3), we take into consideration that $|A - A'| \ll LE' - LE$.

As was noted above, when irrigation is applied, the radiation balance at the earth's surface increases noticeably, because of an increase in albedo.

With ordinary irrigation applications, the increase of heat outgo for evaporation appreciably exceeds the increase in the radiation balance, which results in the difference $T_w - T_w'$ turning out rather large with sufficiently large irrigation amounts.

As a result, the temperature of the active surface of the irrigated site under daytime conditions approaches the air temperature, and with abundant irrigation becomes less than the air temperature. It has been pointed out that irrigation of sufficiently large areas results in substantial changes of the conditions of air-mass transformation, as a consequence of which the regimes of temperature and humidity of the lower layers of air over the irrigated areas are changed. Warm, dry air coming in from outside becomes moist and cool as it moves over the irrigated land.

Changes in air temperature and humidity over irrigated areas can be considered to be a result of transforming air that comes from different outside areas, depending on wind direction. The degree of change is a function of distance from the boundaries of the irrigated oasis, increasing with distance of the site in question from the oasis boundary. In addition, changes in temperature and humidity of the air with irrigation depend on the following factors:

1. The depths of irrigation water applied and the intervals between

applications. The greater the amount of water received and evaporated by the irrigated field in a given interval of time, the larger are the temperature and humidity differences between irrigated and un-irrigated fields.

2. Wind speed and the turbulent exchange coefficient. These two factors are closely interconnected, and determine the thickness of the air layer in which changes of temperature and humidity occur. Essentially, the distributions of temperature and humidity with height within the lower layer of air depend on the same factors.

3. Radiative properties of the underlying surface—mainly its re-flectivity (albedo), this factor having already been discussed.

Empirical study of the effect of these factors taken separately is rather difficult. Therefore, it is more advisable to take the approach of theoretical calculation of changes in temperature and humidity, in conjunction with a test of conclusions with data obtained during experimental investigations at permanent stations and on field expeditions [see Budyko *et al.* (1952)].

On the basis of the theory elaborated, one can rather accurately calculate the changes in temperature and humidity at different altitudes depending on the water loss for evaporation, the changes in albedo, the intensity of tur-bulent exchange, and the distance from the boundary of the oasis. This calculation can be used for designing irrigation systems on areas that have not been irrigated before.

Let us now consider some actual data. Table 40 presents data of observa-tions at meteorological stations situated in the desert and an irrigated oasis, generalized by Sapozhnikova (Budyko *et al.*, 1952). The data are given for one latitude (42°) and altitude above sea level (100 m). Oases with widths that do not exceed 3 km are referred to as small and the others as large. It is seen from the table that the changes in temperature and humidity are maximal (in absolute value) in the summer months, when the water-vapor output from irrigation is the greatest. At this time, the drop in temperature at the level of the meteorological shelter that is caused by the increase in evaporation and transpiration amounts to 2.5–3°, and the absolute humidity in the center of a large oasis, as compared to that of the desert, has grown by approximately 5 mbar. At lower latitudes, the absolute magnitudes of these differences are larger.

In the steppe zone, the effect of irrigation on temperature and humidity of the air is slightly less, which is primarily associated with the smaller addi-tional expenditure of water for evaporation.

It should be mentioned that irrigation of arid lands, lowering temperature on the irrigated fields, increases the mean temperature of the atmosphere. The temperature drop in the irrigated regions is associated with an increased outgo of heat for evaporation, but for the earth as a whole, this change is compensated by an identical increase in the heat of condensation, which occurs in the atmosphere of other regions, where the water vapor from irrigation is condensed.

At the same time, when deserts and dry steppes are irrigated, the albedo of the earth's surface decreases markedly, which increases the amount of radiation absorbed in the earth–atmosphere system.

Let us determine how the presently existing system of irrigation affects the mean temperature near the earth's surface. It is evident from the data presented in Chapter II that with irrigation of arid regions, the albedo of the

TABLE 40

EFFECT OF IRRIGATION ON THE MEAN MONTHLY TEMPERATURE T
AND THE PRESSURE OF WATER VAPOR e AT 2 m HEIGHT

Meteorological element	Apr.	May	June	July	Aug.	Sept.	Oct.	Nov.
Difference T between small oasis and desert	0.0°	−0.5°	−1.6°	−2.4°	−2.5°	−1.7°	−1.4°	−0.4°
Difference T between large oasis and desert	−0.6°	−1.1°	−2.2°	−3.1°	−2.8°	−2.3°	−1.7°	−0.8°
Difference e between small oasis and desert, mbar	1.1	1.8	3.4	3.6	3.7	2.5	1.2	0.4
Difference e between large oasis and desert, mbar	0.4	1.8	4.2	5.4	5.4	3.6	1.6	0.8

earth's surface may decrease by a magnitude of about 0.10. Taking into account the relationship between the albedo of the earth's surface and that of the earth–atmosphere system (Chapter III, section 4), we find that with minimal cloudiness, such a decrease in the surface albedo corresponds to a decrease in the albedo of the earth–atmosphere system equal to 0.07.

Lands now irrigated total approximately two million km², which amounts to about 0.4% of the total area of the earth. Thus, irrigation decreases the earth's albedo by approximately 0.03%.

It was established earlier (Chapter III, Section 4) that a change in the earth's albedo by 1% alters the mean temperature near the earth's surface by 2.3°. Taking this value into account, we find that irrigation raises the mean temperature near the earth's surface by approximately 0.07°.

Such a change in temperature is not of substantial importance for climate, but it is not negligibly small and with expansion of irrigated areas may play a definite role.

Drainage of marsh land usually affects climate in a way opposite to irrigation, that is, because of reduction in soil moisture, the soil temperature rises, evaporation decreases, cultivation of soil can be started earlier in spring, harvesting in autumn becomes easier, and so on [see Budyko *et al.*, (1966)].

One of the means of draining and hence warming oversaturated soils is ridge plowing, applied in the north under the conditions of insufficient heat. As a result of such cultivation, the soil in the plowed layer turns out warmer by 1–1.5° as compared to smooth fields.

A natural bog possesses a number of properties that differ substantially from those of mineral soils. Peat in a damp state contains a great amount of water and therefore possesses high heat capacity with a considerable heat conductivity. In contrast, dry turf and the moss covering it is characterized by low heat conductivity. Strongly heated by day and cooled at night, a dry surface layer of peat allows little heat to pass into the underlying layers of soil. For this reason, at the beginning of summer, the soil under such a peat layer can remain frozen, thawing only after rains saturate it. In summer, bog soil is relatively cold, and in winter, on the contrary, it freezes little and under snow cover it often melts during the course of the winter.

Evaporation from undrained marshes varies over a wide range. If peat is thin (as it usually is on lowland grass marshes), then in summer, the marshes are covered by thick grass, which evaporates an amount of water close to the maximum possible for the given energy resources, provided there is a sufficient supply of moisture. With a thick layer of peat (usually on upland marshes), grass vegetation is replaced by moss. Moss absorbs water well, but evaporates it rather poorly, especially if the marshes are covered by shrub vegetation. The total evaporation from such marshes changes in relation to the degree of water saturation. According to the data of Romanov (1961), marshes situated in the north of the European USSR are saturated by moisture, and evaporate 20–30% more than a dry swale. In the region of Moscow, evaporation from them, on the average for a year, does not exceed that from a dry swale. In more arid places, it may prove to be lower than from fields.

Depending on how and for what purposes drainage is performed, the climate of marshes also changes. Thus, for the purposes of peat production, deep drainage of marshes is undertaken. Because of the small capillary conductivity of peat, the surface of the marshes with deep drainage easily becomes overdry, its vegetation dies, and evaporation diminishes considerably. Diurnal temperature fluctuations increase sharply on the dry peat surface.

Drainage of marshes for the purpose of converting them to agricultural lands is performed in quite another way, and the microclimatic regime changes accordingly. In this case, drainage extends through only the surface layers. Under such conditions, evaporation from vegetation is determined by energy resources and also by the state and phase of vegetation development.

Over a damp surface of peat, no such increase of the diurnal temperature range is observed as on an overdry marsh. At the same time, soil temperature of drained marshes under dense grass vegetation turns out lower than that of dry valleys with loamy soils by 3–6°, and with sandy soils by 4–8°.

Large storage reservoirs on rivers made in the construction of hydroelectric power stations represent water bodies of large area but comparatively shallow depth. Therefore, the influence of such reservoirs on climatic change is similar to that of small bodies of water. It is primarily reduced to a diminution of the roughness of the earth's surface and a corresponding acceleration of wind. In comparison with open, smooth terrain, the wind speed over reservoirs increases by 20–30%. This increase is the greatest during the autumn, when the water is warmer than the air and intensive turbulent exchange is developed over water bodies. In spring, this exchange is relatively weakly expressed, both because of the presence of ice cover on the water bodies, and after its breakup, while the water remains relatively cold. At this time, the increase of wind speed over the reservoir, as compared to an open flat place on land, is hardly noticeable. After creation of a water reservoir, the diurnal temperature fluctuations decline, the radiation balance increases (because of reduction of the albedo), and evaporation averaged over the year increases but during the course of the year has quite a different distribution as compared to the land.

Under conditions of surplus or sufficient moisture, changes in the climatic conditions of the surroundings that accompany the construction of storage reservoirs are small. For example, in the vicinity of the Rybinsk reservoir, one can hardly note any systematic temperature change at stations situated along its present shores.

Substantial changes in shore climate arise when storage lakes are created under conditions of an insufficiently moist climate (Tsimlianskoe, Volgogradskoe, Bukhtarminskoe, and others).

Because of intensive evaporation from a water body as compared to surrounding land (where there is no water for evaporation and from which dry air comes to the near-shore waters of the storage lake), the temperature on the shores of reservoirs in the warm season turns out to be noticeably lower than in regions remote from the reservoir (up to 2–3°). Low temperatures in the daytime contribute to the development of rather strong lake breezes (up to 3–4 m sec^{-1}), whose vertical extent amounts to several hundred meters.

Similar to irrigation, the creation of artificial storage reservoirs results in a decrease of albedo of the earth–atmosphere system and, consequently, in an increase of the amount of absorbed radiation. Thus, storage reservoirs cause a rise in the mean temperature of the atmosphere. This rise, however, is less than the temperature change resulting from irrigation.

When a storage reservoir is built in regions with vegetation cover, the mean albedo of the earth's surface declines in approximately the same way as it does when desert areas are irrigated. However, since the largest artificial reservoirs are built in regions with a comparatively humid climate, where considerable cloudiness exists, the albedo of the earth–atmosphere system in this situation changes less than over irrigated regions, where cloudiness is small. Besides, since the total area of artificial reservoirs is appreciably less than the area of irrigated land, their effect on the mean temperature near the earth's surface turns out to be comparatively small.

Management of vegetation cover

At the beginning of this chapter, it was pointed out that the destruction of forest has for a long time exerted a certain influence on climate. Correspondingly, the planting of forest is also accompanied by changes in meteorological regime, which, however, are mainly limited to the surface layer of air. Among the various forms of forest plantations, forest shelter belts, widely used as an improvement practice, have the greatest effect on climate.

Field-protecting belts usually are tree plantations from several meters up to several tens of meters wide, which border square or rectangular fields having dimensions from several hundreds of meters up to 1–2 km.

Forest belts are more often applied in arid regions, where they promote the maintenance of a more favorable regime of moisture in agricultural fields.

The main factor of the influence of forest belts on the meteorological regime of the surface layer of air is their wind-protection effect, which comes down to a decrease of mean wind speed on the interbelt fields and of the intensity of turbulent exchange in the lowest air layer, next to the surface of the earth.

The weakening of turbulent exchange in the lower layer on the interbelt fields can be explained by the fact that atmospheric eddies moving near the earth's surface are split up and destroyed when they come into the forest belt. As a consequence, the air stream that has percolated through the forest belt is deprived of large eddies, which considerably reduces the intensity of eddy motion in this stream (Iudin, 1950).

It should be noted that such an effect is observed only for a permeable forest belt, through which the air stream passes relatively freely. A dense impermeable forest belt acts on the air stream in quite a different way. Behind such a belt is created a relatively small zone of calm, and then the wind speed rapidly increases and approaches conditions of the wind regime on the open steppe. In this case, no reduction of the size of eddies in the surface layer is observed.

These phenomena are explained by the fact that when the air flow approaches an impermeable forest belt, the air stream rises slightly, skims over it, then sinks at once and comes approximately into its initial state.

Reduction of the intensity of eddy motion in the lower layer of air on fields between the belts has great practical significance. Results of available investigations show that the eddy motion immediately affects the development of two meteorological phenomena—the blowing away of snow, and the formation of dust storms.

The reduction of turbulent exchange near the earth's surface eliminates or weakens dust storms and contributes to preservation of the snow supply on the agricultural fields between belts.

The reduction of turbulent exchange also has great importance for maintenance of the water supply in the soil during the warm season of the year. The value of potential evaporation together with other meteorological factors depends on the intensity of turbulent exchange in the surface layer of air.

All this is indicative of the necessity for quantitative evaluation of the forest-belt effect on turbulent exchange, to determine the hydrometeorological efficiency of various constructions of shelter belts.

This task is associated with significant difficulties. Because of change in the structure of turbulent eddies on fields between shelter belts, application of ordinary methods for determination of the exchange coefficient, based on a generalization of Prandtl's theory, turns out in this case to be impossible. Attempts to use various indirect methods (consideration of changes in wind velocity, and so on) for evaluation of the changes in the exchange coefficient between the forest belts do not yield satisfactory results.

To consider the effect of forest belts on the intensity of turbulent exchange, it is possible to use the method offered by M. I. Iudin and the author, which is based on analysis of the heat-balance components (Budyko *et al.*, 1952). We will give a brief account of its content.

From the equation of turbulent diffusion for water vapor, given in Chapter II, we can derive the following formula for the evaporation rate E:

$$E = \frac{\rho(q_1 - q_2)}{\int_{z_1}^{z_2} dz/k},$$
(10.4)

where q_1 and q_2 are the specific humidities at levels z_1 and z_2.

For the turbulent heat flux P, we can write the formula

$$P = \rho c_p D(T_w - T).$$
(10.5)

In addition, for the sensible-heat flux a relationship similar to Eq. (10.4) can be used:

$$P = \frac{\rho c_p (T_1 - T_2)}{\int_{z_1}^{z_2} dz/k},$$ (10.6)

where T_1 and T_2 are the temperatures at levels z_1 and z_2.

From the above formulas, we derive the relationship

$$D = \frac{E}{\rho} \frac{T_1 - T_2}{(q_1 - q_2)(T_w - T)}.$$ (10.7)

With the use of Eq. (10.7), one can determine the value of the integral coefficient of diffusion D by measuring evaporation, temperature and humidity differences at two levels, and the difference between the temperatures of the underlying surface and the air.

Application of Eq. (10.7) is possible for conditions at some distance from the forest belt, since immediately behind the belt the vertical fluxes of heat and moisture change considerably with height, so that Eqs. (10.4–10.6) cannot be satisfied. Experimental data show that the thickness of a quasistationary sublayer, within which the relative change of fluxes along the vertical is small, increases with distance from the belt. In this situation, the thickness of the sublayer equals $\frac{1}{50}$ to $\frac{1}{100}$ of the distance from the forest belt. It is obvious that measurements of the vertical gradients of temperature and humidity on a field between shelter belts must be taken with consideration of this regularity.

When studying the meteorological effectiveness of forest belts, investigators usually carry out comparative observations on a sheltered field and in open terrain. The problem is put as one of determining the ratio D''/D, where D'' is the integral coefficient of diffusion between the belts, and D is the coefficient in open terrain.

This ratio can be determined by the formula

$$\frac{D''}{D} = \frac{E''(q_1 - q_2)(T_1'' - T_2'')(T_w - T)}{E(q_1'' - q_2'')(T_1 - T_2)(T_w'' - T'')},$$ (10.8)

where the values with two primes relate to meteorological elements on the field between shelter belts.

To calculate the average changes in turbulent exchange for a long interval of time, it is possible to use another approximate method based on application of the equations of heat balance. These equations can be put in the following form:

$$R_0 - 4\delta\sigma T^3(T_w - T) = LE + \rho c_p D(T_w - T) + A,$$
$$R_0'' - 4\delta\sigma T''^3(T_w'' - T'') = LE'' + \rho c_p D''(T_w'' - T'') + A''.$$ (10.9)

For a sufficiently long interval of time, the differences $R_0 - R_0''$, $L(E - E'')$, and $A - A''$ are usually small as compared to the components $\rho c_p D(T_w - T)$ and $\rho c_p D''(T_w'' - T'')$. If we subtract one equation from the other and neglect small differences, we obtain the relationship

$$\frac{D''}{D} = \frac{T_w - T}{T_w'' - T''} - \frac{4\delta\sigma T^3}{\rho c_p D}\left[1 - \frac{T_w - T}{T_w'' - T''}\right]. \tag{10.10}$$

The second term of the right-hand side of this equation is usually far smaller than the first, which permits us to replace the coefficient $4\delta\sigma T^3/\rho c_p D$ by its mean, which, for daytime conditions in the warm season, is approximately equal to $\frac{1}{4}$.

In this case, the last formula can be used in the form

$$\frac{D''}{D} = \frac{5}{4}\frac{T_w - T}{T_w'' - T''} - \frac{1}{4}. \tag{10.11}$$

Equations (10.8), (10.10), and (10.11) have been applied to a series of calculations of the meteorological effectiveness of forest belts of different constructions. The results of these computations corroborate the conclusion that the permeability of a forest belt has great significance for ensuring a sizable decline of the intensity of turbulent exchange.

At the same time, the quantitative data on decrease of the integral coefficient of diffusion D on fields between belts that have resulted from these computations permit the calculation of the effect of field-protecting forest belts on potential evaporation. For this purpose, the combination method for determining potential evaporation was used, based on consideration of data on the heat balance at the earth's surface set forth in Chapter VI.

The principal formulas of this method have the form

$$E_0 = \rho D(q_s - q),$$
$$R_0 - 4\delta\sigma T^3(T_w - T) = L\rho D(q_s - q) + \rho c_p D(T_w - T) \tag{10.12}$$

We would remind the reader that, using the known physical dependence between T_w and q_s, one can derive the value of q_s from the last equation, and then by the first equation find the potential evaporation (potentially possible evaporation from an abundantly moist surface under the given meteorological conditions).

In this case, the value of potential evaporation turns out to be a function of four basic meteorological factors, namely, radiation balance (calculated from the air temperature) R_0, air temperature T, humidity q, and the integral coefficient of turbulent diffusion D. With the use of Eq. (10.12), the character of the relations connecting the value of potential evaporation with the listed factors can be easily investigated.

Among these four basic factors (R_0, T, q, D) that affect potential evaporation in the design of the system of field-protecting forest belts, three (radiation balance calculated from the air temperature, the temperature and humidity of the air) change comparatively little, but the fourth factor (the integral coefficient of turbulent diffusion) changes rather markedly.

Therefore, to clarify the question of the effect of field-protecting forest belts on evaporation, it is necessary to establish the dependence of potential evaporation on the exchange coefficient in the surface layer of air.

The dependence of potential evaporation on the coefficient D, calculated by Eqs. (10.12) for the average conditions of spring, summer, and autumn in the central Ukraine and the North Caucasus, is shown in Fig. 133. It should

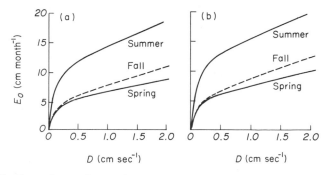

Fig. 133 Dependence of potential evaporation on the integral coefficient of diffusion. a—central Ukraine, b—North Caucasus.

be noted that, as can be seen from the data of this graph, over a broad range of changes in the value of D, the magnitude $(1/E_0)(\partial E_0/\partial D)$ varies comparatively little in different seasons. Hence, it can be inferred that under rather diverse conditions with different absolute magnitudes of D, the effect of a given decrease in the exchange coefficient on the relative decline of potential evaporation will be more or less identical: about 10% with a decrease of D by 0.1 cm sec^{-1} (slightly more in autumn and slightly less in spring and summer).

Thus, if forest belts reduce the exchange coefficient in the surface air layer by 20%, then for the most probable mean values of the coefficient D, the expected decrease in potential evaporation will be of the order of 10%.

Such calculations of the decrease in potential evaporation resulting from the action of field-protecting forest plantations have been used both to evaluate the meteorological effectiveness of forest belts of different construction and to determine the effect of forest belts on irrigation requirements of irrigated interbelt fields.

Besides the decline in potential evaporation, field-protecting forest belts promote an increase of the snow storage on the fields and a certain increase in the amount of precipitation. The effect of all these factors leads to a considerable increase of soil moisture on protected fields.

For a quantitative calculation of the change in soil moisture in fields among shelter belts, it is possible to use the method of simultaneous analysis of water and heat balances at the earth's surface, set forth in Chapter II of this book. Examples of this calculation for several regions with insufficient moisture are given in a series of papers (Budyko, 1956; and others).

These calculations show that the greatest effect on the regime of soil moisture and on average conditions of evaporation in fields in a system of forest belts comes from changes in run-off and the integral coefficient of diffusion.

It has already been noted that numerous observations have proved that the run-off of melt-water from snow from a field with protecting forest belts is noticeably decreased. The decrease is to a great extent explicable by changes in the conditions of snow-cover distribution on protected fields, as compared with unprotected ones. This means that on the fields contained in the forest-belt system, the decrease of wind speed and turbulent exchange in the surface air layer creates conditions for a comparatively even distribution of snow cover, while on open fields, a considerable portion of the snow is piled into ravines or other hollows in the relief, and after melting is essentially lost as run-off. In addition, the high infiltration capacity of soil under the forest belts ensures a somewhat greater retention of melt-water on the fields in the system of shelter belts, as compared to fields in the open. This also reduces spring run-off of snow melt-water under conditions of shelter-belt culture.

It was pointed out above that the integral coefficient of diffusion in the surface layer of air on interbelt fields is usually less than it is on open terrain. This circumstance affects potential evaporation and evaporation noticeably.

A certain influence on the moisture balance of the soil in shelter-belt networks can also arise from a change in the quantity of precipitation, caused by a change in vertical velocity in the atmosphere above the shelter belts, and from a change in evaporation.

For estimating the overall influence of changes in the hydrometeorological factors being discussed upon the soil-water balance, it is possible to make use of the equations of the heat and water balances, considering the values of the integral coefficient of diffusion, run-off, and rainfall corresponding to shelter-belt conditions.

The calculations performed by means of such methods show that on fields protected by forest belts, the soil moisture increases considerably and so does evaporation (though slightly). In this case, the increase of soil moisture has a different character in different seasons, in accordance with the conditions of changes in turbulent exchange, run-off, and precipitation.

If, in addition to considerable retention of melt-water run-off, the shelter-belt system sharply reduces turbulent exchange in summer and simultaneously increases precipitation, then soil moisture increases not only at the beginning of the growing season but also during its second half.

If (as is often the case) the effect of forest belts is expressed essentially in an increase of snow storage and a reduction of spring run-off ("the winter effect"), then soil moisture increases only in spring and at the beginning of summer.

The increase in the quantity of available soil moisture obtained under these conditions may attain the order of 20–40% of the quantity of moisture on fields unprotected by forest belts, other conditions being identical.

These conclusions are well confirmed by observational data from the regions with well-developed forest belts of permeable structure.

A considerable increase in the amount of free moisture in the soil and a slight increase in total evaporation can substantially raise the yield of agricultural crops under average climatic conditions. The increase of yield is determined by the increase in the productivity of plant transpiration (which is also promoted by a decrease in exchange and in wind speed in the surface air layer). Besides, as soil moisture becomes higher, the ratio of the amount of water expended in transpiration to total evaporation increases appreciably, which with the increase of total evaporation also raises the yield of agricultural crops.

Thus, application of shelter-belt forest culture can ensure a considerable change in the water balance of the soil and noticeably raise yield, which, as is well known, is confirmed by the material of numerous experimental works.

Along with the effect that they have on soil-water balance, forest belts play a large role in weakening dust storms that in individual years badly damage the soil cover of arid regions. The significance of forest belts as a factor of protection from dust storms became apparent in the winter of 1968–1969, when a number of severe dust storms took place in the southern part of the European USSR. An examination was undertaken, and showed that damage to winter wheat on fields protected by forest belts was a fraction of that on fields without forest belts.

Forest belts are also used in regions of sufficient moisture, where they simultaneously reduce turbulent mixing and raise the mean temperature of the earth's surface in the warm season. Under such conditions, forest belts produce a favorable effect on the development of heat-loving crops and accelerate the dates of harvest of many agricultural plants (Gol'tsberg, 1952).

Not dwelling on other ways of changing the hydrometeorological regime by means of controlling the vegetation cover, we will only note that man's effect on vegetation cover is a factor allowing him to improve, within certain limits, the climatic conditions in the surface layer of air.

Undirected changes in climate

Along with such measures as irrigation and field-protecting forest belts that are undertaken in order to change the hydrometeorological regime, a constantly growing influence on climate is produced by other aspects of human activity, whose action on climatic conditions is a side effect and a sometimes undesirable result of solving certain questions of production.

One of the consequences of the rapid development in technology and energetics during recent decades has been a progressive fouling of the atmosphere.

A multitude of different admixtures gets into the air in the ejected waste of industrial enterprises, including gaseous admixtures (carbon dioxide, sulfur dioxide, carbon monoxide), solid particles (soot, dust), and other components. During recent decades, the amount of dust received in the atmosphere from agricultural fields has also increased, especially in regions of arid climate, where expansion of cultivated lands is accompanied by intensification of wind erosion.

The enormous influence of human activity on the level of air pollution in many industrial and some agricultural regions is universally known. Less clear is the question to what extent this has a planetary character, that is, to what extent man's activity has changed the properties of the earth's atmosphere as a whole. Some data indicate that atmospheric pollution has already spread over extensive areas and can be considered a factor affecting large-scale atmospheric processes. Thus, in particular, it is highly probable that, as was pointed out in Chapter V, the phenomenon of the reduction in atmospheric transparency over recent decades is in some way associated with man's activity.

The effect of air pollution on climatic conditions has many forms. Well known are the phenomena of a severe reduction of visibility in regions with a high degree of pollution, which is often associated with the development of specific forms of fog ("smog" in Los Angeles and other places). Simultaneously with the reduction of visibility appears a reduction in the amount of short-wave radiation reaching the earth's surface, and light also.

Atmospheric pollution promoting the condensation of water vapor can presumably increase cloudiness and contribute to atmospheric precipitation.

The question of the effect of man-made atmospheric pollution on the thermal regime is rather complicated. Change in the fluxes of short-wave and long-wave radiation in dusty air depends on the dimensions of the dust, its concentration, and its distribution along the vertical. As a result, the effect of dust on the radiation regime and thermal conditions may vary under different conditions. Nevertheless, as can be seen from the data in Chapter V, the tendency for mean temperature near the earth's surface to decrease with an increase of atmospheric dust content presumably prevails. The physical mechanism of this phenomenon has been studied for the most part for fine dust located in the lower layers of the stratosphere. The effect on the thermal regime of coarser dust, which does not ascend above the lower layers of the troposphere, has as yet been insufficiently studied. The question of the effect of increasing the carbon-dioxide concentration in the atmosphere on the thermal regime is also not fully clarified.

Although under natural conditions the atmosphere contains a comparatively small amount of carbon dioxide (about 0.03% by volume), this gas plays a well-known role in absorption of long-wave radiation and maintenance of the "greenhouse" effect that raises the temperature at the earth's surface.

Considering that the increase of carbon dioxide in the atmosphere may change the thermal regime, we should estimate the extent to which the carbon-dioxide content in the air has increased as a result of human activity.

It is known that as a result of consumption of coal alone, about 5×10^9 tons of carbon dioxide enter the atmosphere every year. To this quantity is added the income of carbon dioxide from consumption of other forms of fuel and various industrial processes.

If all the carbon dioxide received as a result of human activity were retained in the atmosphere, a rapid growth of its concentration would have taken place. However, because of the constant exchange of carbon dioxide between the atmosphere and the ocean (which is capable of absorbing an enormous quantity of carbon dioxide), it is difficult to estimate how much the additional amount of carbon dioxide created by man influences its content in the atmosphere.

Although available data on this question are contradictory, many authors tend to think that beginning with the end of the 19th century, the amount of carbon dioxide in the atmosphere has increased by 10–15%.

Such a change in the carbon dioxide content is probably insufficient for any noticeable rise in temperature at the earth's surface. The opinion of several authors that the observed growth of carbon dioxide content may substantially affect the thermal regime is based on calculations in which the effect of carbon dioxide on absorption of long-wave radiation was estimated apart from the effect of water vapor on this process. Simultaneous consideration of both factors has shown (Kondrat'ev and Niilisk, 1963; and elsewhere), that the observed change in carbon-dioxide concentration might change the temperature by a comparatively small value, the evaluations of which by different authors are slightly at variance.

Among other consequences of man's activity that affect climate, we must mention the growth in energy production. All the energy consumed by man is eventually converted into heat, the basic part of this heat being an additional energy source for the earth, which contributes to a rise in its temperature.

Among all the significant components of contemporary energy consumption by man, only hydropower and the energy contained in wood and products of agriculture represent the transformation of solar radiation energy annually absorbed by the earth. The expenditure of such forms of energy does not change the heat balance of the earth and does not lead to additional heating of it.

However, these forms of energy constitute a small part (less than 20%) of the whole sum of energy converted by man. Other forms of energy, such as the energy of coal, oil, natural gas, and also atomic energy, are new sources of heat, independent of the transformation of the energy of solar radiation of the contemporary epoch.

In the author's papers (Budyko, 1962; and others), evaluations of the amount of heat resulting from man's economic activity have been presented. For the unit area of the earth's surface as a whole, this amount is small and approximately equals 0.01 kcal cm^{-2} yr^{-1}. For the most developed industrial regions, this value is two orders greater, that is, it reaches 1–2 kcal cm^{-2} yr^{-1} over areas of tens and hundreds of thousands of square kilometers. In areas of large cities (tens of square kilometers), this value can increase by one more order, up to 10–20 kcal cm^{-2} yr^{-1}.

It can be calculated how this additional heat production affects the mean temperature of the earth.

It was pointed out above that change in the income of energy received by the earth from the sun by 1% changes the mean temperature near its surface by 1.5°. On the assumption that heat production resulting from present human activity is approximately equal to 0.006% of the entire amount of radiation absorbed by the earth–atmosphere system, we find the rise in temperature corresponding to this amount of heat being equal to 0.01°. This value is comparatively insignificant, but with the marked heterogeneity in location of heat sources created by man at the earth's surface, such a rise in temperature may be considerably greater in some regions.

In the absence of atmospheric circulation, the temperature in the most developed industrial regions would have increased by a value having the order of 1°, and in large cities by 10° and more, which presumably would have made life impossible there. The effect of atmospheric circulation weakens these rises in temperature considerably, this weakening being greater, the smaller the area in which the production of additional heat energy is concentrated.

The available observational data show that the mean air temperature in large cities is usually 1–2° higher than in the vicinity. Such a temperature difference may depend on several reasons. Thus, for example, in cities the albedo of the earth's surface is usually less as compared with the country. The heat outgo for evaporation in towns is also lower, since evaporation from pavements and roofs of buildings during rainless periods is insignificant. Although both factors contribute to raising the air temperature, it can be thought that the production of additional heat is in many cases a no less important cause of the heating of the air in large cities.

It can be seen from the data presented here that climatic change appearing as a side-effect of economic activity is small and, with the exception of atmospheric pollution, still has no important effect on natural conditions. However, this change is rapidly intensifying, which makes it very important for an evaluation of future climatic conditions.

2. The Climate of the Future

In Chapter V of this book was discussed the question of changes in past climate produced by natural causes. In discussing future climatic conditions, one should consider both the natural tendencies of climatic fluctuations and the effect of man's activity on climate.

Let us dwell first on those peculiarities of the future climate that are associated with the action of natural factors. As can be seen from the data in Chapter V, climatic conditions are markedly affected by the content of dust in the troposphere and lower layers of the stratosphere.

The present (beginning of the 1970s) amount of dust in the atmosphere is comparatively large, which explains a noticeable decrease of the value of direct radiation incident on the earth's surface. Taking into account the fact that dust located in the stratosphere falls relatively slowly, and considering the effect of thermal inertia of the earth, one can believe that the present negative anomaly of the earth's temperature will remain during the near future.

Further changes in climatic conditions will depend essentially on the level of volcanic activity. A long intensification of volcanism will result in a general cooling trend and advance of glaciers, and an abatement of volcanism in a warming trend and retreat of glaciers.

To work out forecasts of expected changes in climatic regime, it would be necessary to have more detailed information concerning volcanic eruptions, the dust regime of the atmosphere, and the regime of solar radiation. The study of such material may contribute to revealing the regularities of changes in volcanic activity, which will be very important for prediction of the expected fluctuations in the climatic regime.

It should be considered that for time intervals up to several centuries, the natural fluctuations of climate cannot substantially change the meteorological regime of our planet. Taking into account the thermal inertia of oceans, and considering the material on the history of climate in the last millennia, we have to infer that over a duration of several centuries, noticeable fluctuations of climate can occur only in high latitudes, which are sensitive indicators for small changes in climate-forming factors.

Greater changes in climate may take place in the course of several millennia or tens of millennia, which is enough for the appearance and disappearance of large-scale glaciations of planetary significance.

On the assumption that with successive changes of radiation the development of glaciations comparable with the greatest Quaternary glaciation is possible, we cannot exclude the possibility that one of the successive glaciations would reach the critical latitude beyond which complete glaciation of the earth may occur (Budyko, 1968). Such a possibility was presumably close during the epoch of the greatest (Riss) glaciation, when the mean temperature of the earth's surface and the location of the ice cover corresponded to the points plotted on lines T_p and ϕ_0 in Fig. 91 (Chapter V).

It is seen from this figure that under these conditions, the ice cover passed about 75% of the way from the present ice boundary to the critical latitude.

To estimate the probability of a complete glaciation of the earth, one must take into account the principal cause that accounted for the specific climatic conditions of the Quaternary period, that is, change of the meridional heat-exchange conditions in the oceans. Using the paleogeographical maps by Saks (1960) and other authors, it is possible to calculate that at the end of the Jurassic period, the oceans occupied almost half of the parallel of latitude 70° N, which ensured free circulation of sea water between middle and polar latitudes. At the beginning of the Cretaceous period, a gradual expansion of the area occupied by continents in this latitude began, and has continued up to now, as a consequence of which the present-day continents cover five-sixths of this parallel of latitude. Thus, the widths of the straits connecting the seas of middle and high latitudes in the Northern Hemisphere have become one third of their former size.

Correspondingly, a considerable diminution of the meridional heat transfer by marine currents into polar latitudes has occurred, and formed a prerequisite for the development of Arctic glaciation.

There is no reason to suggest that the tendency of the growing isolation of the North Polar basin, which already existed many millions of years ago, will cease in the near future. Continuation of this tendency means that in the future, the probability of new advances of glaciers and the possibility that they will reach the critical latitude will increase. Taking this into consideration, it can be thought that in the latest stage of the history of the earth, there exist two types of stable climatic regime of our planet. The first implies comparatively high temperatures both in low and high latitudes, with a small meridional gradient of temperature and absence of polar glaciations. Such a regime existed throughout the entire Mesozoic era and Tertiary period, that is, for no less than 200 million years. The other type of stable climate relates to the case of complete glaciation of the earth, with extremely low temperatures in all latitudes. This type of climatic regime is presumably much more stable than the first, and its appearance would probably be the end of the long evolution of climates on our planet.

Intermediate types of climate with glaciations covering a considerable part of the earth's surface cannot be stable. This is confirmed by the data of calculations in Chapter V, and also by the history of the climate of the Quaternary period, when abrupt fluctuations of meteorological conditions took place, associated with the pulsations of glaciations.

The question about the stability of the most ancient Paleozoic and pre-Paleozoic glaciations is difficult to discuss, because the location of these glaciations in relation to the poles of the earth is not clear and there is not enough information about the composition of the atmosphere in such a remote time.

As far as Quaternary glaciations are concerned, the material set forth in this book enables us to suggest that the Pleistocene was a comparatively short period of transition from the first stable type of climate, which had been observed over hundreds of millions of years, to the second stable type, which will continue to exist for a long time. (We do not deal here with the possibility that the second climatic regime may change in response to the evolution of the sun, whose luminosity may become noticeably higher over billions of years.)

Thus, evolution of the climate of the earth may result in its complete glaciation within a time that will be very short compared with the long history of our planet.

It should, however, be pointed out that the effect of human activity on climatic conditions makes such a possibility hardly probable.

Among the various ways in which man affects climate, discussed in the previous section, the growth of energy production leading to additional warming of the earth is especially important.

It has already been noted (Budyko, 1962) that maintenance of the present tempo of increase in energy production for one or two centuries is sufficient for a radical change of climatic conditions all over the planet.

Available statistical data show [refer to "Мировое производство атомной энергии (World Production of Atomic Energy)," 1958, and other sources], that the world energy production over recent decades increases by approximately 5% per year. Thus, energy production increases by one order in a time period of less than 50 years.

Taking this estimate into account and considering the current quantity of additional heat income, as was given in the previous section, we find that in a century, warming of the earth as a result of human activity will amount to 1 kcal cm^{-2} yr^{-1}. In two centuries, it will exceed 100 kcal cm^{-2} yr^{-1}, that is, it will be comparable to the income of energy received by the earth from the sun.

In discussing the validity of these estimates, the existence of resources for so great a production of energy and the needs of future society in terms of energy consumption should be taken into consideration.

It is easy to demonstrate that such traditional energy sources as coal, oil, and gas cannot ensure an increase of energy production by several orders as compared to the present level, since in such circumstances they would soon be exhausted. However, specialists in the field of atomic energy consider it probable that in the next decades, highly powerful energy installations using nuclear reactions will be created. Utilization of such devices can lead to a several-fold increase in the tempo of growth of energy production.

The question of the energy needs of future society can be discussed with more or less certainty only in respect to the minimal dimensions of these needs. Presumably, they cannot be less than the level of consumption for a unit-area of the earth's surface that has now been attained in the most developed countries. As was noted above, this level corresponds to an additional income of heat of the order of 1–2 kcal cm^{-2} yr^{-1}, about 1% of the solar radiation absorbed by the earth. With contemporary rates of growth in energy production, such an income of heat would be attained in approximately a century, and in the case of significant progress in the development of atomic energy, it would probably be still sooner.

If polar ice is stable, the effect of this additional heat income on climate would be limited to a rise in the mean air temperature near the earth's surface by 1–$2°$. But because of the instability of the polar ice (see Chapters IV and V), the additional income of heat will cause much more significant changes in climatic conditions.

Using the method set forth in Chapters IV and V, we can compute the distribution of the mean latitudinal air temperature near the earth's surface for an increase of income of heat energy by 1% over present conditions.

The results of this calculation are presented in Fig. 134, where curve T_0 is the temperature distribution in the Northern Hemisphere observed in the contemporary epoch. Curve T_g corresponds to the temperature distribution found by the above-mentioned model for the case of complete glaciation of the earth, when the albedo of the earth–atmosphere system in all latitudes equals 0.80. It is apparent that in this case, the mean air temperature near the earth's surface turns out approximately equal to $-70°$. It should be indicated that this temperature is slightly higher than that of an earth covered by ice with an entirely transparent atmosphere, an evaluation of which is given in Chapter IV. Curves T_1 and T_2 in Fig. 134 characterize the temperature distribution with an increase of energy income by 1%, the second curve relating to conditions of preservation of the Antarctic ice cap and the first to the case of its disappearance.

As follows from this calculation, an increase of 1% in the income of heat energy is sufficient for melting the ice covers surrounding both poles. However, while the principal portion of the Arctic ice cover (sea ice) can melt away in a short period of time in a warming trend, the main part of the Antarctic ice cap, representing a massive terrestrial glaciation, would be destroyed over the course of many years. For this reason, along with the temperature distribution for the stable ice-free regime (curve T_1), this distribution is of interest for intermediate conditions, when, after melting of the

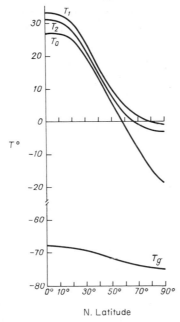

Fig. 134 Latitudinal distributions of temperature in the Northern Hemisphere.

Arctic ice, the Antarctic ice still remains (curve T_2). As seen from this figure, the present thermal regime of the globe occupies an intermediate place between two regimes, the first of which is characterized by curve T_g and the second by curves T_1 and T_2.

The first of these regimes can arise in the course of natural climatic evolution, while the second appears as a result of further progress by human society in the relatively near future.

It can be thought that the thermal regime characterized by curve T_1 (as well as the similar one corresponding to curve T_2) resembles the temperature distribution that was observed in the Northern Hemisphere at the end of the Tertiary period.

Under these conditions, as compared to the present climatic regime, air temperatures in the Arctic will be sharply raised, especially in winter. A smaller but still considerable warming trend extends over the middle latitudes.

It should be borne in mind that with a transition from regime T_0 to regime T_2 in a general warming trend, other changes in climate will also take place, including a redistribution of the amount of precipitation in a number of regions.

Some evaluations of the conditions of water circulation made by Drozdov (1966) show that with a significant warming trend in high latitudes, the amount of precipitation grows in some coastal regions, but in many interior continental areas it decreases. In consequence, moisture conditions over extensive areas will change. Thus, for example, the subtropical arid zone will probably shift to higher latitudes.

After the disappearance of sea ice, melting of the Greenland glacier will begin. Although the process of destruction of this ice cap will be long, it will inevitably result in a certain rise in the level of the world ocean and in flooding of the lowest coastal regions. A similar process will take place in the Antarctic, where the melting of the ice cap will result in a still greater rise in the level of the world ocean.

Thus, as a result, changes in the hydrometeorological regime will occur, which will be partly beneficial and partly harmful for the activity of man.

The massive character of these changes demands detailed study and consideration in planning the development of energy in the next century.

It is highly probable that long before the climatic change caused by the general progress of energy development occurs, it will be possible to carry out some projects aimed at an active impact on climate. In the existing literature, a number of such projects associated with the task of changing climate on areas of different scales are discussed.

One of the biggest projects for acting on climate has as its objective the destruction of the Arctic ice, in order to increase temperatures in high latitudes. In contrast to the aforementioned case, in which the ice is destroyed as a result of additional heating of the planet as a whole, the authors of this project suggest that the polar ice be destroyed under present climatic conditions, on the assumption that it either would not be restored after a single destruction or that its renewal could be warded off by use of available technology.

In considering this question, several research investigations on the interrelations between the regime of polar ice and general climatic conditions were carried out, and their materials set forth in Chapter IV of this book.

The results of this research do not exclude the possibility that an ice-free regime could be maintained after a destruction of the polar ice, but to all appearances indicate the great instability of such a regime.

It might be indicated that the question of actual measures of destroying polar ice has been insufficiently analyzed. In the work of the author (Budyko, 1962), some calculations were carried out, showing that sea ice in the Arctic can melt away in a few years, provided that cloudiness in the northern part of the Atlantic Ocean diminishes and the rate of evaporation from the ocean surface in this region decreases. It is evident that although there exist methods for acting on clouds and on evaporation from the surfaces of water bodies, the possibility of exerting such action on vast spaces appears utterly hypothetical. Borisov (1962) considers that polar ice can be melted by constructing a dam in the Bering Straits and building a powerful system for pumping water from the Bering Sea into the Arctic Ocean. The paper of Fletcher (1966) indicates a possibility that polar ice can be destroyed by the use of atomic energy.

As pointed out above, the effect of the disappearance of polar ice on climate would be complex and furthermore not in all respects favorable for human activity. Therefore, it is by no means evident that with the possibility of ice destruction such a measure is a suitable one to take in the near future.

It is probable that with further development of energetics it will be necessary to work out methods, not for the destruction of polar ice, but for its temporary or long-term preservation. Such methods might be associated with limited consumption of energy in high latitudes or with maintenance of a certain level of dust in the atmosphere.

Taking into account the far-reaching character of the possible effect of destruction of polar ice, it should be considered that the problem of the influence of human activity upon this ice requires detailed study.

Among other ways of acting upon climatic conditions, the possibility of changing atmospheric motion on a large scale, considered in the paper of Iudin (1966), is worthy of attention. It is known that up to now, it has been considered that the motion of air masses is associated with such great expenditures of energy that, at present, man's action upon them cannot yield any results. Iudin pointed out that in many cases, atmospheric motion is unstable, which makes it possible to act upon it at relatively small energy costs. In this regard, he considered the question of change in intensity of a low-level cyclone by means of a system of vertical air jets produced by special devices situated in the area of cyclone formation. It follows from Iudin's calculations that there is, in principle, the possibility of such modification at the present level of energetics, though the technical means for the action were described by the author in the most general terms.

In some investigations, a project is discussed for local action upon climate by means of constructing broad asphalted belts to increase the amount of radiation absorbed by the earth's surface and reduce the conversion of heat for evaporation. The resulting heating of the earth's surface will become much more intense, which may lead to the development of thermal convection and increase of the amount of precipitation. Another project of this kind involves the restoration of vegetation cover in certain arid regions, where it had been once destroyed by man. It is postulated that this measure will reduce the amount of dust in the air of these regions and increase the amount of precipitation (Weather and Climate Modification, 1966).

Widely known projects of climate modification are now in the stage of analysis and have not yet been realized on a large scale. This distinguishes them from projects of weather modification, which in some cases have already made the transition from investigation stage to that of practical application.

We do not dwell here on the problem of weather modification. During recent years, some considerable results have been achieved in this field. Thus, in particular, in the southern regions of the Soviet Union the system of preventing damage by hail by means of dissipating special agents in clouds works successfully. In many countries, large-scale measures are taken to protect plants from frost.

Such methods for modification of atmospheric processes are limited to the brief periods of appearance of dangerous phenomena, and do not deal with large-scale processes forming climate on extensive areas. Nevertheless, the experience of work on weather modification has a certain significance for the support of methods for climate modification and is probably the first stage in solving the problem of human management of atmospheric processes.

Fedorov (1958) pointed out that present methods for weather modification are essentially based on the principle of control of the most unstable atmospheric processes, whose course can be changed with the expenditure of relatively small quantities of energy. Fedorov noted that this principle would have vital significance during analysis of projects for climate modification. In addition, he stressed the special principle of all large-scale measures for climate modification. Effectuating such measures will produce a complex effect on many climatic elements, and it is hardly probable that all aspects of this effect will be favorable for human activity. Therefore, realization of any project of climate modification should be preceded by much research work, resulting in evaluation of every possible consequence of the measure to be taken, both in the region where it is carried out and in surrounding areas. Presumably, for large-scale measures, such research should be done on an international basis.

Since, during the next century, climatic changes due to human activity will become not only possible but also inevitable, it should be considered that study of the possibilities of climate modification is one of the urgent tasks of the contemporary science of the atmosphere.

3. Conclusion

In this book, we have considered the interrelations between climate and different geographical processes developing in the outer envelope of the earth. Among such processes, the biological ones that have a basic effect on the evolution of the atmosphere, the hydrosphere, and the upper layers of the lithosphere occupy an important place. At the same time, the activity of living organisms depends in many respects on climatic conditions.

The appearance of life on the earth turned out to be possible because of a definite combination of the heat regime, moisture, and the chemical composition of the atmospheric air.

Beginning from the first primitive living organisms, which evolved, adjusting themselves to the climatic conditions of their times, biological evolution occurred under the influence of atmospheric factors, which were one of the fundamental elements of the environment in which living organisms existed.

Simultaneously, the living organisms themselves turned out to have a definite influence upon atmospheric conditions. Most noticeably, this effect appeared over long periods of time in respect to changes in the composition of the atmospheric air.

The primary atmosphere, which essentially contained various compounds of hydrogen, was replaced at an early stage in the history of the earth by the secondary atmosphere, which contained oxygen. Accumulation of oxygen in the atmosphere, associated to a considerable degree with the activity of autotrophic plants, had an enormous influence on the further development of living organisms. One of the ways in which this influence was exerted was in the appearance of the ozone screen that protected the earth's surface from the effect of ultraviolet radiation of the sun, which is destructive for many organisms.

Changes in the concentration of carbon dioxide in the atmosphere, which accounted for changes in photosynthetic productivity and intensity of the circulation of biological matter, were very important for the dynamics of biological processes. It can be thought that changes in carbon-dioxide content in the air partially depend on the biosphere developing itself and partially on the course of geologic processes. Fluctuations of carbon-dioxide concentration affected the thermal regime and other elements of climate.

It must be indicated that the interrelations between living organisms and climate were not equally significant. The effect of biological processes on climate either showed itself as a result of slow changes in atmospheric composition or was reduced to changes in the microclimate. Climatic conditions thus depended on biological factors only to a limited extent.

As opposed to this, the existence of living organisms is possible only within relatively narrow limits of climatic conditions. The intensity of biological processes within these limits varies substantially in dependence on climatic factors. As a result, comparatively small climatic changes may produce an enormous influence on living nature.

In Chapters V and IX of this book, data indicative of instability in the earth's climate are presented. It follows from them that comparatively small changes in climate-forming factors may substantially alter the climate. Thus, in the contemporary epoch, a decrease by merely 1% in the amount of solar radiation absorbed by the earth is sufficient for glaciation of a great part of the planet. In pre-Quaternary time, when climate was more stable, abrupt fluctuations of the thermal regime were also possible. Taking into account the limited range of temperature in which active existence of living organisms is possible, a question can be put that earlier was considered trivial: How can the maintenance of climatic conditions permitting the continued existence of life over several billion years be explained?

To answer this question, we must first point to the great plasticity of living organisms, which, in the course of natural selection, have adapted to changes in environmental conditions. It should be also stressed that some groups of organisms were unable to endure severe climatic changes, which were a substantial factor in the extinction of many groups of living things.

Taking these considerations into account, we may still believe that such a long existence of life on our planet is a result of a favorable combination of external climate-forming factors, which include, in particular, the geologic processes that affected the form of the earth's surface and the composition of the atmosphere.

Contemporary knowledge of the regularities of climatic change is insufficient for a quantitative answer to the question about the probability that a meteorological regime favorable for living organisms would be maintained on the planet for several billion years after the time when life appeared. It might be thought, however, that this probability is not very high. In this respect, the aforementioned possibility of a relatively near cessation of conditions favorable for life with the natural evolution of the earth's climate does not seem too paradoxical. More paradoxical is the coincidence of the moment when this possibility arose and the appearance of man, which resulted in an essential change in the interrelation between living nature and climate.

While the influence of biological organisms on climate has so far been limited, in the near future, as noted in the preceding section, the climate will begin to be determined by the conditions of human activity.

Although, as compared to the general history of the biosphere, man appeared very recently, he has already managed to modify greatly the natural conditions on our planet. The present form of man (*Homo sapiens*) sprang up, at most, several tens of thousands of years ago, the age of the most ancient civilizations being no more than 10,000 years. The duration of the period of industrial development is determined as a few centuries, and the duration of the period of the scientific–technical revolution now being experienced, as a few decades. Nevertheless, man has succeeded in the complete modification of many geographical processes over vast areas.

In Chapter IX, data were presented indicative of the fact that as long ago as in the Paleolithic, man exterminated a number of large animals, which substantially modified the fauna of extensive areas.

Later, the animal world has undergone still greater changes, which, in our time, embrace not only the land but also the ocean. Man has profoundly influenced not only the geography of animals but also that of plants, having destroyed the natural vegetation cover on a considerable portion of the surface of the lands and replaced it partially by agricultural plants. Cultivation of the earth was associated with substantial changes in the natural soil cover.

Along with acting on biological processes, man modifies the hydrologic regime of the land on a still growing scale, by regulating stream flow, constructing artificial reservoirs, and carrying out widespread improvement measures.

Large-scale atmospheric processes have so far been less accessible to direct human action, because of the necessity of expending large amounts of energy in their transformation. However, as was pointed out in the previous section, human modification of climate with further progress of technology and energetics in the near future becomes not only possible but inevitable. Such action rules out the possibility of glaciation of the earth, and opens a perspective of the long existence of the biosphere, whose climatic conditions will be regulated by man.

Worth mentioning is the coincidence of the still short period of human activity with the critical epoch in the development of the biosphere, which is the Quaternary period. It has been repeatedly suggested that sudden fluctuations of climatic conditions in the Pleistocene accelerated man's evolution and promoted the appearance of his contemporary form (Gerasimov, 1970; and others). This viewpoint permits the diminution of the role of an element of chance in explaining the appearance of the basic possibility of the survival of the biosphere into an epoch when its further existence was threatened.

It should be borne in mind that for creation of a climatic regime managed by man, further progress of science and engineering is necessary, which would permit considerable increase in the present production of energy. It is beyond doubt that with peaceful development of human society, such progress will be realized in the near future.

REFERENCES

Борисов П. М. (1962). К проблеме коренного улучшения климата. Изв. ВГО, т. 94, вып. 4.

Borisov, P. M. (1962). The problem of the fundamental amelioration of climate. *Izv. Geograf. Obshchestva* **94**, 304–318. MGA 14:249.

Будыко М. И. (1956). Тепловой баланс земной поверхности. Гидрометеоиздат, Л.

Budyko, M. I. (1956). "Teplovoi Balans Zemnoi Poverkhnosti." Gidrometeoizdat, Leningrad; "Heat Balance of the Earth's Surface" (translated by N. A. Stepanova). U.S. Weather Bur., Washington, D.C., 1958. MGA 8.5-20, 13E-386.

Будыко М. И. (1962). Некоторые пути воздействия на климат. Метеорология и гидрология, № 2.

Budyko, M. I. (1962). Some ways of influencing the climate. *Meteorol. Gidrol.* No. 2, 3–8. MGA 14A-43.

Будыко М. И. (1968). О происхождении ледниковых эпох. Метеорология и гидрология, № 11.

Budyko, M. I. (1968). On the origin of glacial epochs. *Meteorol. Gidrol.* No. 11, 3–12. MGA 20.11-383.

Будыко М. И. [и др.] (1952). Изменения климата в связи с планом преобразования природы. Гидрометеоиздат, Л.

Budyko, M. I., Drozdov, O. A., L'vovich, M. I., Pogosian, Kh. P., Sapozhnikova, S. A., and Iudin, M. I. (1952). "Izmenenie Klimata v Sviazi s Planom Preobrazovaniia Prirody Zasushlivykh Rainov SSSR. (Changing the Climate in Connection with the Plan for Transforming Nature in the Drought Regions of the USSR)." Gidrometeoizdat, Leningrad. MGA 4B-296.

Будыко М. И., Дроздов О. А., Юдин М. И. (1966). Влияние хозяйственной деятельности на климат. Сб. «Современные проблемы климатологии». Гидрометеоиздат, Л.

Budyko, M. I., Drozdov, O. A., and Iudin, M. I. (1966). The effect of economic activity on climate. *In* "Sovremennye Problemy Klimatologii (Contemporary Problems of Climatology)" (M. I. Budyko, ed.), pp. 435–448. Gidrometeoizdat, Leningrad. MGA 18.12-397; *Sov. Geogr. Rev. Transl.* **12** (No. 10), 666–679 (1971).

Герасимов И. П. (1970). Природа и развитие первобытного общества. Изв. АН СССР, сер. геогр., № 1.

Gerasimov, I. P. (1970). The nature and development of primitive society. *Izv. Akad. Nauk SSSR Ser. Geogr.* No. 1, 5–8.

Гольцберг И. А. (1952). Экспедиция по изучению атмосферной турбулентности среди полезащитных полос. Труды ГГО, вып. 29.

Gol'tsberg, I. A. (1952). An expedition to study atmospheric turbulence among shelter belts. *Tr. Gl. Geofiz. Observ.* **29**.

Дроздов О. А. (1966). Об изменении осадков северного полушария при изменении температур полярного бассейна. Труды ГГО, вып. 198.

Drozdov, O. A. (1966). On changes in precipitation in the Northern Hemisphere as related to changes in temperature in the Polar Basin. *Tr. Gl. Geofiz. Observ.* **198**, 3–16. MGA 18.1-244.

Дроздов О. А., Григорьева А. С. (1963). Влагооборот в атмосфере. Гидрометеоиздат, Л.

Drozdov, O. A., and Grigor'eva, A. S. (1963). "Vlagooborot v Atmosfere." Gidrometeoizdat, Leningrad. MGA 16.5-48; "Moisture Exchange in the Atmosphere." TT65-501-19. Isr. Program Sci. Transl., Jerusalem, 1965. MGA 17.10-12.

Кондратьев К. Я., Нийлиск Х. Ю. (1963). К вопросу о тепловом излучении углекислого газа в атмосфере. Проблемы физики атмосферы, вып. 2. Изд. ЛГУ.

Kondrat'ev, K. Ia., and Niilisk, Kh. Iu. (1963). Thermal radiation of CO_2 in the atmosphere. *Probl. Fiz. Atmos.* (*Leningrad Gos. Univ.*) **2**, 28–47; *NASA Tech. Transl.* **TTF-208** (1964). MGA 17.3-281.

Мировое производство атомной энергии. (1958). Атомиздат, М.

"Mirovoe Proizvodstvo Atomnoi Energii (World Production of Atomic Energy)." Atomizdat, Moscow, 1958.

Романов В. В. (1961). Гидрофизика болот. Гидрометеоиздат, Л.

Romanov, V. V. (1961). "Gidrofizika Bolot (The Hydrophysics of Marshes)." Gidrometeoizdat, Leningrad. MGA 13.6-9.

Сакс В. Н. (1960). Геологическая история Северного Ледовитого океана на протяжении мезозойской эры. Сб. Международного геологического конгресса. XXI сессия. Доклады советских геологов. Госгеолтехидат, М.

Saks, V. N. (1960). Geologic history of the Arctic Ocean during the Mesozoic Era. *Mezhdunar. Geol. Kongr., 21st*, Copenhagen, *1960. Dokl. Sov. Geol.* Gosgeoltekhizdat, Moscow.

Федоров Е. К. (1958). Воздействие человека на метеорологические процессы. Вопросы философии, № 4.

Fedorov, E. K. (1958). Man's action on meteorological processes. *Vop. Fil.* No. 4.

Юдин М. И. (1950). Влияние лесных полос на турбулентный обмен и оптимальная ширина полос. Сб. «Вопросы гидрометеорологической эффективности полезащитного лесоразведения». Гидрометеоиздат, Л.

Iudin, M. I. (1950). The effect of shelter belts on turbulent exchange and the optimal width of belts. *In* "Voprosy Gidrometeorologicheskoi Effektivnosti Polezashchitnogo Lesorazvedeniia (Problems of the Hydrometeorological Effectiveness of Shelter Belts)" (N. A. Bagrov, ed.), Gidrometeoizdat, Leningrad. Cf. MGA 2.6-82.

Юдин М. И. (1966). О возможностях воздействия на крупномасштабные атмосферные движения. Сб. «Современные проблемы климатологии». Гидрометеоиздат, Л.

Iudin, M. I. (1966). The possibility of controlling large-scale atmospheric motions. *In* "Sovremennye Problemy Klimatologii (Contemporary Problems of Climatology)" (M. I. Budyko, ed.), pp. 393–411. Gidrometeoizdat, Leningrad. MGA 18.12-169.

Fletcher, J. O. (1966). The Arctic heat budget and atmospheric circulation. *Proc. Symp. Arctic Heat Budget and Atmos. Circ., Lake Arrowhead, Calif., 1966* (J. O. Fletcher, ed.), Rep. RM-5223-NSF. Rand Corp., Santa Monica, California.

"Weather and Climate Modification," 1966. Nat. Acad. Sci.-Nat. Res. Council Publ. **1350**, Washington. (Русский перевод: Модификация погоды и климата. Гидрометеоиздат, Л., 1967.)

Subject Index

C
D
E 8
F 9
G 0
H 1
I 2
J 3